Ruminant Toxicology

Guest Editor

GARY D. OSWEILER, DVM, MS, PhD

VETERINARY CLINICS OF NORTH AMERICA: FOOD ANIMAL PRACTICE

www.vetfood.theclinics.com

Consulting Editor
ROBERT A. SMITH, DVM, MS

July 2011 • Volume 27 • Number 2

SAUNDERS an imprint of ELSEVIER, Inc.

W.B. SAUNDERS COMPANY
A Division of Elsevier Inc.

1600 John F. Kennedy Boulevard • Suite 1800 • Philadelphia, PA 19103-2899

http://www.vetfood.theclinics.com

**VETERINARY CLINICS OF NORTH AMERICA: FOOD ANIMAL PRACTICE Volume 27, Number 2
July 2011 ISSN 0749-0720, ISBN-13: 978-1-4557-0523-8**

Editor: John Vassallo; j.vassallo@elsevier.com
Developmental Editor: Don Mumford

Veterinary Clinics of North America: Food Animal Practice (ISSN 0749-0720) is published in March, July, and November by Elsevier Inc., 360 Park Avenue South, New York, NY 10010-1710. Subscription prices are $199.00 per year (domestic individuals), $278.00 per year (domestic institutions), $93.00 per year (domestic students/residents), $225.00 per year (Canadian individuals), $363.00 per year (Canadian institutions), $284.00 per year (international individuals), $363.00 per year (international institutions), and $142.00 per year (international and Canadian students/residents). To receive student/resident rate, orders must be accompained by name of affiliated institution, date of term, and the signature of program/residency coordinator on institution letterhead. *Clinics* subscription prices. All prices are subject to change without notice. **POSTMASTER:** Send address changes to *Veterinary Clinics of North America*: *Food Animal Practice*, Elsevier Health Sciences Division, Subscription Customer Service, 3251 Riverport Lane, Maryland Heights, MO 63043. Customer Service (orders, claims, online, change of address): Elsevier Health Sciences Division, Subscription Customer Service, 3251 Riverport Lane, Maryland Heights, MO 63043. Tel: 1-800-654-2452 (U.S. and Canada); 314-447-8871 (ouside U.S. and Canada). Fax: 314-447-8029. E-mail: journalscustomerservice-usa@elsevier.com (for print support); journalsonlinesupport-usa@elsevier.com (for online support).

Reprints. For copies of 100 or more, of articles in this publication, please contact the Commercial Reprints Department, Elsevier Inc., 360 Park Avenue South, New York, NY 10010-1710. Tel.: 212-633-3812; Fax: 212-462-1935; E-mail: reprints@elsevier.com.

Veterinary Clinics of North America: Food Animal Practice is covered in *Current Contents/Agriculture, Biology and Environmental Sciences, MEDLINE/PubMed (Index Medicus), and Excerpta Medica.*

Printed and bound by CPI Group (UK) Ltd, Croydon, CR0 4YY
Transferred to Digital Print 2011

Contributors

CONSULTING EDITOR

ROBERT A. SMITH, DVM, MS
Diplomate, American Board of Veterinary Practioners; Veterinary Research and Consulting Services, LLC, Greeley, Colorado

GUEST EDITOR

GARY D. OSWEILER, DVM, MS, PhD
Diplomate, American Board of Veterinary Toxicology; Professor, Veterinary Diagnostic Laboratory, Department of Veterinary Diagnostic and Production Animal Medicine, College of Veterinary Medicine, Iowa State University, Ames, Iowa

AUTHORS

KARYN BISCHOFF, DVM, MS
Diplomate, American Board of Veterinary Toxicology; Diagnostic Toxicologist, New York State Animal Health Diagnostic Laboratory; Assistant Professor, Department of Population Medicine and Diagnostic Sciences, Cornell University, Ithaca, New York

SUSAN J. BRIGHT, DVM
Veterinary Medical Officer, Division of Veterinary Product Safety, Office of Surveillance and Compliance, Center for Veterinary Medicine, Food and Drug Administration, Rockville, Maryland

STEVE ENSLEY, DVM, PhD
Clinician, Veterinary Diagnostic and Production Animal Medicine, College of Veterinary Medicine, Iowa State University, Ames, Iowa

TIM J. EVANS, DVM, MS, PhD
Diplomate, American College of Theriogenologists; Diplomate, American Board of Veterinary Toxicology; Toxicology Section Leader, Veterinary Medical Diagnostic Laboratory; Associate Professor, Department of Veterinary Pathobiology, College of Veterinary Medicine, University of Missouri, Columbia, Missouri

THOMAS H. HERDT, DVM, MS
Diplomate, American College of Veterinary Nutrition; Professor, Department of Large Animal Clinical Sciences and Diagnostic Center for Population and Animal Health, College of Veterinary Medicine, Michigan State University, East Lansing, Michigan

BRENT HOFF, DVM, DVSc
Animal Health Laboratory, Laboratory Services Division, University of Guelph, Guelph, Ontario, Canada

BARRY J. JACOBSEN, MS, PhD
Professor and Extension Specialist in Plant Pathology, Department of Plant Sciences and Plant Pathology, Montana State University College of Agriculture, Bozeman, Montana

RANDALL A. LOVELL, DVM, PhD
Diplomate, American Board of Veterinary Toxicology; Veterinary Medical Officer, Division of Animal Feeds, Office of Surveillance and Compliance, Center for Veterinary Medicine, Food and Drug Administration, Rockville, Maryland

SANJA MODRIC, DVM, PhD
Veterinary Medical Officer, Office of New Animal Drug Evaluation, Center for Veterinary Medicine, Food and Drug Administration, Rockville, Maryland

TOMISLAV MODRIC, DVM, PhD
Veterinary Medical Officer, Office of Surveillance and Compliance, Center for Veterinary Medicine, Food and Drug Administration, Rockville, Maryland

SANDRA E. MORGAN, DVM, MS
Diplomate, American Board of Veterinary Toxicology; Associate Professor, Department of Physiological Sciences, Center for Veterinary Health Sciences; Veterinary Toxicologist, Oklahoma Animal Disease Diagnostic Laboratory, Center for Veterinary Health Sciences, Oklahoma State University, Stillwater, Oklahoma

MICHELLE S. MOSTROM, DVM, PhD
Diplomate, American Board of Veterinary Toxicology; Diplomate, American Board of Toxicology; Veterinary Diagnostic Laboratory, Veterinary Diagnostic Services, North Dakota State University, Fargo, North Dakota

MICHAEL J. MURPHY, DVM, JD, PhD
Diplomate, American Board of Veterinary Toxicology; Diplomate, American Board of Toxicology; Veterinary Medical Officer, Division of Surveillance, Office of Surveillance and Compliance, Center for Veterinary Medicine, Food and Drug Administration, Rockville, Maryland

STEVEN S. NICHOLSON, DVM
Diplomate, American Board of Veterinary Toxicology; Louisiana State University School of Veterinary Medicine; Professor, Department of Veterinary Science, Louisiana State University Agricultural Center, Louisiana State University, Baton Rouge, Louisiana

GARY D. OSWEILER, DVM, MS, PhD
Diplomate, American Board of Veterinary Toxicology; Professor, Veterinary Diagnostic Laboratory, Department of Veterinary Diagnostic and Production Animal Medicine, College of Veterinary Medicine, Iowa State University, Ames, Iowa

KIP E. PANTER, PhD
Research Animal Scientist, Poisonous Plant Research Laboratory, USDA-Agricultural Research Service, Logan, Utah

ROBERT H. POPPENGA, DVM, PhD
Diplomate, American Board of Veterinary Toxicology; Professor of Veterinary and Diagnostic Toxicology, California Animal Health and Food Safety Laboratory, School of Veterinary Medicine, University of California at Davis, Davis, California

LYNN O. POST, DVM, PhD, CAPT, USPHS
Diplomate, American Board of Veterinary Toxicology; Veterinarian, Division of Animal Feeds, Office of Surveillance and Compliance, Center for Veterinary Medicine, Food and Drug Administration, Rockville, Maryland

JOSEPH DEEN RODER, DVM, PhD
Diplomate, American Board of Veterinary Toxicology; Global Technical Director, Intervet/ Schering-Plough Animal Health, Canyon, Texas

STACEY SHULTS, DVM
Veterinary Medical Officer, Office of Surveillance and Compliance, Center for Veterinary Medicine, Food and Drug Administration, Rockville, Maryland

MARY C. SMITH, DVM
Diplomate, American College of Theriogenologists; Professor, Ambulatory and Production Medicine, Department of Population Medicine and Diagnostic Sciences, Cornell University, Ithaca, New York

BRYAN L. STEGELMEIER, DVM, PhD
Diplomate, American College of Veterinary Pathologists; Veterinary Pathologist, USDA-Agricultural Research Service, Poisonous Plant Research Laboratory, Logan, Utah

JANICE C. STEINSCHNEIDER, MA, JD
Regulatory Counsel, Office of Surveillance and Compliance, Center for Veterinary Medicine, Food and Drug Administration, Rockville, Maryland

Contents

Preface: Ruminant Toxicology xiii

Gary D. Osweiler

Diagnostic Guidelines for Ruminant Toxicoses 247

Gary D. Osweiler

Management of poisoning is best accomplished when an accurate diagnosis is made and enhanced by attention to five major diagnostic criteria: history, clinical signs, clinical laboratory evaluation, lesions, and chemical analysis. Used properly, all of these factors allow for a better understanding of clinical poisoning. Although not all of these are possible for individual incidents, a systematic approach to support these criteria will bring a more useful assessment of risk and an accurate diagnosis. This article covers key principles of diagnostic toxicology and provides specific suggestions for clinical, laboratory, postmortem, and chemical testing to best suggest and confirm a toxicologic diagnosis.

The Use of Blood Analysis to Evaluate Trace Mineral Status in Ruminant Livestock 255

Thomas H. Herdt and Brent Hoff

This article summarizes effects and evaluation of 8 trace minerals considered significant in ruminant nutrition, both for nutritional deficiencies as well as production-related toxicosis: cobalt, copper, iron, iodine, manganese, molybdenum, selenium, and zinc. Changes in availability, metabolism, and amounts needed for optimum health and productivity in animals are their major effect; frank clinical toxicosis or severe nutritional deficiency are of limited concern in modern production agriculture. The information provided in this article can help to manage the risk of subtle effects that may alter performance and lifetime productivity.

Water Quality for Cattle 285

Sandra E. Morgan

Water is often considered the most important livestock nutrient. It can carry both nutrients and toxic materials and can be a source of poisoning, although death losses are not common. More likely are questions of low-level contaminants or nutrient interactions that affect productivity. This article characterizes the major contaminants of water, their expected effects, and means to evaluate their presence.

Biofuels Coproducts Tolerance and Toxicology for Ruminants 297

Steve Ensley

The rapid growth of the biofuels industry in the Midwest in the past 10 years has created an increased supply of corn coproduct feed for animals. This article discusses the tolerance and toxicology of biofuels coproducts in ruminants, including polioencephalomalacia, sulfur toxicosis, sulfur

metabolism, mycotoxins, antibiotic residue, and biodiesel by-product toxicosis.

Ionophore Toxicity and Tolerance 305

Joseph Deen Roder

The veterinary ionophores are powerful tools to control coccidiosis and enhance the efficiency of ruminants. Intoxication is generally due to the consumption of concentrates, a mixing error, or ingestion by nontarget species. The most common initial clinical sign is anorexia or feed refusal. The primary targets for intoxication are the cardiac and skeletal muscle. Ionophore toxicity should be suspected when a group of animals exhibit acute onset of anorexia, ataxia, or sudden death.

Ruminant Mycotoxicosis 315

Michelle S. Mostrom and Barry J. Jacobsen

Ruminants have the capacity to utilize some mycotoxin contaminated feedstuffs without impact on production or carry-over tissue residues. Despite large investments in crop development to diminish mold invasion and mycotoxin production, grain facilities to dry and store cereals, and use of alternative processing, mycotoxins frequently occur at elevated concentrations that affect ruminants. Fungal invasion by molds can occur in stored forages, silages, and wet bales and toxicity of these mold related mycotoxins is often poorly characterized. Ruminants occupy wide agricultural niches that expose animals to diverse toxins in different conditions, challenging veterinarians making diagnostic interpretations on contaminated forages and grains. This article discusses mycotoxins affecting ruminants in North America.

Diminished Reproductive Performance and Selected Toxicants in Forages and Grains 345

Tim J. Evans

This article discusses reproductive toxicants as the potential, primary causes of observed reproductive abnormalities and other variables that can affect reproductive performance in ruminants. The causes of diminished reproductive performance in ruminants are often multifactorial. It is critical that producers and their veterinarians understand the potential effects of physiologic and genetic predispositions and nutritional, environmental, infectious, and toxic stressors, as well as interactions involving management. The recognition and prevention of the adverse reproductive effects of these enzootic toxic stressors are essential for optimal ruminant reproductive performance and profitability of a ruminant production system.

Commercial and Industrial Chemical Hazards for Ruminants 373

Robert H. Poppenga

There are many potentially hazardous commercial or industrial products used in or around ruminant environments. Although some products are highly toxic, their proper storage and use minimize their hazard to ruminants. Although most exposures to such materials occur via ingestion,

inhalation or dermal exposures also are possible. The diagnosis of intoxication requires both thorough antemortem and postmortem examination of affected animals and thorough investigation of their environment. Fortunately, intoxications from such materials are relatively infrequent. The possibility of residues affecting meat or milk from exposed animals always needs to be considered.

Safety of Antibiotic Drugs in Food Animals: Comparison of Findings from Preapproval Studies and Postapproval Experience in the United States with Safety Information in Published Literature **389**

Tomislav Modric, Sanja Modric, Michael J. Murphy, Susan J. Bright, and Stacey Shults

Antibiotics are among the most widely prescribed drugs and are generally considered safe for the target species. However, their use has been associated with various adverse toxic effects in target animals, such as allergic reactions, gastrointestinal signs, cardiovascular effects, hypoglycemia, hepatic/renal toxicity, thrombocytopenia, and anaphylaxis. This article provides a qualitative summary of the adverse events observed in target animals during the evaluation of antibiotics by the Food and Drug Administration during both preapproval and postapproval periods. As there is a marked scarcity of published data on safety of antibiotics in food animals, more research is needed in this area.

Identifying Plant Poisoning in Livestock: Diagnostic Approaches and Laboratory Tests **407**

Bryan L. Stegelmeier

Plant poisoning is often associated with a variety of livestock diseases and unexplained animal deaths. Although toxic plants commonly poison livestock and it is estimated to cost the livestock industry in the western United States more than $340 million every year, obtaining a definitive diagnosis is difficult and challenging. The purpose of this article is to provide a framework to help veterinarians and diagnosticians make an accurate definitive diagnosis of plant poisoning. We provide suggestions for investigating and sampling field cases of suspected plant poisoning, for where and how to analyze diagnostic samples, and for integrating information and recruiting appropriate expertise.

Pyrrolizidine Alkaloid–Containing Toxic Plants (*Senecio, Crotalaria, Cynoglossum, Amsinckia, Heliotropium, and Echium* spp.) **419**

Bryan L. Stegelmeier

Pyrrolizidine alkaloid (PA)–containing plants are found throughout the world and are probably the most common plant cause of poisoning of livestock, wildlife, and humans. PAs are potent liver toxins that under some conditions can be carcinogenic. This article briefly introduces high-risk North American PA-containing plants, summarizing their toxicity and subsequent pathology. Current diagnostic techniques, treatments, and strategies to avoid losses to PA poisoning are also reviewed.

FORTHCOMING ISSUES

November 2011
Johne's Disease
Michael T. Collins, DVM, PhD,
Guest Editor

March 2012
Evidence-Based Veterinary Medicine for the Bovine Veterinarian
Sébastien Buczinski, Dr Vét and
Jean-Michel Vandeweerd, DVM,
MS, MRCVS, *Guest Editors*

July 2012
Mastitis
Pamela L. Ruegg, DVM, MPVM,
Guest Editor

RECENT ISSUES

March 2011
Therapeutics and Control of Sheep and Goat Diseases
George C. Fthenakis, DVM, MSc, PhD
and Paula I. Menzies, DVM, MPVM,
Guest Editors

November 2010
Production Animal Ophthalmology
David L. Williams, MA, VetMB, PhD,
CertVOphthal, FRCVS, *Guest Editor*

July 2010
Bovine Respiratory Disease
Vickie L. Cooper, DVM, MS, PhD and
Bruce W. Brodersen, DVM, MS, PhD,
Guest Editors

RELATED INTEREST

Veterinary Clinics of North America: Equine Practice
December 2010 (Vol. 26, No. 3)
Pain in Horses: Physiology, Pathophysiology and Therapeutic Implications
William W. Muir, DVM, PhD, *Guest Editor*

Preface
Ruminant Toxicology

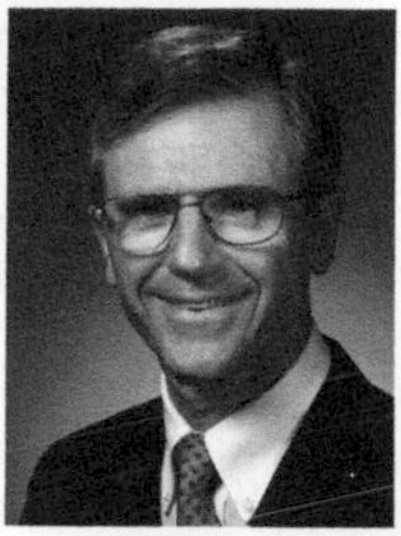

Gary D. Osweiler, DVM, MS, PhD
Guest Editor

Livestock loss from poisoning has long been considered a situation characterized by acute episodes that often result in death or severe clinical disease. Although acute toxicological problems are a limited portion of risk to livestock production, the potential for adverse effects influences some major decisions about livestock production. The previous forty years have seen a dramatic decline in acute losses from poisoning and a change in the types of losses that are experienced. Pest control chemicals have become more specific to the pest and less toxic to mammals. Feed manufacturing technology and quality control have improved accuracy and resulted in less accidental contamination. Livestock increasingly are confined and/or managed tightly by owners and caretakers with generally reduced exposure to dangerous products. In addition, regulatory controls have accounted to some extent for reduced subclinical effects associated with chemicals used in therapy or in the production animal environment.

Despite a reduction in acute risk from toxicants, new technologies and practices challenge our knowledge of the adverse effects that may result. Questions continue about subtle effects of pharmaceuticals and antibiotics, feeds or fermentation byproducts, and environmental chemicals. Recent energy concerns have prompted interest in alternative fuels from grains or cellulose. In addition, recent adverse weather conditions have caused large-scale issues of grain deterioration and mycotoxin contamination. All of these new production issues have raised concern for potential effects on feed efficiency, immune compromise, or reproductive function, which are the same issues of concern for animals managed intensely for maximum production. Thus, accurate evaluation of causes for suboptimal performance or potential interactions of two or more nutrients or chemicals have been more difficult to define. This issue is an attempt to deal with some of the production-related challenges listed.

The objective of the topics covered is to provide review and insight on ruminant toxicoses or toxicant exposures. The authors are experts in their respective areas on a selection of subjects considered of current concern or that are known to be difficult to diagnose, treat, or prevent. Each author has scientific expertise in their topic,

Vet Clin Food Anim 27 (2011) xiii–xiv
doi:10.1016/j.cvfa.2011.03.002

which is enhanced by their direct experience with the subject matter as it affects veterinary practice and production agriculture. This combination of science and experience provides insight that the authors have shared in their work, and in many cases, the need for more information or research is defined as part of the discussion.

This issue is organized into fifteen articles covering four general areas of ruminant toxicology. The initial two articles focus on principles of diagnosis and on an area of growing interest for defining the best approaches to detecting and interpreting micronutrient deficiency or excess. Articles three through eight discuss agents in feed components that affect ruminants through their managed access to water, agronomic crops and forages, or incidental exposures to commercial or industrial chemicals in a relatively controlled environment of the feedlot or dairy farm. These include effects of fermentation byproducts in cattle, risks of contaminated water, issues of evaluating safe and effective ionophore use, effects of mycotoxin consumption on health and immune function, interference with ruminant reproductive performance by agronomic crops, and the effects of specific commercial or industrial products to which production animals may be exposed. The ninth article was included to update veterinary professionals on current issues of antimicrobial risk in food animals, a topic of considerable concern to consumers and others outside the production animal arena. Articles ten through fourteen recognize that a large population of ruminant animals still graze pastures or wooded areas or range across our extensive prairies, plains, and mountain ranges in the United States. These animals continue to have ample access to toxic plants and do experience productivity loss, reproductive failure, or death from those exposures. The plant toxicology contributions outline the unique diagnostic challenges of plant poisoning and then review continuing threats to ruminants either by region of the country or by effects of a specific problem, such as reproductive failure. The final article provides guidance on availability of approved antidotal therapy for food animals with input on available antidotes and the regulatory issues that guide their use.

Modern production agriculture continues to provide a wide range of high-quality products for American consumers and for export. Some production inputs or approaches to ruminant production have been challenged by both consumers and producers, including those times when producers themselves experience livestock problems associated with a potential toxicant. The attending veterinarian has the unique responsibility and opportunity to be the first line of information and response to suspected problems. Judgments to be made include the potential for toxicant–nutrient interactions, best sampling and testing approaches, and the actions needed to reduce or eliminate future threats. The guest editor and authors appreciate the opportunity to provide a measure of input on these selected aspects of contemporary ruminant toxicology.

Gary D. Osweiler, DVM, MS, PhD
2630 Veterinary Diagnostic Laboratory
Department of Veterinary Diagnostic
and Production Animal Medicine
College of Veterinary Medicine
Iowa State University
1600 South 16th Street
Ames, IA 50011, USA

E-mail address:
osweiler@iastate.edu

Diagnostic Guidelines for Ruminant Toxicoses

Gary D. Osweiler, DVM, MS, PhD

KEYWORDS

• Diagnosis • Toxicology • Poisoning • Laboratory • Ruminant

In today's agriculture, many mainstream production units are in well-defined environments, such as confinement buildings, feedlots, dry lots, or intensively grazed improved pasture. In dairy production, forages are commonly harvested and brought to animals in confinement. In other regions of North America, grazing of unimproved pastures or rangelands is still an important and economical approach. Diagnostic evaluation for plant poisonings on rangelands is discussed in more detail elsewhere in this issue (see the article entitled "Identifying plant poisoning in livestock: diagnostic approaches and laboratory tests"). The uses of major diagnostic criteria are discussed in the following pages.

HISTORICAL INFORMATION

Knowledge of circumstances and known exposure to toxicants is often an essential element in effective toxicology diagnosis.[1,2] One must also refrain from basing a diagnosis exclusively on history of exposure. A premise known as the "Post hoc fallacy," as translated from the original Latin, says "After the fact, therefore because of the fact."[3] Often an event associated with loss or illness of animals is assumed to be causal when this is not the case. For example, a recent delivery of feed followed by sickness or death in a herd can lead to a presumption that the feed is the source of the problem, even though animal relocation, changes in water source, or acute infectious disease from mixing animals may be the real cause. Thus, a thorough history, although important to establish possible exposures, is used only as a starting point in the diagnostic process.[1,2,4]

The presence of poisons such as rodenticides, insecticides, drugs, paints, fertilizers, feed additives, and poisonous plants on the premises or in the feed, or a history of their having been used or available, should be determined. Equally important is

The author has nothing to disclose.

2630 Veterinary Diagnostic Laboratory, Department of Veterinary Diagnostic and Production Animal Medicine, College of Veterinary Medicine, Iowa State University, 1600 South 16th Street, Ames, IA 50011, USA
E-mail address: osweiler@iastate.edu

Vet Clin Food Anim 27 (2011) 247–254
doi:10.1016/j.cvfa.2011.02.009 vetfood.theclinics.com
0749-0720/11/$ – see front matter

Box 1
Checklist for information collection in a suspected poisoning

Owner data

Owner:

Manager:

Address:

Phone number:

Fax number:

E-mail address:

Health history:

Illness past 6 months:

Exposure to other animals past 30 days:

Vaccination history:

Medications, sprays, dips, wormers past 6 months:

Last examination by a veterinarian:

Environmental data

- Location: pasture, woods, dry lot, near river or pond, confined indoors
- Building has mechanical ventilation; new construction; recent weather changes
- Recently changed location; recent shows or transport; recent unexplained deaths; access to trash, old construction materials; recent burning of materials
- Access to mining lands, seepage or tailings; access to oil drilling or petroleum storage

Patient data

Species:

Breed:

Age:

Sex:

Pregnancy:

Weight (loss, gain, stable):

Current clinical history

For herds, current size of group:

Other groups on same premises:

Common feed or water among groups:

Morbidity:____________; mortality:____________

Date first observed sick:

Onset and progression of signs (sudden death; acute onset moving to less severe; gradual onset becoming more severe):

Duration of problem in the herd:

If found dead, last seen alive and healthy:

Recent malicious threats:

Changes in exposure

Recent changes in sources of feed, forages, pasture, or lots:

Weed invasion into forage or grain crops; weed seeds in grain or feed; moldy feed or silage:

Specific recent use of pesticides (insecticides, rodenticides, herbicides) and specific types or names if available (ask for tags or bags to identify):

Access to materials used for construction/renovation:

Outside services (eg, lawn care, pasture seeding, tree planting, fertilization, building renovation):

Access to old machinery, automotive products, treated lumber, burn piles, flowing water:

Dietary data

Type of diet:

Recent changes in total diet or a specific feed:

Changes in specific ingredient(s):

Method of feeding (hand-feeding; full-feed, automated or manual):

Feed type (whole grains; sweet feed; pelleted complete feed; total mixed ration):

Type of hay (eg, grass, alfalfa, mixed; weed contaminants):

Presence of molded or spoiled feed or hay:

Pasture type (scant, abundant, weed contamination; trees or brush present):

Recent fertilization or pesticide application:

Water source (flowing stream, pond, well, county or city water):

consideration of the dose of poison that could be obtained. For example, presence of monensin in a newly delivered feed is most pertinent if the feed label or an analysis confirms that the dose is in a toxic range. Thus, exposure alone without attention to the amount encountered is not sufficient for a diagnosis; one should be prepared to approximate the amount or degree of exposure to chemicals in the animal environment.

Fundamental information in a good history should include patient identification and characteristics, important demographic factors about the animals' environment, and the herd characteristics of affected animals.[1] Suggestions for collection of historical information are shown in **Box 1**.

One must remember that the veterinary clinician may see only a short segment of the chronologic development of disease, and therefore historical information should include a discussion with the herd owner or manager to determine the nature or speed of onset of clinical signs. A thorough history combining reported clinical effects and the veterinarian's own examination of animals, feed, and property will lead to a better-informed differential diagnostic list.[1,2,4] The major criteria of history, clinical signs, clinical laboratory evaluation, lesions, and chemical analysis are discussed individually.

CLINICAL SIGNS

Clinical signs are of prime importance to the clinician and toxicologist.[1,4] Both the nature of the signs and their sequence of occurrence may be important. Did signs begin explosively and taper off, or were there mild signs initially that became worse with time? Is one body system primarily affected, or are major signs present in several systems? Details such as these are often important. As an example, problems

Box 2
Checklist of clinical signs pertinent to ruminant poisoning

Neurologic signs

Ataxia

Salivation

Blindness/vision impaired

Depression

Excitement

Seizures

Head pressing

Cerebellar signs

Weakness

Dysphonia

Other (describe)

Gastrointestinal signs

Anorexia

Polyphagia

Polydipsia

Colic

Ruminal tympany

Vomiting

Diarrhea

Melena

Icterus

Respiratory signs

Dyspnea

Cardiovascular signs

Arrhythmia

Bradycardia

Tachycardia

Anemia

Edema

Hemorrhage

Hematuria

Icterus

Hemoglobinuria

Methemoglobinemia

Straining

Fever

Weakness

Dermal signs
Achromotrichia
Alopecia
Photosensitization
Renal/urinary signs
Anuria
Polyuria
Hematuria
Reproductive system
Anestrous
Hyperestrogenism
Agalactia
Abortion
Stillbirth

affecting the central nervous system have a wide range of signs, and a general description of "seizures" or "tremors" is less useful than more detail, including a reasonably accurate chronology of disease progression. Are the signs a typical cranial-to-caudal epileptiform seizure? Is the animal ataxic with cerebellar, vestibular, or peripheral nerve signs? Are parasympathetic signs (vomiting, salivation, urination, diarrhea, and dyspnea) prominent? Are the signs parasympatholytic, such as bloat, dry mouth, mydriasis, hallucinations, or bradycardia? Careful attention to heart rate and rhythm and any change in these can help define several cardiotoxins. Do digestive system effects suggest hypermotility, stasis, tympany, direct irritation, or profuse diarrhea? If respiratory difficulty is present, is there evidence of pulmonary edema, constricted airways, or air hunger from severe anemia? The attending veterinarian may see only one phase of a toxicologic response. Did the owner or caretaker see additional signs?

The entire pattern of changes may be very important to determining diagnosis and prognosis or need for therapy. A list of pertinent clinical signs in poisoning is provided in **Box 2**. Sometimes a list of clinical signs may be difficult to equate to potential toxicologic diagnoses, but attention to the clinical signs and review of potential toxicants associated with them can be enhanced through referencing a database such as CONSULTANT.[5] For example, using "bovine" as the species and entering the signs anorexia, blindness, head pressing, and seizures will provide a differential list of 32 diseases, of which 7 are toxicoses. Using other available clues from the environment and clinical laboratory tests can often pare down the differential list to a few good possibilities that can be closely investigated.

CLINICAL LABORATORY TESTS

There are dangers in making a toxicologic diagnosis based on only clinical signs, because thousands of toxic agents could affect the limited range of clinical responses.[1] One excellent way to extend the evaluation of clinical response is to assess clinical laboratory changes. Some changes are very characteristic of certain toxicants, whereas the absence of organ damage is typical of other toxicants. Clinical

Table 1
Clinical laboratory tests supporting a toxicologic diagnosis

Ammonia (serum)	Nonprotein nitrogen toxicosis, hepatic encephalopathy, excessive protein supplementation
Aplastic anemia	Bracken fern, phenylbutazone, chloramphenicol, gasoline, petroleum solvents, trichloroethylene, T-2 toxin
ALP, GGT	Cholestasis
AST, ALT, LDH increase	Aflatoxin, fumonisins, pyrrolizidine alkaloids, cocklebur, lantana, moldy alfalfa, blue-green algae, amanita mushrooms
Azotemia (BUN, creatinine)	Antifreeze, oak, oxalate plants, arsenic, cadmium
Basophilic stippling	Lead poisoning (inconsistent in ruminants)
Bile acids	Aflatoxin
Carboxyhemoglobin	Carbon monoxide (buildings, trailers)
Cholinesterase	Organophosphates, blue-green algae
CK increase	Ionophores (monensin, lasalocid), white snake root, *Cassia* spp
Coagulopathy (PT, PTT)	Moldy sweet clover, anticoagulant rodenticides, prolonged toxic liver disease
Crystalluria	Antifreeze, oxalate plants
GGT increase	Aflatoxin, fumonisins, pyrrolizidine alkaloids, glucocorticoids
Hematuria	Anticoagulant rodenticides, moldy sweet clover
Hemolysis	Garlic, onion, copper, iron, phenothiazine anthelmintics, zinc
Hypercalcemia	Vitamin D_3, day-blooming jessamine
Hyperkalemia	Digitalis glycosides, oleander, oak poisoning
Hyperosmolarity	Acidosis, antifreeze, aspirin, ethanol, propylene glycol
Hypocalcemia	Antifreeze, oxalate plant poisoning
Hypoproteinemia	Aflatoxin, chronic hepatotoxins
Iron (serum) and TIBC	Iron toxicosis
Methemoglobin	Red maple (unlikely in ruminants), copper, nitrites, chlorate herbicides
Myoglobinuria	*Cassia* spp, ionophores
pH	Lactic acidosis, soybean overload, nonprotein nitrogen/urea toxicosis
Porphyrins	Lead, dioxins, polychlorinated biphenyls
Urinary casts	Aminoglycosides, arsenic, cadmium, mercury, oak
Sodium	Water deprivation/sodium ion toxicosis
Thrombocytopenia	Bracken fern, trichloroethylene, phenylbutazone

Abbreviations: ALP, alkaline phosphatase; ALT, alanine aminotransferase; AST, aspartate aminotransferase; BUN, blood urea nitrogen; GGT, gamma glutamyl transferase; LDH, lactate dehydrogenase; PT, prothrombin time; PTT, partial thromboplastin time; TIBC, total iron-binding capacity.

Data from Osweiler GD, Carson TL, Buck WB, et al. Diagnostic Toxicology. In: Diagnostic and clinical veterinary toxicology, Dubuque (IA): Kendall Hunt; 1985. p. 44–51.

chemistry and complete blood cell count can be part of the clinical filter if there is time to wait for the response. These tests are relatively economical and can also help with the differential diagnosis of other diseases. **Table 1** provides some typical clinical chemistry and hematologic changes that help define various poisons.

NECROPSY LESIONS

Loss of one or more animals in a herd or a single animal at risk provides an invaluable opportunity to increase diagnostic information for toxicology. Evaluation may help improve diagnosis and therapy in the remainder of the herd, or guide the farm in planning forward and eliminating risk for poisoning.[6] Lesions are often absent in certain toxicoses, and lack of lesions should correlate with the indicated clinical signs (eg, lead poisoning may cause few or very subtle lesions whereas oak toxicosis or monensin poisoning provides definite lesions).

Necropsy should include the brain (and a rabies examination) if neurologic signs were present. A thorough selection of organs at necropsy is easier and more inclusive if taken consistently. If legal or insurance claims are likely, a necropsy is usually essential and photographs and detailed notes about the necropsy and premise examination should be taken and preserved. Recommended specimen collections from dead ruminants are summarized in **Box 3**.

CHEMICAL ANALYSIS

Chemical analysis is often indispensible to toxicologic diagnosis. Used properly and in the right context, chemical analysis is often the single best diagnostic criterion. However, it has limitations, and a chemical test without supporting clinical and historical data should never be used alone in making a diagnosis. Factors such as time course of the intoxication, changes since death, or limitations on methodology can render a chemical analysis less useful or ineffective for diagnostic confirmation. In addition, even with tremendous advances in diagnostic technology and instrumentation, tests for all possible poisons are rarely available. Broad spectrum screens using

Box 3
Clinical and necropsy specimens for ruminant toxicology diagnosis

Blood: 5–10 mL in EDTA anticoagulant. Chill and submit on ice.

Serum: centrifuge, remove from clot, store, and submit chilled or frozen

Brain (half frozen, half formalin): leave midline in formalin for pathologist

Cerebrospinal fluid (2–4 mL, chilled): submit in sterile container

Ocular fluid, or entire eye (frozen): useful for electrolytes, ammonia, nitrates, and nitrites

Injection site (100 g, frozen): for identifying drug injection residues

Rumen, abomasal, and intestinal contents (1 kg, frozen): samples of rumen should be taken from several locations; samples may be pooled from the same organ (eg, rumen) but not from different parts of gastrointestinal tract

Colon contents (1 kg, frozen)

Liver (200 g, frozen): biopsy from live animals is useful for evaluating metals, especially copper, and selected organic compounds

Kidney (200 g, frozen)

Urine, if present (100 mL, half chilled, half frozen)

Data from Osweiler GD, Carson TL, Buck WB, et al. Diagnostic toxicology. In: Osweiler GD, Carson TL, Buck WB, et al., eds. Diagnostic and clinical veterinary toxicology, Dubuque (IA): Kendall Hunt; 1985. p. 44–51; and Galey FD. Diagnostic toxicology for the food animal practitioner. Vet Clin North Am Food Anim Pract 2000;16:409–21.

gas chromatography or high-performance liquid chromatography coupled with mass spectrometry provide more latitude for analysis but often are not quantitative and may be less sensitive than more focused assays. Conversely, more generalized tests that include enzyme-linked immunosorbent assay or other immunologic technology can be very sensitive but are limited by cross-reactions or low specificity.

Establishing a relationship with a good laboratory in advance of the need to submit specimens is always a sound practice. Most laboratories welcome phone calls about appropriate sampling and any test limitations, and most laboratories can provide detailed information about their assays and related services. The American Association of Veterinary Laboratory Diagnosticians maintains on their public access page an online listing of accredited laboratories (www.aavld.org). A good laboratory will report when a received sample is inadequate or the test requested is not part of their routine and approved offerings. Any laboratory used should have professional staffing to interpret the veterinary significance of assays conducted. Finally, in some cases, chemical analysis may not be sufficiently developed, or a toxic principle is unknown, and therefore diagnosis must reply on clinical and pathologic confirmation.

SUMMARY

Taken together, the principles and approaches described provide veterinarians and clients a combination of the best efforts, management, and information to provide the greatest value from laboratory assistance. Not all acute or chronic poisonings become a positive diagnosis. In some cases, a toxicology suspect is actually something else that may never be identified, but evaluation of multiple sources of evidence provides the greatest probability for success, and a thorough systematic approach is widely accepted as a standard of practice that is supportable and acceptable in veterinary practice.

REFERENCES

1. Osweiler GD, Carson TL, Buck WB, et al. Diagnostic Toxicology. In: Diagnostic and clinical veterinary toxicology. Dubuque (IA): Kendall Hunt; 1985. p. 44–51.
2. Blodgett DJ. The investigation of outbreaks of toxicologic disease. Vet Clin North Am Food Anim Pract 1988;4:145–58.
3. University of North Carolina at Chapel Hill. Fallacies. Available at: www.unc.edu/depts/wcweb/handouts/fallacies.html. Accessed January 12, 2011.
4. Galey FD. Diagnostic toxicology for the food animal practitioner. Vet Clin North Am Food Anim Pract 2000;16:409–21.
5. White ME. Consultant. Available at: http://www.vet.cornell.edu/consultant/consult.asp. Accessed January 13, 2011.
6. Johnson BJ. Handling forensic necropsy cases. Vet Clin North Am 2001;17:411–8.

The Use of Blood Analysis to Evaluate Trace Mineral Status in Ruminant Livestock

Thomas H. Herdt, DVM, MS[a,*], Brent Hoff, DVM, DVSc[b]

KEYWORDS

• Blood • Analysis • Mineral • Status • Livestock
• Nutrition • Trace mineral

Inorganic elements found in the Earth's crust are often referred to as minerals. Many of these minerals are dietary essentials for optimal growth, physiologic function, and productivity in animals. Of these, 16 are often designated as nutritionally essential trace elements. This classification is based on their small concentrations in animal tissues, which are typically in the submicromolar to micromolar range.[1] Historically, measuring such elements with precision in biologic tissues has been difficult, but modern analytical techniques have made the measurement of these elements in body fluids and tissues practical from a diagnostic standpoint.

This article focuses on 8 trace minerals: cobalt (Co), copper (Cu), iron (Fe), iodine (I), manganese (Mn), molybdenum (Mo), selenium (Se), and zinc (Zn). These trace minerals have been chosen because nutritional deficiencies or disturbances in their metabolism are relatively common, and substantial information is available about their metabolism and the amounts needed for optimum health and productivity in animals. Other biologically active trace minerals, although potentially important, often require special conditions or long periods of deprivation before signs of deficiency are recognized.[2] There are many more mineral elements that are suspected to be essential because when supplemented to the diet they increase weight gain or efficiency of feed use. However, definite biochemical or physiologic roles for these minerals have yet to be determined. Many other minerals occur at trace concentrations in foods

The authors have nothing to disclose.
The authors acknowledge the thoughtful suggestions and input from J.O. Hall and N. F. Suttle.
[a] Department of Large Animal Clinical Sciences and Diagnostic Center for Population and Animal Health, College of Veterinary Medicine, Michigan State University, East Lansing, MI 48824, USA
[b] Animal Health Laboratory, Laboratory Services Division, University of Guelph, Guelph, ON N1H 6R8, Canada
* Corresponding author.
E-mail address: herdt@msu.edu

Vet Clin Food Anim 27 (2011) 255–283
doi:10.1016/j.cvfa.2011.02.004 vetfood.theclinics.com

and tissues of animals but are not suspected to play a useful nutritional purpose and are considered incidental contaminants.

Blood samples are frequently analyzed with the goal of determining the trace mineral status of animals. Blood sampling, or some other direct measure of animal nutritional status, is often desirable because of difficulty in assessing mineral status from diet evaluation. This difficulty arises because it is often impractical or impossible to determine dietary composition or amounts consumed, such as in pasture feeding. The biologic availability of dietary minerals is variable and difficult to predict because mineral availability can be affected by mineral source, chemical form of the mineral, and interactions among dietary constituents. Assessing animals' responses to their diet may add important additional information to dietary assessment. Determination of blood components is one means of assessing animal response; however, it is subject to many limitations and results must be interpreted with care.

Specific evaluation of trace mineral status through blood analysis may involve assessing concentrations or activities of proteins or enzymes that require mineral elements as structural components or cofactors. Examples include the measurement of erythrocyte glutathione peroxidase (GPx) or superoxide dismutase activities for the assessment of selenium and copper status, respectively. Another approach is to measure alterations in specific metabolite concentrations associated with functional deficiencies of certain elements. Measurement of serum concentrations of methylmalonic acid (MMA) as an index of cobalt or vitamin B_{12} deficiency in ruminants is the primary example of this technique. These types of blood analyses for functional disturbances, although specific and diagnostic, are often impractical in the field because of the lack of availability of the tests on a diagnostic service basis, high individual test costs, or excessively rigorous sample handling requirements. Furthermore, functional testing identifies a problem only when it has progressed to the point of dysfunction. Ideally, one wishes to be able to identify nutritional depletion before the existence of dysfunction or disease.

Testing of blood, serum, or tissues for total mineral concentration is a popular and potentially valuable means of assessing trace mineral nutritional status that is generally more practical than the more functional approaches mentioned earlier. Modern analytical techniques make blood trace mineral analysis practical and relatively inexpensive. Of particular importance is the recent application of inductively coupled plasma/mass spectroscopy (ICP/MS) analysis to the diagnostic evaluation of animal samples. This technique is fast, extremely sensitive, precise, accurate, and allows for the simultaneous measurement of a wide array of trace minerals. The reference values given in this article were generated by ICP/MS.

However, direct measurement of trace minerals in blood or tissue is subject to considerable limitations in evaluating nutritional status. Consider the assessment of trace mineral nutriture evaluation in animals as described by Underwood and Suttle[3] and depicted in **Fig. 1**. This conceptual approach recognizes that during periods of inadequate dietary intake depletion of storage pools and transport forms of trace elements occur before the development of measurable dysfunction and/or disease. When the storage pools are accessible for sampling or the transport forms are well defined and accessible, this concept can be readily applied in clinical use. However, from a diagnostic standpoint not all trace elements fit well into this scheme because for some there is no recognizable storage pool and for several the transport and functional pools overlap.

Furthermore, factors other than nutrition are known to affect serum trace mineral concentrations. Most notably homeostatic forces modulate the serum concentrations of most trace minerals within a range of homeostatic set points that vary in widt

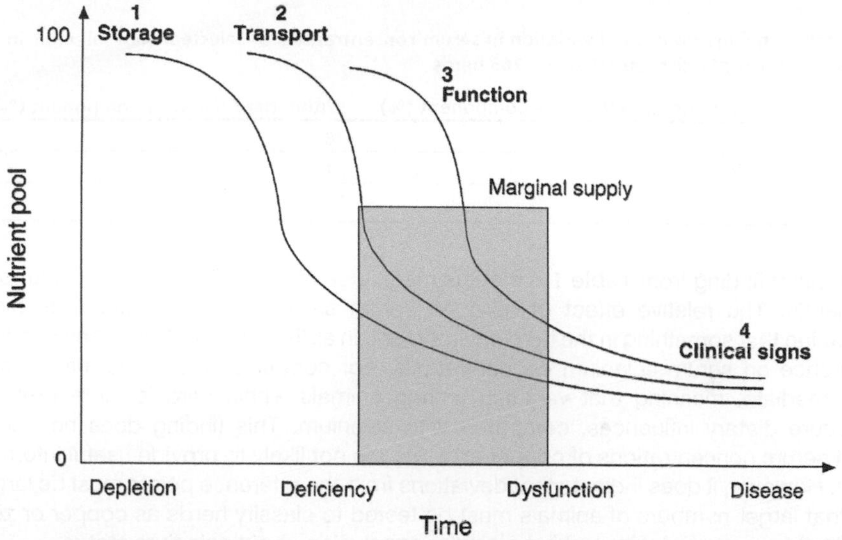

Fig. 1. A chronologic depiction of the events associated with the development of nutritional trace element deficiencies in animals. The figure illustrates 3 pools of the nutrient in the body: storage, transport, and functional. When dietary intake is inadequate the storage pool is depleted first, followed by the transport pool. Functional deficiencies, manifested as clinical disease, do not occur until the storage and transport pools have been depleted. From a diagnostic standpoint it is desirable to sample from the storage pool, when that pool is known and accessible for sampling. (*Reproduced from* Underwood EJ, Suttle N. The mineral nutrition of livestock. 3rd edition. London: CABI Publishing; 1999. p. 52; with permission.)

among the different minerals. Other factors such as physiologic state (eg, pregnancy, lactation, and gestation) may influence serum trace mineral concentrations. As a further example, the presence of inflammation has a large influence on serum concentrations of some minerals. Thus, a wide range of influences may affect serum mineral values. Although nutrition is among these influences, determining its relative influence in a given situation may be difficult.

An important question when considering blood or tissue analysis for trace mineral nutriture assessment is whether or not the effect of dietary intake is likely to be obscured by other influences such as homeostasis, physiologic state, and age. One means of addressing this question is by examining the proportion of population variation in mineral concentration that can be attributed to within-herd and among-herd effects. The assumption is that diet is consistent within herds but that other influences such as physiologic state and random variation within homeostatic set points are likely to be variable within herds. **Table 1** shows within-herd and among-herd variance components for serum selenium, zinc, and copper concentrations. The information was derived from data from herds from which 3 or more samples from separate animals were submitted on the same day to the Diagnostic Center for Population and Animal Health at Michigan State University in 2007 and 2008. The dataset consisted of 165 herds with 1585 animals. Data were analyzed using the mixed procedure of the SAS system.[4] The model included no fixed effects and only herd as a random effect. All animals included were adults, but little other detailed information about the individual animals was available.

Table 1
Proportional distribution of variation in serum concentrations of selected trace minerals in 1585 adult cattle distributed across 165 herds

Mineral	Among-herd Variance Component (%)	Within-herd Variance Component (%)
Selenium	82	18
Copper	49	51
Zinc	65	35

A major finding from **Table 1** is that the magnitude of herd effects is variable among minerals. The relative effect of herd on serum selenium concentrations is high, meaning that something in the herd environment, in all likelihood nutrition, has a strong influence on serum selenium concentrations. For copper and zinc the influence is intermediate, meaning that variation among animals within herd is more likely to obscure dietary influences, compared with selenium. This finding does not mean that serum concentrations of copper and zinc are not likely to provide useful information. However, it does indicate that deviations from the reference points must be larger or that larger numbers of animals must be tested to classify herds as copper or zinc deficient, compared with making a similar conclusion about selenium status.

The following sections discuss individual trace minerals and the most practical approaches to their nutriture assessment.

COBALT

Metabolism and Function

Cobalt functions as an essential component of vitamin B_{12} (cobalamin). In ruminant animals the rumen microflora synthesize cobalamin from inorganic sources of cobalt, and thus the vitamin B_{12} requirements are met from rumen synthesis.[5] Any cobalamin synthesis by the enteric microflora of nonruminant animals occurs distal to the stomach and ileum, organs essential to cobalamin absorption. Thus, nonruminants require dietary cobalt only as a component of preformed vitamin B_{12} and do not have a systemic cobalt requirement per se.[6] Both ruminant and nonruminant animals can absorb inorganic sources of cobalt from the gut. Therefore cobalt in various forms other than vitamin B_{12} can be found and measured in the tissues and blood of all animals. However, there is no known metabolic function for cobalt other than as a component of vitamin B_{12}. In addition to its function in the animal body, vitamin B_{12} is essential to the metabolism of rumen microbes, and biochemical abnormalities in rumen fluid occur in the face of cobalt deficiency.[5] Vitamin B_{12} is stored in the liver and when stores are replete they are normally sufficient to supply all of the animal's needs for periods longer than a year.

Vitamin B_{12} functions in a wide variety of metabolic events across a broad range of tissues. All of these events involve the transfer of methyl groups in biochemical reactions. The metabolism of carbohydrates, lipids, amino acids, and DNA all involve reactions in which vitamin B_{12} is a cofactor.[6] One prominent reaction in which vitamin B_{12} serves as a required cofactor is in the interconversion of succinate and propionate. In ruminant animals this is a particularly important reaction in energy metabolism because it is essential for the synthesis of glucose from propionate.[7] In vitamin B_{12}-deficient animals, propionate accumulates in blood, which may have adverse effects on appetite. In addition, MMA, an intermediate in the conversion of propionate to succinate, accumulates in the blood and is excreted in urine. MMA concentrations in blood and urine are sometimes used in the diagnostic assessment of the cobalt status in ruminants.

Deficiency

Clinical cobalt deficiency is well described and occurs in localized areas worldwide.[3] Generally it is associated with grazing of pastures on well-drained, sandy soils. Grass pastures are more of a problem than legumes, and sheep are more susceptible to deficiency than are cattle. High concentrate, feedlot-type diets are also a potential problem because grains are poor cobalt sources, and the efficiency of vitamin B_{12} synthesis from available cobalt is less on high-grain diets, compared with high-forage diets.[8] However, feedlot diets are more easily supplemented with cobalt or vitamin B_{12} than are pasture diets.

Cobalt deficiency is manifest as a deficiency of vitamin B_{12} in ruminants. Deficiency is associated with decreased feed intake, lowered feed conversion, reduced growth, weight loss, hepatic lipidosis, anemia, immunosuppression, and impaired reproductive function.[9] The overall clinical impression in cases of severe cobalt deficiency is one of inanition and wasting to the point of starvation. In pronounced cases, anemia is severe. Growing animals are at greater risk than adults. Mild cases can seem to be caused by parasitism or poor nutrition. The clinical and pathologic signs of cobalt deprivation are preceded by characteristic biochemical changes in the tissues and fluids of the body.[10] As soon as depletion begins, the concentrations of cobalt and of vitamin B_{12} decrease in the rumen fluid.

Toxicity

Cobalt toxicosis is not a practical problem in animals because the concentrations of cobalt needed to cause toxicosis are higher than those found in animal diets. Errors in formulation of mineral supplements for ruminants could result in cobalt toxicosis, such as with copper, selenium, and iodine. Even although there is a 100-fold margin of safety, field cases of suspected cobalt toxicity in ruminants have been reported.[11]

Evaluation

The cobalt status of ruminant animals may be assessed by the direct measurement of blood or tissue concentrations of vitamin B_{12} or cobalt. Alternatively the accumulation in blood or urine of metabolites associated with vitamin B_{12} deficiency may be monitored. These metabolites include MMA and homocysteine.[12,13]

The normal concentrations of vitamin B_{12} and cobalt in blood serum are low, and specialized assays are necessary to measure them. Measurement of serum vitamin B_{12} concentrations presents an interpretation problem because there are inactive cobalamin analogues in serum that may interfere with some assays.[14] In addition, there are multiple serum proteins to which even the active cobalamin may bind, and these may further confuse the interpretation of serum vitamin B_{12} assays. The most useful serum cobalamin assays seem to be those based on either radioimmunoassay or chemiluminescense.[15,16]

Cobalt concentrations can be measured in serum or tissues. Liver is the tissue of choice because among body tissues it has the largest concentration of cobalt and is the storage site for vitamin B_{12}. Concentrations of cobalt in liver and blood serum are small but may be measured with appropriate equipment such as ICP/MS. The assay procedure for elemental cobalt is more straightforward than the assay for vitamin B_{12}. However, there is a variable and frequently large proportion of cobalt in serum or liver that is not associated with vitamin B_{12}, making the interpretation of serum or liver cobalt concentrations difficult.

The correlation between hepatic cobalt and hepatic vitamin B_{12} concentrations is only moderate ($r^2 = 0.42$),[17] but seems stronger at low hepatic cobalt concentrations relative to higher concentrations. Using the data of Mitsioulis and colleagues[17] a regression can be calculated to estimate the hepatic cobalt concentrations at various hepatic cobalamin concentrations. If it is assumed that adequate bovine hepatic vitamin B_{12} concentrations are in the range of 200 to 400 nmol/kg wet tissue, as suggested by Stangl and colleagues,[12] then bovine hepatic cobalt concentrations less than 0.1 μ/g dry liver tissue are at least suggestive of cobalt and vitamin B_{12} deficiency in cattle. We propose that hepatic cobalt concentrations less than 0.1 μg/g dry tissue be considered as representing potential cobalt deficiency, at least in cattle.

This value applies to growing calves and adults, but not to bovine fetal and neonatal liver cobalt concentrations, which are lower than adult values. For fetal and neonatal liver, cobalt concentrations greater than 0.04 μg/g dry tissue are probably sufficient. The explanation for these lower concentrations is not clear. Vitamin B_{12} is transported across the placenta.[18] Perhaps the placenta presents a selective barrier to the distribution of some of the nonvitamin B_{12}-associated serum cobalt into the fetus.

Serum cobalt concentrations are difficult to interpret relative to vitamin B_{12} adequacy. In most studies the correlation between serum cobalt and serum vitamin B_{12} concentrations has been poor. Optimal serum vitamin B_{12} concentrations in cattle seem to be in the range of 200 to 400 pmol/L or greater.[12] Vitamin B_{12} is 4% cobalt, so cobalamin concentrations in this range represent 0.01 to 0.02 ng/mL of cobalamin cobalt in serum. The serum cobalt concentrations in adult cattle are typically between 0.3 and 1.1 ng/mL. Thus, serum total cobalt concentrations in cattle are an order of magnitude greater than the expected concentration of cobalamin cobalt. Serum cobalt concentrations are influenced by dietary cobalt intake, but even this relationship seems variable and inconsistent. The low proportion of serum cobalt that is present in the form of cobalamin combined with the inconsistent relationship between cobalt intake and serum cobalt concentrations makes the measurement of serum cobalt of little or no value in the assessment of nutritional cobalt (ie, cobalamin) status.

Perhaps the most sensitive means of assessing cobalt status in ruminants is through the measurement of MMA concentrations in serum or urine. MMA accumulates when methylmalonyl coenzyme A fails to be converted to succinate.[12] This conversion is a cobalamin-dependent process. Thus high MMA concentrations are a functional indication of cobalamin deficiency. MMA assays are not readily available on a diagnostic basis.

COPPER

Function

Copper is an essential trace element in livestock and has 2 major functions. It can be a structural component in macromolecules acting as a coordination center. It is also a component of several enzymes in which it serves a catalytic function. These enzymes include cytochrome oxidase, which plays a role in production of adenosine triphosphate; superoxide dismutase, which plays a role in immune defense and inactivation of toxic oxygen radicals; tyrosinase, which is responsible for melanin synthesis; and lysyl oxidase, which is important in connective tissue formation. Several other enzymes containing copper promote vital functions in growth, immunocompetence, and proper functioning of the nervous system.[19] In cattle, copper deficiency is a more common and economically important disease than copper toxicosis. Copper toxicosis is more common in sheep.

Deficiency

Soils in many midwestern states and provinces are deficient in copper. Grazing young livestock are most likely to be copper deficient.[20] Copper deficiency may be primary or secondary dependent on whether there is an absolute deficiency of copper in the diet (primary deficiency) or copper availability is reduced by presence of interfering substances. Primary copper deficiency is caused by consumption of diets or forages that have inadequate copper. Forages for cattle are copper deficient if copper concentration is less than 7 ppm dry weight (DW)[21] and total rations deficient if the concentration is less than 10 ppm.[2] Secondary copper deficiency occurs when the overall concentration of copper in the diet seems adequate, but biologic availability is insufficient because of the presence of interfering substances. The bioavailability of copper is influenced by the concentration of other trace elements, especially molybdenum and sulfur. The effect of these elements in ruminants is such that nutritional copper requirements cannot be adequately defined without knowledge of the dietary molybdenum and sulfur concentrations. In addition, dietary excesses in iron, zinc, and calcium also interfere with copper absorption.[22] These elements may induce secondary copper deficiency by either reducing copper absorption or by interfering with its use at the cellular level.

An early and dramatic sign of copper deficiency is loss of hair color in dark-haired breeds of cattle. In a study of beef cattle in most regions of the United States, 36% of all animals were marginally deficient in copper.[20] Marginal copper deficiency causes lost production, which is clinically characterized by increased feed intake per body weight gain, decreased weight gain, alterations in estrous cycle length, anestrous, early embryonic loss, increased prevalence of ovarian cysts, suboptimal immune function, and increased incidence of disease. Increased abomasal ulceration is another characteristic of marginal copper deficiency in cattle.

Toxicity

Copper toxicosis is frequently diagnosed in sheep. Blood is not a suitable sample for diagnosis of copper poisoning in sheep or any other species. This disease is characterized by acute release of copper after a prolonged period of consuming a diet high in copper. The liver has the capacity to accumulate copper and maintain plasma copper concentration within the normal range. Consequently, monitoring serum copper concentration to determine copper toxicosis is not recommended. Plasma copper concentration is only increased when stressful events such as transportation, extreme weather conditions, advanced pregnancy, or lactation cause the liver to release copper suddenly. Usually, such animals are weak and have hemoglobinuria, which is the result of hemolysis caused by sudden massive release of copper from the liver into the circulation. Only in these clinically ill sheep is plasma copper analysis recommended for diagnosis of copper toxicosis. Plasma copper concentrations greater than 1.35 μg/mL indicate copper poisoning in sheep.[23] Because the disease is acute, there is little chance to take blood samples for animals that die suddenly, and copper poisoning is often diagnosed post mortem using liver and kidney samples. One must remember the liver accumulation of copper in interpreting potentially toxic liver content. It is only toxic on release. Thus, high liver copper should be accompanied by increased kidney copper content (as it is being eliminated from blood) and/or compatible clinical signs or lesions for a diagnosis of copper toxicosis.

Copper toxicosis is rare in adult cattle, but it has been reported.[24,25] It is more common in calves than in adults. Excessive but sublethal liver copper content is a relatively common finding in adult dairy cattle, likely caused by oversupplementation. Feeds containing more than 100 ppm of copper can cause copper toxicosis in adult cattle.[24] Because calves are more sensitive to copper poisoning than adults, feeds containing more than 50 ppm of copper DW are toxic to calves. As in sheep, blood of no value in diagnosing copper poisoning in cattle. In sheep feed, the ideal copper/molybdenum ratio is 6:1 and a ratio greater than 10 is likely to cause copper toxicosis. Sheep feed should not contain more than 20 ppm of copper.

Evaluation

Fig. 1 should be carefully reviewed when considering the evaluation of copper status. The liver represents the storage pool of copper and it reflects the long-term availability of dietary copper to the animal. Thus, hepatic copper concentrations within the adequate range are reliable indications that animals have been receiving sufficient dietary copper in an available form. Because their stores of copper are replete, it can generally be assumed that copper status is also functionally adequate. However, within the range of adequate hepatic copper stores, liver copper concentration is not a functional measure of status. There is no reason to believe that an animal with a liver copper concentration of 100 μg/g dry tissue is any less healthy than an animal with a liver copper concentration of 300 μg/g dry tissue. Nor is there any reason to believe that the animal with 100 μg/g hepatic copper would benefit from additional dietary copper. Both animals have adequate copper nutriture.

Depletion of hepatic copper concentration is the earliest sign of inadequate copper consumption. Therefore, liver biopsy samples are the most sensitive means of copper nutriture evaluation. Copper concentrations can be reliably determined on liver samples as small as 50 to 75 mg of fresh tissue weight. Such samples are easily obtained with Tru-Cut–style biopsy instruments. Samples taken with a 14-G Tru-Cut needle (Products Group International, Lyons, CO, USA) are about the diameter of a pencil lead. For shipment to the laboratory they can be transferred directly from the biopsy needle into any test tube that is also appropriate for blood collection for trace mineral analysis. Ideally they should be delivered to the laboratory within 24 hours, but sample stability is not a large concern.

Blood samples are frequently taken for the evaluation of copper status. Blood copper concentrations reflect the transport pool, but are also to some degree a part of the functional pool. Approximately 80% of copper in blood is present in ceruloplasmin, a protein secreted by the liver. Smaller but functionally important portions are present in association with albumin and perhaps other transport proteins.[19] Regulation of blood copper concentrations is not well understood, but is presumably under homeostatic control at the level of the hepatic copper stores; while hepatic stores are adequate blood copper concentrations remain relatively stable. Inflammation has an upregulating effect on blood copper concentrations. This effect is because ceruloplasmin concentrations respond in the manner of a positive acute-phase protein, increasing during conditions of a generalized inflammatory response.

Dietary sulfur and molybdenum may in some cases create a paradoxic effect relative to the evaluation of blood copper concentrations and functional copper status. These elements, when present in the rumen in sufficient concentrations, combine to form soluble oxythiomolybdate molecules. These molecules can be absorbed into the body, where they have a copper chelating effect, mobilizing copper from tissue stores in a form that is not functional biologically. Thus, in situations in which there are significant concentrations of circulating oxythiomolybdates, blood copper concentrations may seem adequate even although there is a functional copper deficiency.[26] Oxythiomolybdates can be removed from serum or plasma by treatment with trichloroacetic acid (TCA). When their presence is expected, serum or plasma copper concentrations should be evaluated both before and after TCA treatment of the samples.

Blood serum is commonly used for copper assessment because it is convenient to collect and separate, and because it is a versatile sample that may be used for multiple laboratory analyses. However, plasma seems to be a superior sample for copper assessment. Ceruloplasmin and perhaps other copper-containing serum proteins seem to become incorporated into the clot such that serum copper concentrations are always lower than plasma concentrations. Furthermore, the proportion of blood copper that becomes incorporated in the clot is not consistent among animals, so there is no reliable means by which to estimate plasma concentrations from serum concentrations.[27,28] The reference values given in this article are for serum copper concentrations because it is for serum concentrations that most data are available. However, we encourage the development of databases for the evaluation of plasma copper concentrations.

The relationship between liver and blood copper concentrations is curvilinear. At hepatic concentrations greater than 30 to 50 μg/g DW there is little correlation between liver and blood concentrations. Low blood (serum or plasma) concentrations are generally not observed until liver concentrations decrease to less than approximately 25 μg/g DW.[29,30] However, even at low hepatic copper concentrations the relationship of blood to liver values is inconsistent; some animals with plasma copper values in the adequate range may be observed even at low hepatic copper concentrations. This situation does not reduce the usefulness of assessing blood concentrations for herd-level assessment of copper status, but does emphasize the need for sampling a sufficient number of animals. Depending on the level of confidence desired for the interpretation, at least 10 to 15 blood samples should be analyzed for herd-level assessment of copper status. See the "Strategies for assessment" section later in this article or a previous article in this series[31] for a discussion of sample size calculations.

IODINE

Function

The primary role of iodine is the synthesis of hormones by the thyroid gland. Thyroid gland hormones actively regulate energy metabolism, thermoregulation, reproduction, growth and development, circulation, and muscle function.

Deficiency

Soils in many parts of the world, including much of North America, are iodine deficient. Deficiency signs vary depending on the animal species and the severity of the deficiency. Calves may be born hairless, weak, or dead. Fetal death can occur at any stage of gestation. Reproductive failures have been reported in both male and female cattle, sheep, and pigs suffering from goiter.[3] Goitrogenic substances in feed may increase iodine requirement 2-fold to 4-fold depending on the amount and type of these natural toxicants.[32] These goitrogens impair iodine uptake by the thyroid gland or by inhibiting thyroperoxidase. They include thiocyanates from white clover and glucosinolates in *Brassica* seeds and forages such as kale, turnips, and canola seeds.[33]

Toxicity

Problems caused by excess iodine intake have been reported with a great variety of tolerable doses in various species. The horse seems to be exceptionally vulnerable to iodine toxicity, with goiter being reported in mares and their foals given large amounts of seaweed.[34] Toxicosis has been caused by misuse of ethylenediamine dihydroiodide in the treatment of foot rot.

Evaluation

Evaluation of iodine status is of interest because of the large potential for dietary deficiency, the possibility of toxicity, and also because of the transfer of iodine to human food products, especially dairy products. Evaluation is also important because dietary requirements are not well defined and vary with ambient temperature, selenium status, and the presence of goitrogens.

Overt iodine deficiency is manifested as goiters, which are enlargements of the thyroid gland. Goiters may occur in utero and not be observed until birth. Such congenital goiters may occur in the offspring of dams that are not themselves suffering from overt iodine deficiency. For postmortem diagnosis of iodine deficiency the tissue of choice is thyroid gland. Adequate thyroid iodine concentrations in most mammals are in the range of 2 to 5 g/kg DW. In cattle and sheep concentrations less than 1.2 g/kg DW indicate iodine deficiency.[3] At high iodine intakes liver concentrations may increase more than normal, but hepatic concentrations are not useful in diagnosing iodine deficiency.

For the antemortem diagnosis of iodine deficiency evaluation of thyroid function is the most suitable means of evaluation. This evaluation involves at minimum the determination of serum thyroxin concentrations (T_4) and ideally should include measurement of thyrotropin-releasing hormone and thyroid-stimulating hormone. Direct measurement of serum iodine is less sensitive and specific for the diagnosis of iodine deficiency, relative to thyroid evaluation.

Direct measurement of serum iodine concentrations may include total serum iodine, protein-bound iodine (PBI), and/or plasma inorganic iodine (PII). PBI is composed primarily of T_4 and in adult cattle is normally in the range of 10 to 25 ng/mL. Both T_4 and PBI tend to be relatively stable and do not respond rapidly to changes in iodine intake. This situation is because the thyroid gland buffers the effect of changes in dietary iodine intake on the plasma concentrations of T_4 and PBI, as long as overall iodine status is adequate. In contrast, PII fluctuates rapidly with changes in iodine consumption. Although PII does not reflect the iodine status of the animal, it does reflect the dietary iodine intake, at least in the short-term. Blood serum concentrations of PII in cattle receiving diets of adequate iodine concentration are in the range of 100 to 200 ng/mL.[35] Because PII contributes most serum iodine in typical feeding situations, serum total iodine may be used as a general index of short-term iodine intake. However, the finding of low serum total iodine concentrations (<80 ng/mL in cattle) does not indicate iodine deficiency because there may be adequate thyroid iodine reserves in the face of a short-term insufficiency of dietary iodine.

IRON

Function

Iron is an essential nutrient that is required in a wide variety of metabolic processes and is found in all body cells. The largest portion is found as a necessary component of the protein molecules hemoglobin and myoglobin. As an essential component of these proteins it is involved in the electron transport chain and oxygen transport. Iron is essential for normal cellular function of all cell types and is found in plasma (transferrin), milk (lactoferrin), and liver (ferritin and hemosiderin).[36]

The iron content of animal feeds is variable. The amount of iron in herbage plants is determined by the species and type of soil in which the plants grow. Iron deficiency in livestock is associated with reduced growth, poor immune function, weakness, and anemia.[3] The clinical manifestation of iron deprivation is preceded by depletion of storage iron present as ferritin in liver, kidney, and spleen, a decrease in serum iron concentration, an increase in serum total iron binding capacity (TIBC) and a decrease in serum iron binding saturation.[37]

Deficiency

Lack of dietary iron is of limited practical significance in farm livestock. Confinement increases the possibility of iron deficiency in young suckling animals or animals reared largely on a diet of milk or milk products. Infection as a cause of anemia is also possible because bacteria also need iron and have a variety of systems for removing iron from the host. Severe blood loss from a parasitic infestation and variety of causes of blood loss also produces secondary iron deficiency. A variety of factors in feeds can have an enhancing or inhibiting effect on iron bioavailability. Inhibitors of nonheme iron absorption include phytate, polyphenols, and calcium.[38] Trace mineral interaction may also alter bioavailability. An excess of 1 trace mineral may impair the absorption or transportation of another mineral with similar divalent form, possibly by competing for intestinal binding sites on the mucosa.[39] Excessive dietary cobalt or manganese may interfere with iron availability.

Toxicity

Iron toxicosis is not a common problem in most domestic animals, probably because of the limited absorption and uptake of iron when intakes are high. Systemic iron uptake is generally well regulated at the point of intestinal absorption. Iron toxicosis may occur in animals given excessive supplements to prevent deficiencies, or if they consume large amounts of iron over a long period. This situation can result in tissue overload, with excessive free iron levels becoming sufficient to cause peroxidative damage, especially in the liver.[3] Animals can tolerate considerably higher daily exposure of iron when it is consumed in feed rather than when it is delivered in the water or in a fasting state. Calcium is an important factor in modulating iron toxicity.[40] The maximum tolerable concentration of dietary iron has been set at 500 mg/kg for cattle and sheep. Young animals absorb iron more efficiently than older animals and have a lower tolerance. High iron exposure can cause accumulation in liver, spleen, and bone marrow, the major sites for iron storage.

Evaluation

Both liver and serum concentrations are commonly used to diagnose iron deficiency and toxicosis. Iron deficiency can be determined from the reduced concentrations of iron in serum that precedes development of anemia. When using serum to measure iron deficiency, samples that have any evidence of hemolysis should not be used, because they have artificially increased iron concentrations from the lysed red blood cells. Ideally all serum iron concentrations should be determined by methods that do not detect iron in heme molecules. Such methods are commonly available, but are not suited to techniques that measure multiple elements in a single analytical procedure, such as ICP techniques. Other factors that can be used to assist with the diagnosis of iron status include serum iron binding saturation, status of the erythron (ie, red blood cell count, blood hemoglobin concentration, or packed cell volume) and serum ferritin concentration.[37] Of these factors, serum ferritin may be the most sensitive for the determination of iron status. However, serum ferritin assays are immunologically based and dependent on species-specific antibody. Few species-specific ferritin assays are available for domestic livestock. Inflammatory diseases can alter serum and liver iron concentrations because the body both tries to limit availability of iron to growing organisms and increases the availability of iron to the body's immune cells. Transferrin, the primary iron-carrying protein in blood serum, behaves as a negative acute-phase protein, with concentrations diminishing substantially in the presence of inflammation.[41] Interpretation of the iron status should therefore be made with consideration of the overall health of the animal. See **Table 2** for reference values for serum iron, TIBC (transferrin), unbound iron binding capacity (UIBC), and percent saturation. Low total iron with normal TIBC and low percent saturation suggest iron deficiency.

MANGANESE

Function

Manganese is involved in a broad array of enzyme systems in the body and affects a wide variety of biochemical processes including carbohydrate, fat, and protein use. It is also involved in proper bone development and maintenance. Manganese is required by glycosyltransferases, which are involved in the synthesis of the glycocoaminoglycans and glycoproteins of bone and cartilage matrix.[42] Through its role in mitochondrial superoxide dismutase, manganese plays an important role in free-radical quenching and protection against oxidative tissue damage.

Manganese is distributed widely throughout the body but is one of the least abundant trace minerals in the animal body. Highest concentrations are found in liver, pancreas, and kidney. The homeostasis of manganese seems to be tightly controlled via both absorption and excretion. The absorption of manganese from the gut is normally less than 10% in most species, but within the range of dietary concentrations between 1% and 10% the absorption efficiency is strongly influenced by body needs. Manganese absorbed in excess of requirements is excreted primarily via bile. There does not seem to be a storage pool for manganese, probably because it is so widely distributed throughout the body. Homeostasis is tightly regulated and animals maintain tissue concentrations over long periods of insufficient intake. Fetal liver concentrations of manganese are typically lower or equivalent to those of the dam; thus it seems that there is no fetal accumulation of manganese as occurs for several other nutritional trace elements.[42,43]

Pasture grasses and legumes are typically good sources of manganese, whereas corn silage frequently is not. Cereal grains, especially corn, are generally poor sources, although by-products containing substantial amounts of bran may have substantially higher concentrations than base grains from which they were derived. However, the availability of manganese from high phytate sources such as brans is low, especially for monogastrics.

Deficiency

Manganese deficiency in domestic animals is associated with impaired growth, skeletal abnormalities, ataxia of the newborn, disturbed or depressed reproductive

Table 2
Reference values for serum iron concentration, TIBC, UIBC, and percent saturation. Equine and bovine data are from the Animal Health Laboratory, Guelph; other species are from Suttle[36]

Species	Iron[a] (μmol/L)	TIBC (μmol/L)	UIBC (μmol/L)	Saturation (%)
Horses	15–44	45–93	14–74	33–47
Cattle	14–37	48–80	34–43	29–46
Swine	16–35	43–70	27–35	37–50
Sheep/goats	33–36	56–63	23–27	57–59
Poultry	17–36	N/A	N/A	N/A

[a] Values can be converted from SI units (μmol/L) to conventional units (μg/dL) by multiplying by 5.59.

function, defects in lipid and carbohydrate metabolism, and productivity problems.[44] Severe manganese deficiency has also been shown to impair immunity.[45] From a practical standpoint clinical manganese deficiency has its greatest risk in poultry, in which deficiency causes musculoskeletal abnormalities including slipped tendon and nutritional chondrodystrophy.

Cases of well-documented manganese responsive disorders in mammalian livestock are rare. Recently there has been concern that congenital abnormalities of bone formation have occurred in cattle in association with manganese deficiency. In a controlled study of Holstein heifers those fed a low-manganese diet throughout growth and gestation gave birth to calves that had lower blood manganese concentrations than controls and abnormalities of bone growth, including superior brachygnathism (parrot mouth), unsteadiness, disproportionate dwarfism, and swollen joints.[46] In clinical observations it has been noted in the Utah Veterinary Diagnostic Laboratory that cattle of the dairy breeds seem to have generally lower tissue manganese concentrations than do cattle of beef breeds.[47] This situation may in part be because of high calcium and phosphorus concentrations in dairy rations, which can be antagonistic to the bioavailability of manganese. Furthermore, the National Research Council recently lowered the recommended dietary manganese concentration from 40 mg/kg to approximately 20 mg/kg, which might place some pregnant animals at risk for fetal manganese deficiency.[2]

Toxicity

Manganese is considered to be one of the least toxic of the essential elements.[48] Although manganese excess can produce toxic effects, the levels needed to produce toxicosis are high. Generally, depressed iron status and hematologic changes were the most common signs of manganese toxicosis, even in animals fed adequate iron. The chemical form of manganese can play an important role in potential toxic effects. Water-soluble, reduced manganese is highly red-ox reactive and can have adverse effects on the rumen microbial flora, resulting in poor feed conversion.

Evaluation

Evaluation of manganese status is difficult and subject to some degree of controversy. Liver, whole blood, and serum are the most frequent samples tested for manganese concentration. Liver and whole blood are frequently recommended as the samples of choice because of their higher manganese concentrations relative to serum; however, their manganese concentrations are poorly responsive to supplementation and have remained constant in the face of prolonged intake of manganese-deficient diets. Whole-blood manganese concentrations less than 20 ng/mL and liver concentrations less than 1.0 μg/g wet weight are generally considered evidence for manganese deficiency.[49] Blood serum, at least in sheep, seems to be the matrix most responsive to sustained intake of manganese-deficient diets.[50] Care must be exercised in the collection and handling of serum samples for manganese analysis because red blood cells have a higher manganese concentration than serum (usually 10-fold to 20-fold).[51] Therefore, hemolysis or prolonged contact of the serum with the clot results in the escape of red cell manganese into the serum and a false increase in serum manganese concentrations. Manganese seems to leach from red cells soon after sample collection, so not only should hemolysis be avoided but serum should be separated from the clot quickly, optimally within 2 to 3 hours of collection. Serum manganese concentrations are low and many laboratories do not offer this analysis because of inadequate sensitivity of analytical methods. ICP/MS is the analytical method of choice for serum manganese.

MOLYBDENUM

Function

Early nutritional interest in molybdenum was centered on its antagonistic effect on copper availability in ruminants. An essential role for molybdenum came from the discovery that the flavoprotein enzyme, xanthine oxidase, contains molybdenum and that its activity depends on the metal.[52] Molybdenum is required for nitrogen fixation and for the reduction of nitrate to nitrite in bacteria.[53]

Deficiency

Although molybdenum is probably essential for all higher animals, the requirements are low and clear signs of deficiency have been shown in few species. Primary molybdenum deficiency has been reported in goats,[54] with depressed growth, impaired reproduction, and death of kids and dams. Secondary molybdenum deficiency was produced in chickens fed high levels of tungsten.[55]

Toxicity

The tolerance of livestock to high dietary molybdenum intakes varies with the species, the amount and chemical form of the ingested molybdenum, the copper status of the animal, and the diet and the forms and concentration of sulfur in the diet. Cattle are the least tolerant species, followed by sheep, whereas pigs are the most resistant.[36] The clinical signs of molybdenum toxicity also vary among species. Growth retardation, weight loss, and anorexia are common and diarrhea is typical only in cattle.[36] Ruminants have typical clinical signs that mimic copper deficiency if they have less severe exposure, as a result of ruminal formation of oxythiomolybdates, which can diminish copper absorption and bind systemic copper and render it nonfunctional.

Evaluation

Assessment of molybdenum status is usually concerned with molybdenum toxicity or conditioned copper deficiency. Molybdenum in soluble dietary forms is readily absorbed and serum, whole-blood, milk, liver, and kidney values reflect dietary intake.[56] Assessment of serum and hepatic molybdenum concentrations is useful as a reflection of potentially excessive intake with concomitant secondary copper deficiency.[57] High serum molybdenum concentrations should cause concern for the presence of oxythiomolybdates, which should affect the interpretation of serum or plasma copper concentrations (see section on copper).

SELENIUM

Metabolism and Function

Some of the exact physiologic functions of selenium are still not clear, but much has been elucidated since the discovery of selenium as an integral part of cellular GPx.[58] Although the biologic significance of selenium was initially recognized through its toxicity to livestock, selenium deficiency is a more widespread practical problem. In mammals, selenium is an essential component of at least 12 enzymes: 4 GPxs that use glutathione to break down hydroperoxides; 3 iodothyronine 5′-deiodinases that catalyze the deiodination of *l*-thyroxine to the biologically active thyroid hormone 3,3′5-triiodothyronine; 3 thioredoxin reductases that reduce oxidized proteins; a selenophosphate synthetase 2 that is involved in selenium activation of selenocysteine synthesis; and a methionine-R-sulfoxide reductase.[59] There are 3 characterized selenium-containing proteins: selenoprotein P, which accounts for 60% of selenium in plasma; selenoprotein W, which may be related to white muscle disease; and a 15-kDa selenoprotein that may be related to cancer.[60] Recent work has also shown that deficiencies in either selenium or vitamin E can in certain cases increase viral pathogenicity by changing relatively benign viruses into virulent ones.[61]

For both ruminants and nonruminants, various forms of selenium are readily absorbed in the small intestine. Selenocysteine and selenomethionine are absorbed via an active amine acid transport mechanism, whereas selenite is absorbed by simple diffusion, and selenate by sodium-mediated carrier shared with sulfate.[62] No homeostatic control of selenium absorption has been identified or presumably exists because dietary selenium concentrations or body selenium status has no apparent effect on its absorption efficiency.[63] Cattle and sheep have lower absorption of selenium with greater variation than nonruminants. High dietary sulfur, lead, alfalfa hay, and dietary calcium reduce selenium absorption in ruminants.[64]

Deficiency

Forages in many areas of the world do not provide adequate dietary selenium for livestock, whereas in other areas selenium concentrations in some plants are high and can result in animal toxicosis. The major biochemical lesions associated with selenium deficiency are low GPx and iodothyronine 5'-deiodinase activities.[61] Excess cellular free-radical damage can be the initial underlying factor leading to widespread disease. The simultaneous deficiencies of other antioxidants, such as vitamins A and E, amplify the signs of selenium deficiency. Selenium deficiency directly affects the free-radical scavenging system, which can be expressed as clinical disease. Nutritional muscular dystrophy is a selenium-responsive disorder that mainly affects young farm animals. The myopathy is typically associated with excessive peroxidation of lipids, resulting in degeneration, necrosis, and eventually fibrosis of skeletal and cardiac myofibrils. This myopathy may be associated with cardiac involvement and, depending on the species, hepatic necrosis.[65]

In cattle, mastitis has been shown to be selenium responsive.[66] Testicular degeneration and impaired sperm production, infertility, abortion, and weak and stillborn young and retained placenta have all been shown to be responsive to selenium supplementation. There are also negative effects of selenium deficiency on immunocompetence, but the biochemical lesions underlying this effect have not been delineated. Anemia is also associated with selenium deficiency and it seems to involve a depression in GPx activity with Heinz body formation.[66]

Toxicity

Selenium is the most toxic of the essential trace elements. Problems can arise naturally or from careless administration of selenium supplements and accidental acute and chronic problems have become more common, even in seleniferous areas.[67] Selenium toxicosis occurs in livestock in seleniferous areas of many countries, including the Great Plains of the United States and Canada, as well as many areas in Russia, Israel, and China. The tolerance of livestock toward high-selenium intake varies with the form in which the selenium is ingested, the duration and continuity of the exposure, animal genotype, and the interactions between these factors. The precise tolerance of grazing cattle and horses on seleniferous range is difficult to establish, because selenium intakes from forages vary widely because of palatability and accessibility.

Three types of selenium toxicity have been identified in livestock: acute toxicosis, blind staggers, and chronic alkali disease.[48] However, blind staggers has never been reproduced with pure selenium deficiency. Blind staggers was likely miscategorized as a selenium toxicosis because of its occurrence in alkali seleniferous areas.

Blind staggers is more likely a disease or diseases caused by poisonous plant or high dietary sulfur that can occur in these environments. Abnormal movement and posture, respiratory distress, and diarrhea with sudden death characterize acute selenium toxicosis. Alkali disease occurs when animals consume high-selenium diets for a prolonged period. Alkali disease is characterized by emaciation, lack of vitality, cardiac atrophy, hepatic cirrhosis, anemia, and erosion of the long bones.[48]

Evaluation

Selenium seems to be absorbed from the gut based on its dietary availability, with little homeostatic regulation at the level of absorption. Dietary availability seems to be affected by factors such as the valence state of selenium and whether it is in an organic or inorganic form. Different chemical forms of selenium have significantly different availabilities, which influence absorption efficiency, but absorption does not seem to be controlled by homeostatic regulation. After absorption, a high proportion of selenium is transferred to the liver,[68,69] which seems to function as a clearinghouse for the distribution of selenium in the body. When in excess of body needs, some of the liver selenium pool is excreted in bile, but much of it is cycled back to the serum for renal excretion. Serum is therefore the major transport pool for selenium disposal, making the concentration of selenium in serum a good indicator of dietary intake.[68] The half-life of selenium in the plasma compartment of slowest turnover is 6.6 hours in humans and is probably similar in other mammals. The kinetics of serum selenium concentration is fairly rapid, and short-term changes in serum selenium are to be expected. Increasing dietary selenium uptake in cattle resulted in a significant increase in serum selenium within 2 to 6 days, depending on the amount of selenium intake.[70] The major drawback of serum selenium concentration as a nutritional assessment tool may be its short-term sensitivity to dietary intake, resulting in rapid fluctuations with small changes in intake.

Assessing selenium status is of great interest. When measured in blood, selenium may be determined in whole blood or serum. Whole blood contains both the erythrocyte and serum selenium fractions. The kinetic and homeostatic patterns of each of these fractions, or pools, are different. Selenium in erythrocytes of most domestic animals is present primarily as GPx,[71] the concentration of which is affected by dietary selenium availability. GPx is formed at the time of erythrocyte development,[72] which results in a buffering effect on the rate of change in erythrocyte selenium concentrations, relative to dietary intake. The half-life of erythrocytes in most domestic species, including cattle, is roughly 100 days. After changes in dietary availability of selenium occur, changes in the selenium concentration of circulating erythrocytes can happen no faster than the rate of erythrocyte turnover. The contribution of erythrocyte selenium to whole-blood selenium in cattle is roughly 60%, although this varies with species and individuals.[73,74] Both the rapidly changing serum pool and the more slowly changing erythrocyte pool consequently affect whole-blood selenium concentration. This combination of short-term and long-term effects makes whole-blood selenium generally more desirable than serum selenium for the determination of selenium nutrition, although either is effective.

Variability factors other than dietary selenium concentration and availability that affect whole-blood and serum selenium concentrations include gestation-lactation stage and age, at least in cattle. Selenium is preferentially partitioned to the fetus during midgestation to late gestation.[73] In late gestation, this characteristic seems to lower serum selenium concentrations in the dam, without measurably affecting whole-blood selenium concentration. This finding is reflected in low serum selenium concentrations at calving, which increase progressively during at least the first month of lactation.[75] In the fetus, selenium in blood is mostly in the erythrocyte pool, with a smaller proportion in serum than in adult animals.[73] This general trend is apparent after birth, with newborn animals having lower serum selenium than adults, although whole-blood concentrations are more similar. Serum selenium concentrations in young animals remain low during the suckling period because the selenium concentration in milk is low. Serum selenium concentrations increase after consumption of solid feed.

Liver from biopsies or postmortem samples is useful for the evaluation of status. However, for appropriate diagnosis of status, one must know the age of the animal being tested. Late-term feti and early neonates have a higher normal range than adults. This situation is because of maternal movement of significant stores to the fetus during gestation. The stores help prevent deficiency during the time period of a predominantly milk diet. Thus, an early neonate with liver selenium near the low end of the normal range for an adult likely suffers deficiency before significant grazing.

ZINC

Metabolism and Function

Zinc is the most abundant intracellular trace element and second only to iron in overall abundance in the body. Zinc is a component of several enzymes and serves catalytic, structural, and regulatory functions within the body. Zinc is important in cell division and interpretation of the genetic code but its functions go beyond that. Zinc seems to be particularly important in regulation of appetite, growth, and immune function. The physiologic functions of zinc seem to be protected in a hierarchical fashion, with some functions being more sensitive to dietary zinc insufficiency than others. In general it has been difficult to tie the signs of zinc deficiency to any 1 specific biochemical function.[76]

Monogastric livestock (swine and poultry) are at greatest risk of zinc deficiency because dietary phytate, especially in combination with excess dietary calcium, severely reduces the availability of dietary zinc. Reducing dietary calcium and including phytase as a diet supplement can improve zinc availability for poultry and swine. Zinc deficiency is less of a clinical problem in ruminants because phytate is digested by rumen microbes. The risk of zinc deficiency in ruminants is generally associated with zinc-deficient forages. Successive cuttings of hay crops within a season seem to be associated with diminishing zinc concentrations. Highly mature forages including straws generally have low zinc concentrations.[77] Cow's milk is a poor source of zinc, as is generally true for all nutritional trace elements. Both ruminant and monogastric animals suffering from diarrhea are at risk of zinc deficiency, especially if the condition is prolonged.

Zinc may have pharmacologic properties beyond its nutritional requirement. In swine, poultry, and cattle supplementing zinc at dietary concentrations beyond those generally recognized as the nutritional requirement can result in improved growth performance and feed efficiency.

Zinc homeostasis is primarily controlled at the level of absorption, and the efficiency of absorption is largely dependent on the zinc status of the animal.[78] Homeostasis is tightly regulated, and tissue concentrations remain relatively constant across a wide range of zinc intakes. There is no clear storage pool of zinc in the body, and homeostasis depends on a continual pool of zinc in the gut lumen and intestinal epithelium. Under conditions of ample intake, zinc absorption is reduced and a portion of the absorbed amount is sequestered in the intestinal epithelium as a complex with the metal-binding protein metallothionein. This protein effectively removes zinc from the active metabolic pool and seems to be a major point of homeostatic regulation of zinc status.

Deficiency

Initial signs of clinical zinc deficiency are usually poor feed intake, poor growth, and lesions of the integument. Disturbances of several facets of immune function[79,80] as well as reproductive performance are also common. Skin abnormalities generally include hair loss, skin thickening, cracking, and fissuring.

Evaluation

Evaluation of zinc status is difficult because there is no well-defined storage pool of zinc in the body. From necropsy specimens zinc can be evaluated from pancreatic tissue, bone, liver, and reproductive organs, especially testes. Liver zinc concentrations are generally not reflective of zinc intake, but do decline after sufficient periods of dietary deficiency.

For antemortem evaluation, analysis of blood serum zinc concentration is the most practical means for assessing zinc status in livestock. Serum zinc concentrations are reduced in zinc deficiency, but functional alterations such as reductions in feed efficiency may occur before a decline in serum zinc concentrations. Reduced feed efficiency in cattle has been observed in as little as 21 days after the introduction of a zinc-deficient diet. This finding occurred in the face of stable serum zinc concentrations,[81] indicating that functional deficiencies may occur before reductions in serum zinc. Thus the finding of low serum zinc is significant, but finding adequate serum zinc concentration does not rule out deficiency.

Factors other than zinc deficiency may influence serum zinc concentration. Low serum zinc can be associated with hypoalbuminemia because about two-thirds of zinc in serum is bound to albumin. Inflammation also results in reduced serum zinc concentration because of increased hepatic zinc recruitment. Artifacts caused by errors in sample handling can lead to high serum zinc concentration. If serum is left in contact with the clot for too long zinc can leach from the red cells, increasing serum zinc concentrations. For best results serum should be separated from the clot within 4 to 6 hours. Rubber stoppers in many blood collection tubes are lubricated with a zinc-containing substance. Thus unless tubes specifically designed for trace mineral sampling are used serum zinc concentrations may be artificially increased.

Measurement of serum alkaline phosphatase activity is a potential means of indirect assessment of zinc status. Alkaline phosphatase is a zinc-dependent enzyme and its serum activity diminishes in zinc deficiency. There are several disease conditions, including biliary stasis, that may also influence alkaline phosphatase activity, although in most disease states the activity is increased rather than reduced. Interpretation of alkaline phosphatase and other serum enzymes should be based on reference values established by the reporting laboratory.

STRATEGIES FOR ASSESSMENT OF MINERAL STATUS FROM BLOOD ANALYSIS IN LIVESTOCK

Choice of Sample

The best choice of sample (tissue, blood, or other fluid) for analysis varies with the mineral under investigation and the purpose of the testing. Blood, urine, and saliva have the advantage of accessibility by simple, minimally invasive procedures. Liver is a valuable sample for copper, iron, and cobalt evaluation, but veterinarians are often reluctant to take liver biopsies. Some of this reluctance may stem from the need for large samples of liver tissue that were required by older analytical techniques.

ICP/MS techniques can successfully measure trace-element concentrations in samples obtained by Tru-Cut biopsy instruments (usually 50–70 mg of fresh liver). These samples are easily and quickly obtained, with little or no risk to the patient or operator. Hair samples have generally been disappointing, although they may be useful for some evaluations of excess mineral exposure. Surveys of soil-plant-animal relationships indicate that soil and plant samples rarely give information that would be sufficient for diagnostic purposes in animals.[36]

Blood

Whole blood, serum, and plasma are widely sampled, and serum is usually chosen for analytical analysis because it is easy to obtain and it avoids the cost and possible analytical complications of adding an anticoagulant, and gives a more stable form for transportation as long as it is free of products of hemolysis. Results for plasma and serum have been assumed to be the same, but serum invariably contains less copper than plasma.[82] Results for serum or plasma samples generally reflect the mineral status of the transport pool of the element, and low values indicate onset of the deficiency phase (see **Fig. 1**). Whole blood is used in cases in which the erythrocyte concentration of the mineral in question enhances ability for interpretation, as is the case for selenium.

Herd-level Approaches

Taking samples from multiple animals reduces the effect of random and unexplained variation. This strategy means taking a herd level approach, which should be the aim when nutritional evaluation is the goal. The major questions arising from herd-level sampling are the number of animals to be sampled, the statistical approach to data analysis, the reference ranges to be used for interpretation, and the confidence that can be placed on the results.

Reference ranges have typically been established based on individual animal values. A specific critical value that indicates deficiency is generally difficult to define because clinical manifestations of deficiency do not occur at uniform blood mineral concentrations. Deficiency is usually defined as the concentration less than which clinical signs of deficiency disease are likely to occur. Adequate refers to the range of blood or serum mineral concentrations commonly found in randomly selected healthy animals. The minimum extreme of adequate values is usually higher than the critical value for deficiency. The range between the critical value for deficiency and adequate is sometimes referred to as mild, moderate, or marginal deficiency. Reference ranges for adequate blood and blood serum mineral concentrations in cattle and sheep are listed in **Tables 3** and **4** and for hepatic mineral concentrations in **Tables 5** and **6**. These ranges are adequate, or normal, with respect to blood serum concentrations. As discussed earlier, for some minerals adequate blood concentrations do not necessarily signify adequate nutritional status. In general, blood or serum mineral concentrations should be considered sufficiently specific indicators of deficiency, but are generally poorly sensitive.

Assessing the mineral status of populations (or herds) of animals presents considerations beyond those of assessment of individuals. Trace mineral concentrations in blood, serum, or tissues are subject to multiple sources of biologic variation. Therefore, testing multiple animals is always indicated to better identify the nutritional status of the group. However, the methods by which values from several animals should be evaluated to assess the status of the group are not well defined.

These observations bring up important questions relative to the evaluation of herd data, which is usually the situation in livestock evaluation. How many animals per

Table 3
Reference ranges for bovine trace mineral concentrations in serum and whole blood

	Adults and Growing Calves	Neonates
Cobalt (ng/mL)	0.17–2.0	0.18–2.3
Copper (μg/mL)	0.6–1.1	0.3–1.0
Iron (μg/mL)	1.1–2.5	0.25–1.7
Manganese (ng/mL)	0.9–6.0	1.0–4.0
Molybdenum (ng/mL)	2.0–35	1.0–15
Selenium (ng/mL)	65–140	20–70
Whole-blood selenium (ng/mL)	120–300	100–250
Zinc (μg/mL)	0.6–1.9	0.6–1.75

Table 4
Reference ranges for ovine trace mineral concentrations in serum and whole blood

	Adults and Growing Lambs	Neonates
Cobalt (ng/mL)	0.18–2.0	NA
Copper (μg/mL)	0.75–1.7	NA
Iron (μg/mL)	0.9–2.7	NA
Manganese (ng/mL)	1.0–6.0	NA
Molybdenum (ng/mL)	1.0–50	NA
Selenium (ng/mL)	60–200	50–100
Whole-blood selenium (ng/mL)	120–350	NA
Zinc (μg/mL)	0.55–1.2	NA

Table 5
Reference ranges for bovine hepatic trace mineral concentrations. Values are expressed on a dry tissue basis

	Adults and Growing Calves	Neonates
Cobalt (μg/g)	0.10–0.4	0.06–0.4
Copper (μg/g)	50–600	125–650
Iron (μg/g)	140–1000	160–1000
Manganese (μg/g)	5–15	3.5–15
Molybdenum (μg/g)	1–4	0.6–3
Selenium (μg/g)	0.7–2.5	1.5–3.5
Zinc (μg/g)	90–400	120–400

Table 6
Reference ranges for ovine hepatic trace mineral concentrations. Values are expressed on a dry tissue basis

	Adults and Growing Lambs	Neonates
Cobalt (μg/g)	0.08–.35	NA
Copper (μg/g)	200–600	NA
Iron (μg/g)	250–1000	NA
Manganese (μg/g)	3.5–20	NA
Molybdenum (μg/g)	0.9–7.5	NA
Selenium (μg/g)	0.8–3	NA
Zinc (μg/g)	80–300	NA

herd should be tested and how the group data should be analyzed and evaluated are important questions that have received little attention. Calculating means and standard deviations within herds and populations of herds may have merit, but appropriate comparisons among herds using these parameters are dependent on normal distribution of the serum mineral values, which for several minerals is not the case. Furthermore, reference ranges generated from means of populations of known healthy herds are not available.

An alternative approach is to dichotomize the values based on predetermined cut points. Based on the binomial distribution and the central limit theorem the herd-level proportion of animals outside the cut points can be estimated. Critical considerations in using this approach are the reference cut points, the proportion of animals outside the cut points that are considered important, and the confidence we wish to place in the estimation of that proportion. In the following discussion animals with values outside the cut points are referred to as positive and the proportion of positive animals at which we become concerned is referred to as the action-level proportion. **Tables 7** and **8** illustrate considerations for sample size, action-level proportions, and confidence values. For example in the central cells of **Table 8** we see the 75% confidence limits for number of positive animals found when sampling 15 animals from a population with a true positive proportion of 20%. That confidence limit range is 1 to 3. Any number of positive animals between 1 and 3 leads us to conclude that the proportion of positive animals in the herd is not different from 20% and action such as modifying the diet should be taken. If zero positive animals or more than 3 positive animals were found we would conclude that the true proportion was less than or

Table 7
Upper (U) and lower (L) limits for 90% confidence estimation (*P*<.1) of herd proportions of animals less than reference range. Individual cell values represent numbers of animals outside a reference range. Cells with "less than" operators (<) indicate there is no lower limit. See text for examples of use of the table

	Numbers of Animals Tested					
	10		15		20	
Action-level Proportion (%)	L	U	L	U	L	U
10	<0	3	<0	3	0	4
20	<0	4	0	4	1	7
30	1	5	0	5	2	9

Table 8
Upper (U) and lower (L) limits for 75% confidence estimation (*P*<.25) of herd proportions of animals less than reference range. individual cell values represent numbers of animals outside a reference range. Cells with "less than" operators (<) indicate there is no lower limit. See text for examples of use of the table

	Number of Animals Tested					
	10		15		20	
Action-level Proportion (%)	L	U	L	U	L	U
10	<0	2	0	2	0	4
20	0	3	1	3	1	6
30	1	5	2	5	4	8

Box 1
Useful mass unit concentration conversions

ng/mL = μg/L= parts per billion (ppb)

μg/mL = mg/L = parts per million (ppm)

ng/g = μg/kg = parts per billion (ppb)

μg/g = mg/kg = parts per million (ppm)

Table 9
Useful molar unit to mass unit conversions. These formulas may be modified so long as the same changes in metric units or prefixes are made on each side of the equation. For example liters (L) could be changed to kilograms (kg) or nano units (n) could be changed to micro units (μ)

Cobalt	nmol/L = (ng/L)/59
Copper	μmol/L = (μg/L)/63.5
Iodine	nmol/L = (ng/L)/127
Iron	μmol/L = (μg/L)/55.8
Molybdenum	nmol/L = (ng/L)/96
Manganese	nmol/L = (ng/L)/55
Selenium	nmol/L = (ng/L)/79
Zinc	μmol/L = (μg/L)/65.4

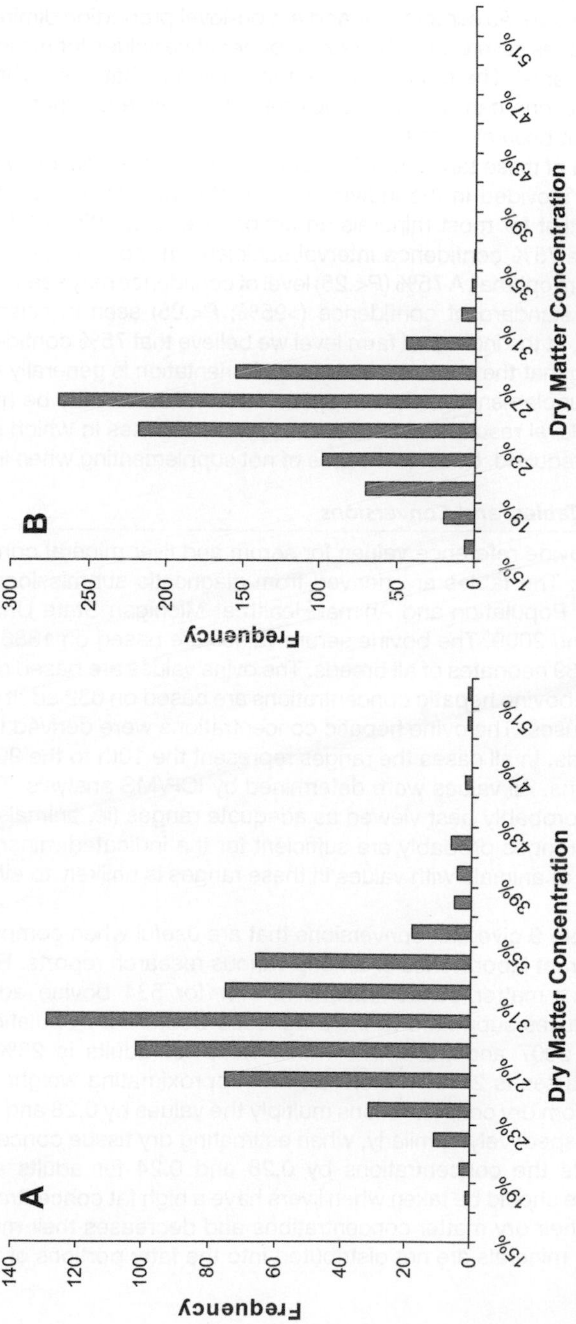

Fig. 2. Distribution of hepatic dry matter concentrations in adult (*A*) and fetal and neonatal bovine liver samples (*B*).

greater than 20%, respectively. The values in these tables are affected by herd size, but that effect is small.

Further examination of these tables shows some of the important considerations relative to sample size. As sample size and action-level proportion diminish and confidence level increases several cells have zero or negative values for the lower bound of the confidence interval. The ramification of this finding is that even when no positive animals are found one can still not conclude with confidence that the action-level proportion has not been exceeded.

The application of these tables must be approached in conjunction with the physiologic information provided in the individual mineral narratives in this document. The authors suggest that for most minerals an action-level proportion of 10% or 20% is appropriate and a 75% confidence interval sufficient. In most cases sample sizes of 15 to 20 animals are optimal. A 75% ($P<.25$) level of confidence may seem low compared with the general standard of confidence (>95%; $P<.05$) seen in scientific research reports. However, at the individual farm level we believe that 75% confidence is appropriate considering that the cost of mineral supplementation is generally moderate and the cost of not supplementing when supplement is indicated may be high. Using the 75% confidence level results in a moderate number of cases in which supplement is added when not required, but in few cases of not supplementing when indicated.

Practical Values, Tables, and Conversions

Tables 3 to **6** provide reference values for serum and liver mineral concentrations in cattle and sheep. The tables are derived from diagnostic submissions to the Diagnostic Center for Population and Animal Health at Michigan State University during the years 2008 and 2009. The bovine serum values are based on 1386 adult animals of all breeds and 39 neonates of all breeds. The ovine values are based on 143 animals of all breeds. The bovine hepatic concentrations are based on 632 adult cattle and 255 neonates and fetuses. The ovine hepatic concentrations were derived from 143 adult sheep of all breeds. In all cases the ranges represent the 10th to the 90th percentiles for the distributions. All values were determined by ICP/MS analysis. The intervals in these tables are probably best viewed as adequate ranges (ie, animals with concentrations in those ranges probably are sufficient for the indicated mineral). Increasing supplementation of animals with values in these ranges is unlikely to elicit a favorable clinical response.

Box 1 and **Table 9** give unit conversions that are useful when comparing reported results from different laboratories or among various research reports. **Fig. 2** gives the distribution of dry matter concentrations in liver for 534 bovine adults, and 523 neonates and fetuses submitted to the Diagnostic Center for Population and Animal Health between 2007 and 2009. The mean value for adults is 28% and that for neonates and fetuses is 24%. Therefore when approximating weight tissue mineral concentrations from dry concentrations multiply the values by 0.28 and 0.24 for adults and neonates, respectively. Similarly, when estimating dry tissue concentrations from wet values divide the concentrations by 0.28 and 0.24 for adults and neonates, respectively. Care should be taken when livers have a high fat concentration. This situation increases their dry matter concentrations and decreases their mineral concentrations because minerals are not distributed into the fatty portions of the cells.

SUMMARY

A variety of samples can be tested for mineral content, but may not provide any indication of the overall mineral status of the animal. It is therefore important to involve groups of animals in the diagnostic process. This evaluation should include a through clinical history, ration and supplementation history, and evaluation of several animals for mineral status.

Animal responses are a useful means of evaluating and assessing nutritional status. Blood trace mineral concentrations represent responses that may be of value, although there are important limitations. The nutritional value in monitoring blood trace mineral concentrations varies with the specific mineral, being generally most valuable for those minerals in which homeostasis is regulated primarily by excretion, as opposed to regulation by variable absorptive efficiency. Examples of trace minerals for which blood concentrations are good measures of nutritional intake are selenium and iodine. Blood concentrations of copper, iron, and zinc are specific, but generally insensitive measures of dietary sufficiency. For copper, iron, and cobalt liver biopsy samples are more sensitive measures of status than are blood concentrations.

Blood trace mineral concentrations are affected by multiple variability factors. Sampling adequate numbers of animals aids in reducing the effect of extraneous variation.

Care should be taken to use the proper sampling protocol, so as to not cause artifacts that result in variation. Removal of the serum from the clot within 2 hours of sample collection is an important step, as well as using the proper trace mineral sampling vial.

Dietary mineral evaluation should augment the trace mineral evaluation of animal groups. If the trace minerals are deemed to be adequate in the diet, but the animals are found to be deficient, antagonistic interactive effects of other dietary components needs to be investigated. High sulfur or iron levels are examples of minerals that can cause deficiencies in copper and selenium, even although there are adequate concentrations of the latter in the diet.

REFERENCES

1. Fraga CG. Relevance, essentiality and toxicity of trace elements in human health. Mol Aspects Med 2005;26(4–5):235–44.
2. National Research Council. Nutrient requirements of dairy cattle. 7th edition. Washington, DC: National Academy Press; 2001.
3. Underwood EJ, Suttle N. The mineral nutrition of livestock. 3rd edition. London: CABI Publishing; 1999.
4. Littell RC, Milliken GA, Stroup WW, et al. SAS System for Mixed Models. Cary (NC): SAS Institute; 1996.
5. Tiffany ME, Fellner V, Spears JW. Influence of cobalt concentration on vitamin B12 production and fermentation of mixed ruminal microorganisms grown in continuous culture flow-through fermentors. J Anim Sci 2006;84(3):635–40.
6. Stabler SP. Vitamin B12. In: Bowmann BA, Russell RM, editors. 9th edition, Present Knowledge in Nutrition, vol. 1. Washington, DC: International Life Sciences Institute; 2006. p. 302–13.
7. Kincaid RL, Socha MT. Effect of cobalt supplementation during late gestation and early lactation on milk and serum measures1. J Dairy Sci 2007;90(4):1880–6.
8. Sutton AL, Elliot JM. Effect of ratio of roughage to concentrate and level of feed intake on ovine ruminal vitamin B 12 production. J Nutr 1972;102(10):1341–6.
9. Judson GJ, McFarlane JD, Mitsioulis A, et al. Vitamin B12 responses to cobalt pellets in beef cows. Aust Vet J 1997;75(9):660–2.
10. Somers M, Gawthorne JM. The effect of dietary cobalt intake on the plasma vitamin B 12 concentration of sheep. Aust J Exp Biol Med Sci 1969;47(2):227–33.

11. Dickson J, Bond MP. Cobalt toxicity in cattle. Aust Vet J 1974;50(5):236.
12. Stangl GI, Schwarz FJ, Müller H, et al. Evaluation of the cobalt requirement of beef cattle based on vitamin B12, folate, homocysteine and methylmalonic acid. Br J Nutr 2000;84(5):645–53.
13. Furlong JM, Sedcole JR, Sykes AR. An evaluation of plasma homocysteine in the assessment of vitamin B12 status of pasture-fed sheep. N Z Vet J 2010;58(1): 11–6.
14. Herrmann W, Obeid R, Schorr H, et al. Functional vitamin B12 deficiency and determination of holotranscobalamin in populations at risk. Clin Chem Lab Med 2003;41(11):1478–88.
15. Zhou YK, Li H, Liu Y. Determination of vitamin B12 by chemiluminescence analysis. Yao Xue Xue Bao 1989;24(8):611–7.
16. Kumar SS, Chouhan RS, Thakur MS. Enhancement of chemiluminescence for vitamin B12 analysis. Anal Biochem 2009;388(2):312–6.
17. Mitsioulis A, Bansemer PC, Koh TS. Relationship between vitamin B12 and cobalt concentrations in bovine liver. Aust Vet J 1995;72(2):70.
18. Smith CH, Moe AJ, Ganapathy V. Nutrient transport pathways across the epithelium of the placenta. Annu Rev Nutr 1992;12:183–206.
19. Prohaska JR. Copper. In: Bowman BA, Russell RM, editors. 9th edition, Present knowledge in nutrition, vol. 1. Washington, DC: International Life Sciences Institute; 2006. p. 458–70.
20. Dargatz DA, Garry FB, Clark GB, et al. Serum copper concentrations in beef cows and heifers. J Am Vet Med Assoc 1999;215(12):1828–32.
21. Corah LR, Dargatz DA. Forage analyses from cow/calf herds in 18 states. Ft Collins (CO): USDA report N199.396, APHIS - Centers for Epidemiology and Human Health; 1996.
22. Graham TW. Trace element deficiencies in cattle. Vet Clin North Am Food Anim Pract 1991;7(1):153–215.
23. Osweiler GD, Carson TL, Buck WB. Clinical and diagnostic veterinary toxicology. 3rd edition. Dubuque (IA): Kendall/Hunt Publishing; 1985.
24. Perrin DJ, Schiefer HB, Blakley BR. Chronic copper toxicity in a dairy herd. Can Vet J 1990;31(9):629–32.
25. Laven RA, Livesey CT, Offer NW, et al. Apparent subclinical hepatopathy due to excess copper intake in lactating Holstein cattle. Vet Rec 2004;155(4):120–1.
26. Suttle NF. The interactions between copper, molybdenum, and sulphur in ruminant nutrition. Annu Rev Nutr 1991;11:121–40.
27. Laven R, Smith S. Copper deficiency in sheep: an assessment of relationship between concentrations of copper in serum and plasma. N Z Vet J 2008;56(6): 334–8.
28. Laven RA, Lawrence KE. Analysis of the value of measurement of the activity of caeruloplasmin as an alternative to measurement of the concentration of elemental copper in plasma and serum of farmed red deer. N Z Vet J 2010; 58(4):207–12.
29. Claypool DW, Adams FW, Pendell HW, et al. Relationship between the level of copper in the blood plasma and liver of cattle. J Anim Sci 1975;41(3):911–4.
30. Mulryan G, Mason J. Assessment of liver copper status in cattle from plasma copper and plasma copper enzymes. Ann Rech Vet 1992;23(3):233–8.
31. Herdt TH, Rumbeiha W, Braselton WE. The use of blood analyses to evaluate mineral status in livestock. Vet Clin North Am Food Anim Pract 2000;16(3):423–44.
32. Bell JM. Nutrients and toxicants in rapeseed meal: a review. J Anim Sci 1984; 58(4):996–1010.

33. Tripathi MK, Mishra AS. Glucosinolates in animal nutrition: a review. Anim Feed Sci Technol 2007;132(1):1–27.
34. Driscoll J, Hintz HF, Schryver HF. Goiter in foals caused by excessive iodine. J Am Vet Med Assoc 1978;173(7):858–9.
35. Hemingway RG, Fishwick G, Parkins JJ, et al. Plasma inorganic iodine and thyroxine concentrations for beef cows in late pregnancy and early lactation associated with different levels of dietary iodine supplementation. Vet J 2001; 162(2):158–60.
36. Suttle NF. The mineral nutrition of livestock. 4th edition. London: CABI Publishing; 2010.
37. Harvey JW. Iron metabolism and its disorders. In: Kaneko JJ, Harvey JW, Bruss ML, editors. Clinical biochemistry of domestic animals. 6th edition. Oxford (UK): Elsevier; 2008. p. 259–85.
38. Hallberg L, Hulthén L. Prediction of dietary iron absorption: an algorithm for calculating absorption and bioavailability of dietary iron. Am J Clin Nutr 2000; 71(5):1147–60.
39. Hill CH, Matrone G. Chemical parameters in the study of in vivo and in vitro interactions of transition elements. Fed Proc 1970;29(4):1474–81.
40. Institute of Medicine. Dietary reference intakes for vitamins and minerals. Washington, DC: National Academy Press; 2000.
41. Andrews NC. Anemia of inflammation: the cytokine-hepcidin link. J Clin Invest 2004;113(9):1251–3.
42. Leach RM, Harris DH. Manganese. In: O'Dell BL, Sunde RA, editors. Handbook of nutritionally essential mineral elements. New York: Marcel Dekker; 1997. p. 335–56.
43. Aschner JL, Aschner M. Nutritional aspects of manganese homeostasis. Mol Aspects Med 2005;26(4–5):353–62.
44. Keen CL, Ensunsa JL, Clegg MS. Manganese metabolism in animals and humans including the toxicity of manganese. Met Ions Biol Syst 2000;37:89–121.
45. Hurley LS, Keen CL. Manganese. In: Underwood EJ, Mertz W, editors. 5th edition, Trace elements in human and animal nutrition, vol. 1. San Diego (CA): Academic Press; 1987. p. 185–214.
46. Hansen SL, Spears JW, Lloyd KE, et al. Feeding a low manganese diet to heifers during gestation impairs fetal growth and development. J Dairy Sci 2006;89(11): 4305–11.
47. Hall J. Appropriate methods of diagnosing mineral deficiencies in cattle. Proceedings of the 2006 Tri-State Dairy Nutrition Conference; 2006. p. 43–50. Available at: http://tristatedairy.osu.edu.
48. National Research Council. Mineral tolerance of animals. 2nd edition. Washington, DC: National Academy Press; 2005.
49. Hidiroglou M. Manganese in ruminant nutrition. Can J Anim Sci 1979;59(2): 217–36.
50. Masters D, Paynter D, Briegel J, et al. Influence of manganese intake on body, wool and testicular growth of young rams and on the concentration of manganese and the activity of manganese enzymes in tissues. Aust J Agric Res 1988;39: 517–24.
51. Milne DB, Sims RL, Ralston NV. Manganese content of the cellular components of blood. Clin Chem 1990;36(3):450–2.
52. Johnson JL. Molybdenum. In: O'Dell BL, Sunde RA, editors. Handbook of nutritionally essential minerals. New York: Marcel Dekker, Inc; 1997. p. 413–38.
53. Williams RJ, Fraústo da Silva JJ. The involvement of molybdenum in life. Biochem Biophys Res Commun 2002;292(2):293–9.

54. Anke MB. Essentiality, toxicity, requirement and supply of molybdenum in human and animals. In: Mills CF, editor. Trace elements in man and animals. Slough (UK): Commonwealth Agricultural Bureaux; 1985. p. 154–7.
55. Nell JA, Annison EF, Balnave D. The influence of tungsten on the molybdenum status of poultry. Br Poult Sci 1980;21(3):193–202.
56. Kincaid R. Assessment of trace mineral status of ruminants: a review. J Anim Sci 2000;77:1–10.
57. Turnlund JR, Keyes WR. Plasma molybdenum reflects dietary molybdenum intake. J Nutr Biochem 2004;15(2):90–5.
58. Rotruck JT, Pope AL, Ganther HE, et al. Selenium: biochemical role as a component of glutathione peroxidase. Science 1973;179(73):588–90.
59. Gladyshev VN, Kryukov GV, Fomenko DE, et al. Identification of trace element-containing proteins in genomic databases. Annu Rev Nutr 2004;24:579–96.
60. Brown KM, Arthur JR. Selenium, selenoproteins and human health: a review. Public Health Nutr 2001;4(2B):593–9.
61. Beck MA. Selenium and vitamin E status: impact on viral pathogenicity. J Nutr 2007;137(5):1338–40.
62. Barceloux DG. Selenium. J Toxicol Clin Toxicol 1999;37(2):145–72.
63. Vendeland SC, Deagen JT, Butler JA, et al. Uptake of selenite, selenomethionine and selenate by brush border membrane vesicles isolated from rat small intestine. Biometals 1994;7(4):305–12.
64. Spears JW. Trace mineral bioavailability in ruminants. J Nutr 2003;133(5 Suppl 1): 1506S–9S.
65. Arthur JR. Free radicals and diseases of animal muscle. In: Reznick AZ, editor. Oxidative stress in skeletal muscle. Basel (Switzerland): Birkhauser Verlag; 1998. p. 317–26.
66. Spears JW. Micronutrients and immune function in cattle. Proc Nutr Soc 2000; 59(4):587–94.
67. O'Toole D, Raisbeck MF. Pathology of experimentally induced chronic selenosis (alkali disease) in yearling cattle. J Vet Diagn Invest 1995;7(3):364–73.
68. Janghorbani M, Young VR. Selenium metabolism in North Americans: studies based on stable isotope tracers. Paper presented at: Selenium in Biology and Medicine, 3rd International Conference. New York, 1984. p. 450–71.
69. Patterson BH, Zech LA. Development of a model for selenite metabolism in humans. J Nutr 1992;122(Suppl 3):709–14.
70. Ellis RG, Herdt TH, Stowe HD. Physical, hematologic, biochemical, and immunologic effects of supranutritional supplementation with dietary selenium in Holstein cows. Am J Vet Res 1997;58(7):760–4.
71. Koller LD, South PJ, Exon JH, et al. Comparison of selenium levels and glutathione peroxidase activity in bovine whole blood. Can J Comp Med 1984;48(4):431–3.
72. McMurray CH, Davidson WB, Blanchflower WJ. Factors other than selenium affecting the activity and measurement of erythrocyte glutathione peroxidase. Paper presented at: Selenium in Biology and Medicine, 3rd International Symposium. New York, 1984. p. 354–9.
73. Van Saun RJ, Herdt TH, Stowe HD. Maternal and fetal selenium concentrations and their interrelationships in dairy cattle. J Nutr 1989;119(8):1128–37.
74. Maas J, Galey FD, Peauroi JR, et al. The correlation between serum selenium and blood selenium in cattle. J Vet Diagn Invest 1992;4(1):48–52.
75. Miller GY, Bartlett PC, Erskine RJ, et al. Factors affecting serum selenium and vitamin E concentrations in dairy cows. J Am Vet Med Assoc 1995;206(9): 1369–73.

76. Cousins RJ. Zinc. In: Bowman BA, Russell RM, editors. 9th edition, Present knowledge in nutrition, vol. 1. Washington, DC: International Life Sciences Institute; 2006. p. 445–57.
77. White CL. The zinc requirements of grazing animals. In: Robson AD, editor, Zinc in Soils and Plants, vol. 55. London: Kluwer Academic Publishers; 1993. p. 197–206.
78. Cousins RJ, Liuzzi JP, Lichten LA. Mammalian zinc transport, trafficking, and signals. J Biol Chem 2006;281(34):24085–9.
79. Fraker PJ, King LE. Reprogramming of the immune system during zinc deficiency. Annu Rev Nutr 2004;24:277–98.
80. Nagalakshmi D, Dhanalakshmi K, Himabindu D. Effect of dose and source of supplemental zinc on immune response and oxidative enzymes in lambs. Vet Res Commun 2009;33(7):631–44.
81. Engle TE, Nockels CF, Kimberling CV, et al. Zinc repletion with organic or inorganic forms of zinc and protein turnover in marginally zinc-deficient calves. J Anim Sci 1997;75(11):3074–81.
82. Laven RA, Livesey CT. An evaluation of the effect of clotting and processing of blood samples on the recovery of copper from bovine blood. Vet J 2006; 171(2):295–300.

Water Quality for Cattle

Sandra E. Morgan, DVM, MS[a,b,*]

KEYWORDS

• Water • Cattle • Food animal • Quality

Water is the most critical factor in the diet of food animals and is involved either directly or indirectly in virtually every physiologic process essential to life.[1,2] Performance factors such as growth, reproduction, and milk production have a positive relationship with access to clean water.[2] When cattle do not drink enough safe water every day, feed intake and production drop, affecting their health, resulting in the producer losing money.[3,4] Water quality is important in maintaining water consumption of cattle, but it is often disregarded and may not even be considered until a problem occurs.[5] Surface and ground water should be protected against contamination from microorganisms, chemicals, and other pollutants.[6] An extensive review of the literature of inorganic compounds pertaining to health effects in livestock and wildlife was done by Raisbeck and colleagues.[1]

The consumption of water varies with age, weight, breed, species, ambient temperature, humidity, lactation status, diet, and level of production.[1] Dry cows need 8 to 10 gallons of water per day, whereas cattle in their last 3 months of pregnancy may drink up to 15 gallons a day. Lactating cows require approximately 5 times as much water as the volume of milk they produce. This is why they are usually the first to die when a mixed group of cattle is deprived of water. Weaned calves require more water than unweaned calves.[4]

An equation for water intake of feedlot steers has been developed by Hicks[7]:

$$\text{Water intake (gallons/day)} = -4.939 + (0.1040 \times MT) + (0.2923 \times DMI) - (2.5971 \times PP) - (1.1739 \times DS)$$

- MT is the weekly maximum temperature in degrees Fahrenheit
- DMI is dry matter intake in pounds fed daily
- PP is weekly mean precipitation in inches
- DS is the percentage of dietary salt in %

The author has nothing to disclose.

[a] Department of Physiological Sciences, Center for Veterinary Health Sciences, Oklahoma State University, McFarland & Farm Road, Stillwater, OK 74078, USA
[b] Oklahoma Animal Disease Diagnostic Laboratory, Center for Veterinary Health Sciences, Oklahoma State University, 1812 Farm Road, Stillwater, OK 74078, USA
* Oklahoma Animal Disease Diagnostic Laboratory, 1812 Farm Road, Stillwater, OK 74078.
E-mail address: sandra.morgan@okstate.edu

Vet Clin Food Anim 27 (2011) 285–295
doi:10.1016/j.cvfa.2011.02.006 vetfood.theclinics.com

Some criteria considered for assessing water quality for humans and livestock are odor, taste, pH, total dissolved solids (TDS), total dissolved oxygen, hardness, heavy metals, toxic minerals, organophosphates, hydrocarbons, nitrates, sodium, sulfates, iron, and bacteria.[8] Most veterinary diagnostic laboratories have routine water quality tests. The parameters vary somewhat, but the basic tests usually include TDS, sodium, sulfates, nitrates, nitrites, and blue-green algae. Conductivity, pH, hardness, and minerals are also tested, but not always included in a routine test. Some laboratories include coliform counts. It is worth a phone call to make sure the laboratory you are using can do the analysis you need. The cost for these tests is usually minimal and well worth the expense when considering potential loss of production or life.

TDS

TDS are all of the organic and inorganic substances in water that can pass through a 2-μm filter.[1] It is a measurement that does not specify what it is made up of. The organic substances include pollutants, hydrocarbons, and pesticides. Elevated TDS adversely affect the palatability of water, which affects water consumption and indirectly feed consumption and performance. Raisbeck and colleagues[1] recommend not relying on TDS alone for evaluation of water quality. If no other information is available, then TDS concentrations less than 500 mg/L should ensure safety from almost all inorganic constituents. If the level is above 500 mg/L, the individual components should be identified, quantified, and then evaluated. TDS are approximated by the electrical conductance of the water. TDS and conductivity are complementary.[2]

SALINITY

Salinity is often used synonymously with TDS based on the assumption that all of the dissolved solids are saline.[9] Salinity is the saltiness or dissolved salt content of a body of water and is expressed as total soluble salts (TSS). This includes sodium, chloride, carbonates expressed as oxides, bromide and iodine expressed as chlorine and calcium, magnesium, bicarbonate, and sulfate.[10] The guidelines for TDS published in 1974 by the National Academy of Sciences have not changed and are widely accepted in the livestock industry (**Table 1**).[10,11] The concentration of salts in water are usually expressed as parts per million (ppm), micrograms per milliliter (μg/mL), and milligrams per liter (mg/L) and are all considered equivalent.[10]

SODIUM CHLORIDE

The toxicity of sodium chloride (NaCl) is directly related to the availability of water. It is difficult to separate the chronic effects of sodium chloride from those attributed to TDS in the literature, because they are the major constituents of salinity under natural conditions. Sodium is responsible for the toxic effects of "salt poisoning."[1] High levels of sodium depress water intake and result in weight loss and diarrhea.[2] Chronic health effects, such as decreased production, have been reported at water concentrations as low as 1000 mg Na^+/L in dairy cows.[1]

Toxic levels of sodium can be detected in brain, cerebrospinal fluid, and rumen contents of cattle that have died after ingestion of saltwater associated with oil well drilling. Rumen contents greater than 9000 ppm and brain sodium levels greater than 1800 ppm confirm salt poisoning in these cattle. In spite of this, oil field brine has been used for livestock drinking water if the owner is amenable to using this source. There are few if any regulations, but a rule of thumb is to limit the TDS to 6000 mg/L.[12]

Table 1
Guide to use of saline water for cattle

Total Dissolved Solids (TDS), Equivalent to mg/L or ppm[10]	Expected and/or Documented Health and Performance Effects
<1000 ppm: fresh water	Acceptable with no reported side effects.
1000–2999 ppm: slightly saline	Few health or performance effects but may cause temporary mild diarrhea and/or production loss in dairy cows. At 2500 ppm TDS, water intake increased as much as 7% while feed consumption and milk yield was reduced.[27]
3000–4999 ppm: moderately saline	May cause diarrhea, especially on initial consumption. Young dairy heifers had reduced water intake at TDS drinking water concentration of 3500 ppm.[28]
5000–6999 ppm: saline	Can be used with reasonable safety for adult ruminants; risk is increased if sulfate is a high proportion of the TDS. Generally should be avoided for pregnant cattle and young milk-fed calves.
7000–10,000: very saline	Avoid if possible; pregnant, lactating, stressed, or young animals can be affected.
>10,000 ppm: brine	Unsafe under any conditions. Concentrations of 12,500 ppm caused sodium ion toxicosis in cattle.[29]

Data from Academy of Sciences. Salinity of water as related to livestock production. In: Nutrients and toxic substances in water for livestock and poultry. Washington, DC: National Academy of Sciences; 1974. p. 49.

SULFATE

Toxic sulfur concentrations have been shown to reduce the feed and water intake of animals, resulting in reduction of growth and performance.[1,13] The most common form of sulfur (S) in water is sulfate (SO_4^{2-}). Once sulfate is dissolved in water, it cannot be removed unless it is released as hydrogen sulfide, incorporated into organic matter, or reduced to sulfide by anaerobic organisms and precipitated in sediments. Reverse osmosis, distillation, and ion exchange can be used to remove sulfate from water, but are generally cost prohibitive.[1,13] Elevated sulfate in water is reported to decrease copper absorption at concentrations as low as 500 mg/L.[1]

Outbreaks of polioencephalomalacia (PEM, polio) have occurred when water has been a source of sulfur. During droughts, the sulfate becomes more concentrated and with high ambient temperatures the cattle consume more water. Changing from one well to another with higher sulfate levels has also caused these outbreaks. It is recommended that water for livestock consumption contain less than 500 ppm sulfate. The maximum safe level is considered to be 1000 ppm for cattle exposed to moderate dietary sulfur levels or high environmental temperatures. The threshold for taste discrimination and reduced performance in feedlot cattle is considered to be 2000 ppm sulfate or higher.[14] Other reports show PEM and sudden death in cattle from water containing 2000 ppm sulfate. Elevated sulfate in water results in decreased water intake experimentally. It is believed that cattle are able to adapt to elevated levels of sulfate if they are gradually introduced to them over a period of days to weeks. Feedlot and range cattle performance (ADG, feed efficiency) have been affected by sulfate levels as low as 500 to 1500 mg/L in the water.[1]

The sulfate levels in water combined with the sulfur levels in feed have created the need for calculations to decrease the incidence of clinical polio.[15] The water, grain, and forage can be tested for sulfates and/or sulfur and be used accordingly.[16] (See also article by Steve Ensley elsewhere in this issue.) The amount of sulfate that an animal consumes depends on the type of feed, the environmental temperature, and the condition of the animal. The National Research Council recommends that sulfur content of cattle diets be limited to the requirement of the animal, which is 0.2% dietary sulfur for dairy and 0.15% in beef cattle and other ruminants.[1]

Sulfates can be removed from drinking water by water purification using a process of reverse osmosis. Some feedlots have gone to great expense to desulfonate their water, which has resulted in an increased availability of copper and increased weight gains.[14]

Raisbeck and colleagues[1] indicate that assuming normal feedstuff sulfur concentrations, keeping water sulfate concentrations less than 1800 mg/L should minimize the possibility of acute death in cattle. Concentrations less than 1000 mg/L should not result in any easily measured loss in performance.

NITRATES AND NITRITES

Nitrate and nitrite contamination of water can result in death and/or abortion in ruminants.[1,16] Because nitrates are soluble, they can move with percolating soil, water, or surface runoff water.[6] Sources of nitrate/nitrite contamination of water include supplemental water hauled in fertilizer tanks, nitrogenous fertilizer contamination of ponds, deep wells filled with seepage from highly fertile soils, effluent from butcher shops and meat processors that use sodium nitrate or nitrite in meat-pickling brine, effluent from cheese manufacturers if the whey contains potassium nitrate, water holes made by explosives if nitrate is left in the holes when the water fills up, or industrial contamination from rubber-processing plants. Open storage tanks collecting rain runoff from roofs may contain nitrites from the plant debris on the bottom; juices from silage made from plants high in nitrates and water from condensate in barns may trap ammonia and eventually contain 8000 to 10,000 ppm nitrate.[14] Nitrates in water are additive to nitrates in feedstuffs.

Raisbeck and colleagues[1] reviewed the literature of inorganic contaminants of water that affected the health of livestock and wildlife. They noted that acute nitrate toxicity and acute poisoning from water occurred less often but was more potent than ingestion of nitrate from feed. Chronic toxicity from low doses of nitrate was indicated as controversial, but water concentrations less than 400 mg/L should not be a hazard to a well-managed herd.[1] They also noted that more research needs to be done on the maximum safe concentration of nitrite but based on the existing knowledge base, 100 mg/L of nitrite (as the nitrite ion) should not cause poisoning in livestock.

BLUE-GREEN ALGAE

Cyanobacteria, commonly called toxic blue-green algae, have become increasingly problematic in livestock water sources because of the increased use of fertilizers and their subsequent eutrophication of ponds, lakes, and ditches. Because of the "fast death factor," the common history is often "found dead in the pond." There are many species with different toxic effects. Muscle tremors and liver damage and death are common clinical signs.[6] If cattle survive initial ingestion, they may develop photosensitivity secondary to liver damage.[9] *Microcystis* and *Anabaena* are 2 common species found in water sources in the Midwest (**Fig. 1**). *Oscillatoria* and *Nodularia* have also been identified. Other species are common depending on the geographic area where they occur. Water can be analyzed for specific toxins, but may be cost prohibitive for smaller livestock operations, and chemical assays are available only at a limited number of veterinary laboratories. Microscopic identification of a toxic genus in a water bloom is helpful to veterinarians and producers. Producers are advised to remove the cattle from access to the water source. They can then decide if they want to treat the pond or lake with copper sulfate at 20 to 40 g/50,000 L (target concentration: 0.2–0.4 ppm).[17] Treatment kills the cells, potentially releasing more toxins. Treating the water will not guarantee prevention of another algae bloom in the future.

To control algae in storage tanks, light should be excluded and organic pollutants should be reduced. Water tanks can be disinfected by adding 1 ounce of chlorine bleach per 30 gallons of water, holding for 12 hours, then draining and refilling with clean water. Certain bacteria can also be killed by chlorination.[4]

MINERALS

As caretakers of food-producing animals, it is our responsibility to provide them with a constant source of fresh, clean water. The minerals in water generally contribute to but do not meet the dietary requirements of ruminants.[5] Guidelines for acceptable levels of minerals in water for livestock are listed in **Table 2**.[18] Different areas of the country have had to deal with various minerals in their water, owing to the geological environment through which the water passes.[3] The complex interactions of the various minerals make mineral supplementation more challenging. In most situations, the naturally occurring minerals in water lead to chronic conditions of poor performance and increased health problems instead of acute toxicosis.[3] Because of the complex metabolic interactions of dietary minerals, it is difficult to determine if animal health problems are caused by mineral toxicity without proper blood and tissue analysis. Toxicity from a specific mineral is a function of its concentration and the relative levels of other minerals with which it interacts.[16] Water sources of minerals can be additive with minerals in feedstuffs or forages, so analysis of the total ration and water supply will provide the best estimate of risk.

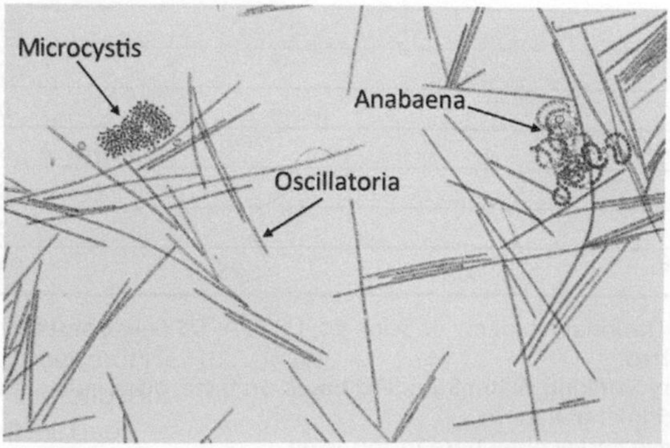

. 1. *Microcystis, Oscillatoria,* and *Anabaena* are 3 common species found in water sources he Midwest.

Table 2
Recommended concentration limits for selected potentially toxic substances in drinking water for livestock

	Safe Upper Limit of Concentration (mg/L)			
Element	**US EPA (for humans)**	**US EPA (for livestock)**	**NAS[10] (for livestock)**	**Canada[18] (for livestock)**
Alkalinity	30–500			<2000[18]
Aluminum		5.0		5.0
Arsenic	0.05	0.2	0.2	0.5 5.0 (if not in feed)
Barium	1.0		NE[a]	
Beryllium		NE		0.1
Boron		5.0		5.0–30
Cadmium	0.01	0.05	0.05	0.02
Calcium				1000
Chromium	0.05	1.0	1.0	0.10[18] 1.0
Cobalt		1.0	1.0	1.0
Copper	1.0[b]	0.5	0.5	1.0 (cattle) 5.0 (avian, swine) 0.5 (sheep)
Cyanide				0.20[18]
Fluoride	2.0	2.0	2.0	2.0
Hardness				2000[18]
Iron	0.3[b]	NE	NE[a]	0.4[18]
Lead	0.015	0.1	0.1	0.1
Magnesium				35–250
Manganese	0.05[b]	NE[a]	NE[a]	0.05
Mercury	0.002	0.001	0.01	0.01[18]
Molybdenum	0.05–2.50	NE[a]	NE[a]	0.5 0.25[18]
Nickel			1.0	1.0
Nitrate	45	100	440	100
Nitrite		33	33	10
pH				5.5–8.3[18]
Phosphate				0.7[18]
Radium				1.0 Bq/L[18]
Salinity (TDS)	500[b]			3000
Selenium	0.01	0.05		0.05
Silver				0.05
Sulfate	250[b]			500–1000[c]
Uranium				0.2[18]
Vanadium				0.1[18]
Zinc	5.0[b]	25.0	25.0	25.0[18]

Abbreviations: NAS, National Academy of Sciences; US EPA, US Environmental Protection Agency.
[a] No limit established.
[b] US EPA Secondary Drinking Water Standard based on taste, odor, color, and certain other non-aesthetic effects of drinking water.
[c] See article by Steve Ensley elsewhere in this issue.
Data from Carson TL. Current knowledge of water quality and safety for livestock. In: Osweiler G[illegible] Galey FD, editors. The Vet Clin N Amer: Food Animal Practice 2000;16:455–64.

A few examples of mineral interactions in water are included here. An increased incidence of urothiliasis in feedlot animals is reported from water with high levels of sodium or calcium bicarbonate.[19] Copper added to water (2–3 mg copper per liter of water) has been effective in controlling copper deficiency in cattle.[14] Copper sulfate is commonly used to kill blue-green algae. Water from deep wells or artesian bores has been the source of fluorine intoxication. Minor teeth lesions have occurred at 5 mg/kg of fluorine. Excessive tooth wear occurs when the level is greater than 10 mg/kg and more systemic effects are observed at 30 mg/kg.[14] Water that is in contact with seleniferous rocks and soils may also accumulate selenium. Alkali disease (chronic selenosis) resulting in loss of mane and tail with separation of hoof from coronary band, can occur in horses and cattle. Research indicates that horses are more sensitive to oral selenium than cattle. Therefore, water that is safe for horses should be safe for other livestock.[1]

pH

The normal pH of water is usually described as between 5.5 to 6.5 and 8.0 to 9.0. The pH controls the solubility and concentrations of elements in water. This is important because many metals dissolve in acidic water and precipitate out of alkaline water. A high pH reduces the effectiveness of chlorination, whereas a low pH may precipitate or inactivate medications in drinking water.[1]

The preferred pH for dairy cattle is 6.0 to 8.0 and for other livestock the preferred pH is 5.5 to 8.3.[20] Animals may refuse to drink water with extremes in pH, even though cattle have become poisoned by drinking acid that has leaked out of holding tanks used in oil well drilling. Besides damaging the gastrointestinal (GI) tract, these extremes in pH may dissolve material from pipes, thus leaching the metals from the plumbing, which can then contribute to excessive exposure.

It has been suggested that the pH of water could be between 3.0 and 7.0 without causing problems in normally managed animals, but research has not been done to prove it. Feedlot animals may not be able to handle the more acidic water because they are marginally acidotic from their diet.[1]

MICROBIOLOGICAL AGENTS

Bacterial, viral, and protozoan microbiological agents can be spread through water and cause disease.[17,21] There are no regulations governing the number of microorganisms or bacteria in water used for livestock production with the exception of a Grade A dairy. These dairies must have a safe and sanitary water supply with no fecal coliforms.[6] Some laboratories routinely include a coliform count in their water quality panel. The desired range of total bacteria/100 mL is less than 200 with more than 1,000,000 being the problem range.[17] Studies of fecal coliforms in creeks with and without cattle clearly shows that when cattle are present, fecal coliform levels are elevated and after cattle are removed, the fecal coliform numbers decline to near background levels.[21] The US Environmental Protection Agency recommends that livestock water contain less than 5000 coliform organisms per 200 mL with fecal coliforms near zero.[6] Suggestions to reduce the amount of *Escherichia coli* 0157:H7 contamination at the water trough include chlorination, ozonization, frequent cleaning, and screens to reduce organic solids. Field studies of chlorination found that the prevalence of *E coli* 0157:H7 was not altered at the troughs or in the feces of cattle in those pens.[14]

Salmonella typhimurium has been isolated in water supplies of dairy calves in California dairy herds. The continuous water tank–filling method was a risk factor compared with a water pH greater than 8.0 and a valve on-demand system. Contamination of irrigation water by human sewage has been a source of *Salmonella* found in crops used for livestock feed.[14] *Leptospira* spp. are not uncommon contaminants of water sources, especially ponds, causing late-term abortions and decreased milk production. Fusobacterium from contaminated water has resulted in chronic lameness and possible sepsis.[17] Tuberculosis (*Mycobacterium bovis*) has been transmitted by communal drinking water, but a large infective dose is required. A running stream has not spread the disease to animals downstream, but stagnant water has caused infection up to 18 days after its last use by an infected animal.[14] Occasional outbreaks of botulism have occurred after drinking water contaminated with carcasses of dead animals. The carcasses of ducks and other waterfowl that have died from *Clostridium botulinum* are a common source.[14]

HARDNESS

The hardness of water is primarily the sum of calcium and magnesium reported in equivalent amounts of calcium carbonate. Animal performance and water intake have not been shown to be affected by hardness, but washing of milking equipment and "liming up" of water heaters becomes a water quality and sanitation factor.[6,8]

TEMPERATURE

Arias and Mader[22] determined that ambient temperature was the primary factor that influenced drinking water intake in finishing cattle, whereas solar radiation and dry matter intake had a smaller influence on drinking water intake. Drinkable water should be between 40°F and 60°F. Steers drinking cool water will gain 0.3 to 0.4 pounds per day more than those drinking warm water.[23] Water heaters should be checked regularly. Water heaters left on in the summer months caused decreased milk production, dehydration, and general ill thrift in dairy cattle.

When water temperatures increase, dissolved oxygen levels decline, lowering the oxygen-holding capacity of water. Decomposing algae and fecal material have a high oxygen demand. Algal blooms also deplete oxygen that normally occurs by respiration at night. The lowered oxygen environment affects the survival of aquatic species often resulting in "fish kill."[21] The fish kill can affect palatability of the water for cattle.

OTHER FACTORS

A variety of factors and conditions can affect suitability of water for livestock. Stray voltage has caused decreased water consumption.[23,24] The color of a pond could be indicative of a problem. A rapid change in color could be a blue-green algae bloom. Other color changes could indicate chemical treatment, turbidity, or tannic acid from leaves.[25] High iron content in a well can result in iron bacteria forming a red, slimy mass that can clog well screens and require treatment with chlorine.[6] Cattle readily drink petroleum hydrocarbons that leak from ruptured pipelines. Water supplies are often contaminated with petroleum products. Ingestion causes aspiration pneumonia and damage to the GI tract. Grease or tall oil has also been a contaminant of livestock water supplies from illegal dumping of restaurant waste. The water supply can be condemned for livestock consumption depending on the amount dumped. Pesticides, arsenicals, other metals, and chemicals have contaminated water supplies and poisoned livestock.

Cows given free access to water produce more milk than cows allowed to drink only 2 times a day.[23] Increased cleaning of watering troughs may improve milk production. Heifers with access to water pumped from a well or stream gained 23% more weight than heifers drinking pond water.[2] Most livestock ponds and streams should be completely fenced to prevent soil erosion, damage to the vegetation on the dam, fecal contamination of the water, and excess sediment in drinking water.[26] To obtain the best water from a pond, a grassed watershed should be provided where no chemicals or manure have been applied. A screened pipe intake should float about 2 feet below the surface. Water can then be pumped or gravity fed to a watering tank.[6] This has also been used to help prevent blue-green algae ingestion by getting water from deeper parts of the pond. If fencing the entire pond is not practical, then fencing the dam would prevent destruction.

SAMPLING

When investigating illness and death in cattle associated with water, a thorough history is needed, along with accurate observations, intelligent questions, and samples of suspected water.[6] Water samples are generally taken with any container that is readily available. To avoid contamination, water samples should be taken in clean glass jars. These jars can be rinsed with acetone (nail polish remover) then dried thoroughly for extremely sensitive tests. Two liters should be obtained from each site and promptly delivered to a qualified laboratory.[23] In most cases, sampled water should be chilled and kept at refrigerator temperature during shipping. Proper labeling is necessary for all samples, especially legal cases. Communication with personnel at the receiving laboratory is important because not all laboratories run all tests.

Turbidity of water can affect sulfate testing. For blue-green algae identification, either a fresh sample or a small amount mixed half-and-half with 10% neutral buffered formalin can be examined microscopically.[24] Large 5-gallon buckets can be used for collection of blue-green algae if the toxin is to be identified.

WATER TREATMENTS

Treatment of water must be cost effective. Chlorine is the most inexpensive way to reduce microorganisms. Ultraviolet light can also disinfect water if it is not cloudy or discolored. Distillation, reverse osmosis, and ion exchange can be used to reduce sulfates, nitrates, and minerals in water. Ion exchange systems will also reduce water hardness and TDS.[12]

Table 3
Safe levels for basic water tests

Test Procedure	Acceptable Range
pH	5.5–9.0[1]
Nitrate	<100 mg/L <400 mg/L (in a well-managed herd)[1]
Nitrite	<33 mg/L[20] <100 mg/L (NO_2^-/L as the nitrite ion)[1]
Sulfate	<500 mg/L[14] <1000 mg/L (maximum safe level for cattle exposed to moderate dietary sulfur levels or high ambient temperatures)[14]
Total salts	<1000 mg/L (is ideal, more is tolerated)[10]

SUMMARY

In general, cattle health problems are not caused by poor water quality, but by stress resulting from lack of water or from unpalatable water with high levels of dissolved substances.[6] Testing water sources is the only way to know if they are acceptable for livestock use (Table 3).[3] Continual monitoring and observation of best management practices for water management are inexpensive and effective ways to improve animal performance.[2]

REFERENCES

1. Raisbeck MF, Riker SL, Tate CM, et al. Water quality for Wyoming livestock and wildlife, a review of the literature pertaining to health effects of inorganic contaminants. University of Wyoming Department of Veterinary Sciences, UW Department of Renewable Resources, Wyoming Game and Fish Department, Wyoming Department of Environmental Quality, B-1183; 2008. Available at: http://ces.uwoy.edu/search_start.asp. Accessed December 1, 2010.
2. Brew MN, Carter J, Maddox MK. The impact of water quality on beef cattle health and performance. University of Florida: IFAS Extension; 2009. Publication #AN187. Available at: http://edis.ifas.ufl.edu/an187. Accessed April 6, 2011.
3. Mineral tolerance of animals. 2nd revised edition. Washington, DC: National Research Council of the National Academies, The National Academies Press; 2005. p. 372–9, 470–6.
4. Faries FC Jr, Sweeten JM, Reagor JC. Water quality: its relationship to livestock. Texas Agricultural Extension Service; 1998. L-2374. Available at: http://lubbock.tamu.edu/irrigate/documents/2074410-L2374.pdf. Accessed April 6, 2011.
5. Subcommittee on Beef Cattle Nutrition, Committee on Animal Nutrition, Board on Agriculture, & National Research Council. Vitamins in water. In: Nutrient requirements of beef cattle, Update 2000. 7th revised edition. National Research Council, Washington, DC: National Academy Press; 1996. p. 80–2.
6. Pfost DL, Fulhage CD. Water quality for livestock drinking. University of Missouri Extension; 2001. EQ381. Available at: http://extension.missouri.edu/publications/DisplayPub.aspx?P=EQ381. Accessed April 6, 2011.
7. Hutcheson D. Water quality and guidelines, beef briefs. Montana State University Extension Service; Oct. 2001. Available at: http://www.animalrangeextension.montana.edu/articles/beef/wklynwsltr/10-23-01.htm. Accessed April 6, 2011.
8. Subcommittee on Dairy Cattle Nutrition, Committee on Animal Nutrition, Board on Agriculture and Natural Resources & National Research Council. Water. In: Nutrient requirements of dairy cattle. 7th revised edition. National Research Council, Washington, DC: National Academy Press; 2001. p. 180–2.
9. Carlson MP, Ensley S. Water quality and contaminants. In: Gupta RC, editor. Veterinary toxicology: basic and clinical principles. Boston: National Academy Press, Elsevier; 2007. p. 1045–54.
10. National Academy of Sciences. Salinity of water as related to livestock production. In: Nutrients and toxic substances in water for livestock and poultry. Washington, DC: National Academy of Sciences; 1974. p. 49.
11. Corporate Document Repository FAO. Water quality for livestock and poultry. 1994. Available at: http://www.fao.org/docrep/003/t0234e/T0234E07.htm. Accessed December 1, 2010.
12. Global Petroleum Research Institute Designs. Conversion of oil field produced brine to fresh water. 2003. Available at: http://www.pe.tamu.edu/gpri-new/home/BrineDesal/Uses.htm. Accessed December 1, 2010.

13. Linn SJ, Raeth-Knight M. Water quality and quantity for dairy cattle. Department of Animal Science. Minneapolis: University of Minnesota; 2010. Available at: Manitowoc.uwex.edu/files/2010/11/WaterDairyCattle.pdf. Accessed February 28, 2011.
14. Radostits OM, Gay CC, Hinchcliff KW, et al, editors. Veterinary medicine. 10th edition. New York: Saunders Elsevier; 2007.
15. Niles G, Morgan S, Edwards W. Case report: Sulfur-induced polioencephalomalacia in beef steers consuming high sulfate water. Bov Pract 2002;36:101–4.
16. Runyan C, Bater J, Mathis C. Water quality for livestock and poultry. Las Cruces New Mexico: New Mexico State University Cooperative Extension Agency; 2009. Guide M-112.
17. Brahmbhatt DP. Water quality issues. In: Haskell SRR, editor. Blackwell's five-minute veterinary consult: ruminant. Ames (IA): Wiley-Blackwell; 2008. p. 119, 954–5.
18. Carson TL. Current knowledge of water quality and safety for livestock. In: Osweiler GD, Galey FD, editors. The Veterinary Clinics of North America: Food Animal Practice. Philadelphia: WB Saunders Co; 2000. p. 16, 455–64.
19. Doyle JC, Chirase NK, Huston JE. Mineral supplementation of beef cattle: rangeland and feedlot. In: Howard JL, Smith RA, editors. Current veterinary therapy IV, food animal practice. Philadelphia: WB Saunders; 1999. p. 181.
20. Bagley C, Kotuby-Amacher M, Farrell-Poe K. Analysis of water quality for livestock. Logan (UT): Utah State University Cooperative Extension; 1997. AH/Beef/28.
21. Alkire D. The Samuel Roberts Noble Foundation, Inc. The importance of monitoring livestock water quality. Available at: http://www.noble.org/ag/livestock/waterquality/index.html 1997–2010. Accessed December 1, 2010.
22. Arias RA, Mader TL. Environmental factors affecting daily water intake on cattle finished in feedlots. J Anim Sci 2010; DOI: 10.2527/jas.2010-3014. Available at: www.asas.org. Accessed December 1, 2010.
23. Natural Resources Conservation Service. Georgia—Livestock water quality. Available at: http://www.nrcs.usda.gov/feature/buffers/georgia.html. Accessed December 2, 2010.
24. Boyles S. Ohio State University Extension. Available at: http://beef.osu.edu/library/water.html. Accessed December 2, 2010.
25. Wynne F. Kentucky State University Cooperative Extension Program. Available at: http://ces3.ca.uky.edu/westkentuctyaquaculture/info/waterq.pdf. Accessed December 2, 2010.
26. Galey FD. Diagnostic toxicology. In: Plumlee KH, editor. Clinical veterinary toxicology. St Louis (MO): Mosby; 2004. p. 22–3.
27. Jaster EH, Schu JD, Wegner TN. Physiologic effects of saline drinking water on high producing dairy cows. J Dairy Sci 1978;61:66.
28. Wegner TN, Schu JD. Effect of highly mineralized livestock water supply on water consumption and blood and urine electrolyte profiles in dairy cows [abstract]. J Dairy Sci 1974;57:608.
29. United States Environmental Protection Agency. National primary drinking water standards. Washington, DC: US EPA; 1999.

Biofuels Coproducts Tolerance and Toxicology for Ruminants

Steve Ensley, DVM, PhD

KEYWORDS

- Corn coproducts • Distillers grain • Polioencephalomalacia
- Sulfur toxicosis

The rapid growth of the biofuels industry in the Midwest in the past 10 years has created an increased supply of corn coproduct feed for animals.[1,2] Corn coproducts are a by-product of the dry and wet corn-milling ethanol manufacturing industry. The dry mill corn coproduct includes distillers grain and solubles feedstuffs. Distillers grain can be further categorized into dry distillers grain (DDG), dried distillers grain with solubles (DDGS), wet distillers grain with solubles (WDGS), modified WDGS, and corn syrup (solubles). Wet mill ethanol production produces 2 main feedstuffs: corn gluten (wet and dry) and heavy steep water. A second type of biofuel, biodiesel, has a feed by-product called glycerol, which can also be used for cattle feed.[3]

CORN COPRODUCTS

During production of ethanol from corn, sulfuric acid is added during fermentation to balance the pH. Sulfuric acid also is used to flush the distillation columns to keep them clear of precipitate. This added sulfur can increase sulfur concentration in corn coproducts to a level that can induce sulfur toxicosis in ruminants. Exposure to high levels, greater than 0.4% dietary sulfur, can induce polioencephalomalacia (PEM) in ruminants.[4–12] Total dietary sulfur concentration is used to assess risk of developing sulfur toxicosis in ruminants. This includes sulfur in feed and water sources.

The daily sulfur requirement for growing and adult beef cattle is 1500 to 2000 ppm of the ration on a dry matter basis. Recommended dietary sulfur concentrations are 0.20% of diet dry matter for most dairy cattle (NRC 2001).[13] Higher amounts (0.29%) are recommended for calves consuming milk or milk replacers. The maximum tolerated dietary sulfur concentration is 0.4% of the diet in cattle other than feedlot cattle (NRC 2001).[13] Feedlot cattle should have a diet with sulfur concentration less than 0.3%.

Vet Diagnostic & Production Animal Med, Iowa State University College of Veterinary Medicine, 1600 South 16th Street, Ames, IA 50011, USA
E-mail address: sensley@iastate.edu

Vet Clin Food Anim 27 (2011) 297–303
doi:10.1016/j.cvfa.2011.02.003 vetfood.theclinics.com
0749-0720/11/$ – see front matter

PEM is a descriptive term for the lesions observed in the brain and is not pathognomonic for sulfur toxicosis. These lesions can be caused by lead poisoning and water deprivation, as well as excess dietary sulfur.[7,11,14–16] Grain overload has also been associated with PEM.[17,18] Historically, PEM was thought to be caused solely by thiamine deficiency.[19–23] Now that the association has been made with sulfur toxicosis and PEM, the explanation of PEM being solely induced by thiamine deficiency should be rethought. Reports of PEM or cerebrocortical necrosis have been in the veterinary literature since the 1950s. Impaired thiamine metabolism in ruminants was investigated as the cause for PEM in the 1970s. Additional research was done during this time to determine if thiaminase compounds in plants or pharmaceuticals like amprolium could contribute to thiamine deficiency resulting in the development of PEM. It was not until the 1980s that elevated dietary sulfur was linked to PEM. Investigators in Missouri discovered that when sulfate salts used as feed limiters were removed from herds and feedlots experiencing PEM, cases of PEM decreased.[20] At that time it was not known if PEM was caused by the sulfur in the diet, or if the sulfur in the diet was blocking thiamine production in the rumen, or if there was something toxic present in the sulfate salt used in the feed.[20] Since this original observation, several investigators have clearly demonstrated that PEM can be caused by the direct action of elevated rumen sulfur.[5,7,8,11,14,24–27] Many historical cases of blind staggers in Colorado and Wyoming have now been recognized to have most likely been caused by elevated dietary sulfur and not selenium.[28]

SULFUR TOXICOSIS

Hydrogen sulfide inhibits the electron transport chain and interferes with metabolism in the mitochondria.[29] Hydrogen sulfide blocks cytochrome aa3, which blocks ATP.[14,25,29,30] The brain is the target organ of sulfur toxicosis because of the high energy demand, high lipid content, and low amount of antioxidants.[27] The laminar cortical necrosis associated with PEM can sometimes be detected grossly using fluorescence from a UV light at 365 nm. The fluorescence is a result of ceroid lipofuscin present in areas of the brain that are damaged. Fluorescence is not always observed with PEM but is helpful if observed. Sulfides are also potent oxidants and can bind superoxide dismutase and glutathione peroxidase. Hydrogen sulfide toxicosis can also cause a rapid respiratory paralysis associated with inhalation of hydrogen sulfide that is attributable to paralysis of the carotid body.[25,29]

RUMINAL SULFUR METABOLISM

Bacteria in the rumen can metabolize sulfur as elemental, inorganic, and organic sulfur. Sulfur-metabolizing bacteria have been classified as assimilatory or dissimilatory.[8] Assimilatory bacteria reduce sulfate (SO_4) and produce amino acids containing sulfur. Dissimilatory bacteria use sulfur for an energy source but produce sulfide instead of amino acids. Dissimilatory bacteria include *Desulfovibrio* and *Desulfotomaculum*. Most sulfide production in the rumen is from dissimilatory bacteria (**Fig. 1**). The amount of hydrogen sulfide production in the rumen is limited by the amount in the rumen gas cap.[31] This has been demonstrated in vitro using hydrogen sulfide generation tubes and measuring the gas in the headspace. As the gas cap is eliminated in the tubes, the bacteria are able to produce more hydrogen sulfide. This would suggest that as rumen gas is eructated, more hydrogen sulfide is produced in the rumen. The numbers of dissimilatory bacteria do not increase but their ability to produce more sulfide does.[31,32] Non–sulfate-reducing rumen bacteria include *Veillonella, Megasphaera, Wolinella, Selenomonas, Anaerovibrio,* and *Clostridium* spp. These bacteria contain

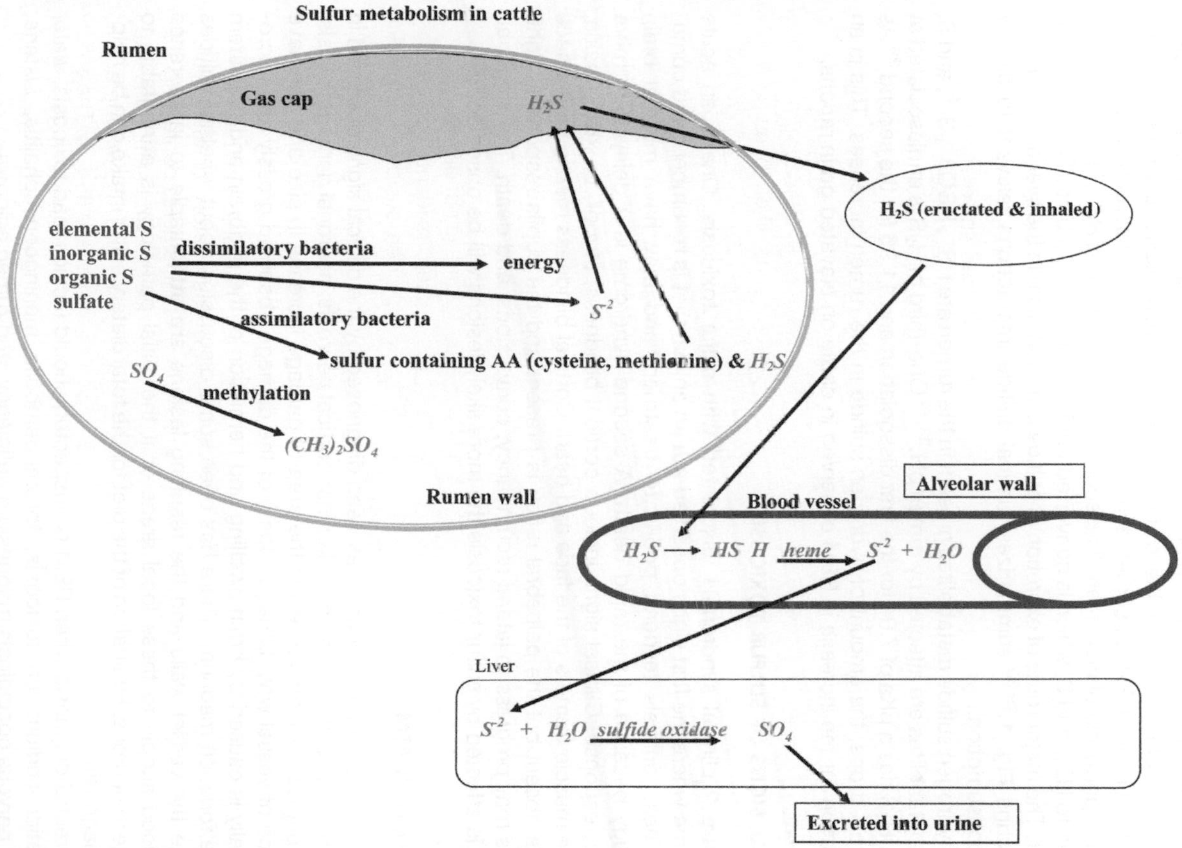

Fig. 1. The ruminal sulfide interactions relevant to dietary sulfur consumption.

cysteine desulfhydrase, an enzyme that metabolizes sulfur-containing proteins and produces sulfide.

To summarize hydrogen sulfide metabolism in the rumen, there is oxidation to sulfate (SO_4), methylation of sulfate, and reaction with metalloproteins. Dissimilatory bacteria use inorganic sulfur for energy and produce sulfide(S^{-2}), which can then be used by assimilatory bacteria to produce sulfur-containing amino acids and sulfide.[14] Other rumen bacteria can use these sulfur-containing amino acids to produce sulfide. Hydrogen sulfide (H_2S) is absorbed across the rumen wall or absorbed via the lungs, enters the portal circulation, then disassociates to hydrogen and HS^-. HS^- is oxidized by heme to H2O and S, which is converted back to sulfate (SO_4) by sulfide oxidase in the liver. The major route of excretion of sulfide is metabolism in the liver and excretion in the urine **Fig. 1**.[29,30] summarizes ruminal sulfide interactions relevant to dietary sulfur consumption.

The hydrogen sulfide metabolites present in the rumen are HS^-, $HSO3^-$, S^{-2}, and S. These metabolites are affected by rumen pH.[33,34] One-third of H_2S is undissociated at pH 7.4. H_2S has a pKa of 7.04 for the first dissociation and 11.96 for the second.[29] As rumen pH drops, the amount of hydrogen sulfide in the rumen increases. This is an explanation for the increase in PEM observed in cattle on elevated grain rations.

CLINICAL SIGNS OF SULFUR TOXICOSIS

There are 2 clinical syndromes associated with sulfur toxicosis. One is an acute syndrome where the first signs observed are an animal that is recumbent and comatose. These animals respond poorly to treatment and may have minimal brain pathology because of the rapid death. A second syndrome is a delayed or more chronic response. Clinical signs include cortical blindness, stupor, bruxism, ataxia, and fine muscle tremors of the face and head. Cortical blindness means the menace reflex is absent but the palpebral reflex is present and the pupils respond to light. Animals may progress to lateral recumbancy, convulsions, and death. The longer an animal is affected by sulfur toxicosis the more likely lesions will be observed.

DIAGNOSIS OF PEM

PEM caused by sulfur toxicosis has been diagnosed by the clinical signs observed in addition to microscopic lesions of laminar cortical necrosis, neuronal damage, gliosis, and spongiosis. Blood vessels in the area of damage increase in size and can have evidence of vessel wall damage. Some of the damage observed grossly and microscopically is caused by brain swelling and herniation of the midbrain and brainstem into the foramen magnum. There has been some discussion about whether sulfides damage the vessel walls and the resulting lesions are attributable to interference with blood supply to these local areas or if the initial pathology is attributable to damage to neurons. Evaluation of the diet for the total dietary sulfur intake can be helpful in diagnosis.

Differential diagnosis when PEM is suspected should include lead toxicosis, water deprivation–sodium ion toxicosis, thromboembolic meningoencephalitis, *Listeria*, rabies, nervous coccidiosis magnesium deficiency, and rumen acidosis.

Treatment of PEM is symptomatic because there is no specific antidote for sulfur toxicosis. Removing the animal from more exposure to the toxin is always one of the first intervention steps to take. Sulfur toxicosis is still a thiamine responsive condition even though it is not a thiamine deficiency. The more rapid the treatment is initiated the more likely there will be a response to treatment. Thiamine at 10 mg/kg twice a day for 3 days can be effective. A broad-spectrum antibiotic and steroids are also used as adjunctive therapy.

BIOFUELS AND MYCOTOXINS

During ethanol production, the concentration of mycotoxins increases 3 times in the final product.[35] One-third of the corn is used for ethanol production, one-third produces carbon dioxide, and the remaining one-third produces the corn coproduct. Mycotoxin concentration in corn coproducts can be a significant issue when mycotoxins are elevated in the corn that is used to produce ethanol. With wet corn coproducts there is the possibility of production of mycotoxins when they are stored on the producer's site; this is called post production of mycotoxins. Corn coproducts are good substrates for mycotoxin growth, especially when the moisture concentration is elevated.

BIOFUELS AND ANTIBIOTIC RESIDUE

Why is antibiotic residue an issue in corn coproducts? Ethanol fermentation containers can become contaminated with bacteria and interfere with the yeast production of ethanol. The lactic acid–producing bacteria, *Lactobacillus*, *Pediococcus*, *Leuconostoc*, and *Weissella,* can affect ethanol yields significantly. Yeast converts starch to ethanol, but bacteria convert those same sugars to lactic or acetic acid. Ethanol production yields can drop up to 5%, which causes economic problems for ethanol producers. Virginiamycin is the only antibiotic that is approved for use during ethanol fermentation. Analysis of corn coproducts by the Food and Drug Administration (FDA) has shown the presence of virginiamycin, penicillin, tylosin, and tetracyclines. In 2008, the FDA tested 60 DDGS samples for residues of virginiamycin, tylosin, and erythromycin. Of the 45 samples analyzed, 24 came back positive, according to Dr Daniel McChesney,[36] director of the FDA/Center for Veterinary Medicine's (CVM) Office of Surveillance and Compliance. Fifteen of the samples contained virginiamycin, 12 contained erythromycin, and 5 contained tylosin. Some were detected at levels exceeding 0.5 ppm, the limit established for virginiamycin, the only antibiotic the FDA regulates in corn coproducts. Dr Linda Benjamin[36] of FDA/CVM indicated that in this survey DDGs contained residues in 17 of 27 samples. In the 17 samples, 10 contained virginiamycin and 7 contained erythromycin; 4 of the 17 samples also contained tylosin. In wet distillers grains, 6 of 14 contained residues. Five of the samples contained virginiamycin and 1 contained erythromycin. In 4 samples of corn solubles, 1 of the 4 samples contained tylosin.

There are many alternatives to the use of antibiotics during fermentation to control bacterial growth. Most ethanol producers do not have antibiotic residue in their corn coproducts.

BIODIESEL BY-PRODUCT TOXICOSIS

Glycerol is a by-product of the production of biodiesel via transesterification. Triglycerides are reacted with an alcohol such as ethanol or methanol with a catalytic base to give ethyl esters of fatty acids and glycerol. There are 2 forms of glycerol on the market: crude and purified. Crude glycerol, which is used in livestock feed, is 85% glycerin and 15% other impurities. Purified glycerol, which is more expensive, is used for human products. Methanol is included in the impurities found in glycerol. Methanol is a substance used in the production of biodiesel. Additional impurities include salts and heavy metals. Methanol is toxic and the FDA does not recognize glycerol with more than 150 ppm to be generally recognized as safe. Generally recognized as safe (GRAS) means the FDA recognizes a given substance as safe for its intended use. Crude glycerol is GRAS for use in livestock feed, but only if methanol levels are at or below 150 ppm. Crude glycerol has been shown to be a safe feed additive for cattle.[37]

REFERENCES

1. Clemens R. Steady supplies or stockpiles? Dried distillers grains and U.S. beef production. Iowa Ag Review 2008;14:4–5 11.
2. Winterholler SJ, Holland BP, McMurphy CP, et al. Use of dried distillers grains in preconditioning programs for weaned beef calves and subsequent impact on wheat pasture, feedlot, and carcass performance. Professional Animal Scientist 2009;25:722–30.
3. Bart JCJ, Palmeri N, Cavallaro S. In: Bart JCJ, Palmeri N, Cavallaro S, editors. Biodiesel science and technology: from soil to oil. Number 7. Woodhead Publishing Series in Energy; 2010. p. xviii + 840.
4. Maxie GM, Youssef S. Polioencephalomalacia of ruminants. In: Maxie GM, editor. Jubb, Kennedy and Palmer's pathology of domestic animals. 5th edition. Philadelphia: Elsevier; 2007. p. 351–4.
5. Niles GA, Morgan S, Edwards WC, et al. Effects of increasing dietary sulfur concentration on the incidence and pathology of polioencephalomalacia in weaned beef calves. Animal science research report—agricultural experiment station. Stillwater (Oklahoma): Oklahoma State University; 2000. p. 55–60.
6. Niles GA, Morgan SE, Edwards WC. Sulfur-induced polioencephalomalacia in stocker calves. Vet Hum Toxicol 2000;42:290–1.
7. Gould DH. Polioencephalomalacia. J Anim Sci 1998;76:309–14.
8. Gould DH. Update on sulfur-related polioencephalomalacia. Vet Clin North Am Food Anim Pract 2000;16:481–96, vi–vii.
9. Gould DH, Cummings BA, Hamar DW. In vivo indicators of pathologic ruminal sulfide production in steers with diet-induced polioencephalomalacia. J Vet Diagn Invest 1997;9:72–6.
10. Gould DH, Dargatz DA, Garry FB, et al. Potentially hazardous sulfur conditions on beef cattle ranches in the United States. J Am Vet Med Assoc 2002;221:673–7.
11. Gould DH, McAllister MM, Savage JC, et al. High sulfide concentrations in rumen fluid associated with nutritionally induced polioencephalomalacia in calves. Am J Vet Res 1991;52:1164–9.
12. Hamlen H, Clark E, Janzen E. Polioencephalomalacia in cattle consuming water with elevated sodium-sulfate levels—a herd investigation. Can Vet J 1993;34:153–8.
13. Nutrient requirements of dairy cattle. 7th edition. Washington, DC: National Academy Press; 2001.
14. Loneragan GH, Gould DH, Callan RJ, et al. Association of excess sulfur intake and an increase in hydrogen sulfide concentrations in the ruminal gas cap of recently weaned beef calves with polioencephalomalacia. J Am Vet Med Assoc 1998;213:1599–604 1571.
15. Padovan D. Polioencephalomalacia associated with water deprivation in cattle. Cornell Vet 1980;70:153–9.
16. Sager R, Hamar D, Gould D. Clinical and biochemical alterations in calves with nutritionally induced polioencephalomalacia. Am J Vet Res 1990;51:1969–74.
17. Brent BE. Relationship of acidosis to other feedlot ailments. J Anim Sci 1976;43: 930–5.

18. Owens FN, Secrist DS, Hill WJ, et al. Acidosis in cattle: a review. J Anim Sci 1998; 76:275–86.
19. Niles G. The relationship between sulfur, thiamine and polioencephalomalacia—a review. Bov Pract 2002;36:93–9.
20. Raisbeck MF. Is polioencephalomalacia associated with high-sulfate diets? J Am Vet Med Assoc 1982;180:1303–5.
21. Nyack B, Mobini S, Padmore CL, et al. Polioencephalomalacia (thiamine deficiency) in a calf. Vet Med Small Anim Clin 1983;78:583–6.
22. Loew FM, Dunlop RH. Induction of thiamine inadequacy and polioencephalomalacia in adult sheep with amprolium. Am J Vet Res 1972;33:2195–205.
23. Loew FM, Dunlop RH. Blood thiamin concentrations in bovine polioencephalomalacia. Can J Comp Med 1972;36:345–7.
24. Loneragan GH, Wagner JJ, Gould DH, et al. Effects of water sulfate concentration on performance, water intake, and carcass characteristics of feedlot steers. J Anim Sci 2001;79:2941–8.
25. McAllister MM, Gould DH, Hamar DW. Sulphide-induced polioencephalomalacia in lambs. J Comp Pathol 1992;106:267–78.
26. McAllister MM, Gould DH, Raisbeck MF, et al. Evaluation of ruminal sulfide concentrations and seasonal outbreaks of polioencephalomalacia in beef cattle in a feedlot. J Am Vet Med Assoc 1997;211:1275–9.
27. Olkowski AA. Neurotoxicity and secondary metabolic problems associated with low to moderate levels of exposure to excess dietary sulphur in ruminants: a review. Vet Hum Toxicol 1997;39:355–60.
28. O'Toole D, Raisbeck M, Case JC, et al. Selenium-induced "blind staggers" and related myths. A commentary on the extent of historical livestock losses attributed to selenosis on Western US rangelands. Vet Pathol 1996;33:104–16.
29. Beauchamp RO. A critical review of the literature on hydrogen sulfide toxicity. Crit Rev Toxicol 1984;13:25.
30. Kandylis K. Toxicology of sulfur in ruminants: review. J Dairy Sci 1983;67: 2179–87.
31. Cummings B, Caldwell D, Gould D. Identity and interactions of rumen microbes associated with dietary sulfate-induced polioencephalomalacia in cattle. Am J Vet Res 1995;56:1384–9.
32. Haven T, Caldwell D, Jensen R. Role of predominant rumen bacteria in the cause of polioencephalomalacia (cerebrocortical necrosis) in cattle. Am J Vet Res 1983; 44:1451–5.
33. De Oliverira L, Jean-Blain C, Komisarczuk-Bony S. Microbial thiamin metabolism in the rumen simulating fermenter (RUSITEC): the effect of acidogenic conditions, a high sulfur level and added thiamine. Br J Nutr 1997;78:599–613.
34. Kung L, Bracht J, Hession A. High sulfate induced PEM in cattle examined. Feedstuffs 1998;16:12–7.
35. Zhang Y, Caupert J, Imerman PM, et al. The occurrence and concentration of mycotoxins in U.S. distillers dried grains with solubles. J Agric Food Chem 2009;57:9828–37.
36. Olmstead J. Fueling Resistance? Antibiotics in ethanol production. Minneapolis (MN): Minnesota Institute for Agriculture and Trade Policy; 2009.
37. Parsons GL, Sheller MK, Drouillard JS. Performance and carcass traits of finishing heifers fed crude glycerin. J Anim Sci 2009;87:653–7.

Ionophore Toxicity and Tolerance

Joseph Deen Roder, DVM, PhD*

KEYWORDS

• Cation • Cardiomyopathy • Anorexia • Feed-related

GENERAL

The carboxylic acid ionophores are anticoccidials and growth promoters that are extensively used in animal production in North America. These chemotherapeutic agents exhibit complex behaviors within biologic systems and their actions represent a dynamic interplay of drug, animal, nutritional, and environmental factors. The term, *ionophore* (literally meaning ion bearer),[1] is a descriptive and dynamic definition of antibiotics with the ability to bind and transport ions across biologic membranes. The carboxylic ionophores (nigericin, monensin, dianemycin, salinomycin, lasalocid, and A23187) are open-chained oxygenated heterocyclic rings with a single terminal carboxyl group. All of these compounds are byproducts of fungal fermentation, specifically the *Streptomyces* spp.[2] These compounds are of moderate molecular weight (200–2000) with the ability to form lipid-soluble transport complexes with polar cations (potassium, sodium, calcium, and magnesium). The 3-D structures of the ionophores of veterinary clinical significance (monensin, lasalocid, and salinomycin) may explain their affinity for certain cations. Both monensin and salinomycin have a structure that resembles a doughnut with the cation-binding site at the area of the doughnut hole. This confers some degree of cation selectivity (sodium, potassium) for these ionophores. In contrast, lasalocid forms a dimer and has a shape that resembles a potato chip or catcher's mitt. This open configuration may explain the ability of lasalocid to bind with and a variety of monovalent and divalent cations.[3]

MECHANISM OF ACTION

Each ionophore has a characteristic ion affinity and transport capacity described by in vitro complexation and transport studies. The transport of specific ions (potassium, sodium, calcium, and magnesium) across membranes accounts for the pharmacologic effects of the ionophores. The ensuing transport is electrically neutral involving a cation-for-proton exchange. The carboxylic ionophores mediate concentration-dependent,

Intervet/Schering-Plough Animal Health, Summit, NJ, USA
* Intervet/Schering-Plough Animal Health, 19601 FM 2590, Canyon, TX 79015.
E-mail address: jdroder@gmail.com

Vet Clin Food Anim 27 (2011) 305–314
doi:10.1016/j.cvfa.2011.02.012 vetfood.theclinics.com

pH-sensitive transport of ions independent of membrane potential. These compounds act as exchange diffusion carriers, transporting a cation during both stages of the exchange cycle. The kinetics of ion transport by ionophores is rapid with turnover rates in biologic membranes shuttling across the membrane several thousand times per second.[3]

APPROVED IONOPHORE PRODUCTS

In 1971, monensin was approved for use as a coccidiostat in chickens (Coban) and later (1975) was approved for use in cattle (Rumensin).[4,5] Lasalocid was approved for use as a coccidiostat in chickens (Avatec) in 1977 and as a growth promoter in cattle (Bovatec) in 1982.[6,7] Salinomycin (Bio-Cox)[8] was approved for use as a coccidiostat in chickens in 1983.[9] The most recent ionophore approved is laidlomycin proprionate (Cattlyst).[10] All of the ionophores are approved in multiple combinations and most for multiple species. In the United States, monensin is labeled for use in the following species: beef cattle feedlot, beef cattle pasture, beef calves (not veal), dairy cows, dairy heifers, confined goats, chickens, quail, and turkeys. Lasalocid is approved for use in beef cattle feedlot, beef calves (not veal), beef cattle pasture, dairy heifers pasture, domestic rabbits, partridges, turkeys, and chickens. Salinomycin is approved for use in broiler chickens and quail whereas laidlomycin is approved for use in beef feedlot cattle.

IONOPHORE USE AND BENEFITS

The ionophores of veterinary significance (monensin, lasalocid, and salinomycin) are used to control and treat coccidiosis, especially Eimeria spp, to increase feed efficiency in ruminants and to control bloat in cattle. The actions of ionophores on coccidia relate to the ionphore's ability to transport ions across biologic membranes. Coccidia are intracellular parasites that depend upon the host cell for energy (ATP). Ionophores mediate cation influxes that require coccidial energy to maintain ionic homeostasis. The ionophores alter ionic balance within coccidia, which leads to cell dysfunction and death. In vitro incubation of coccidia with ionophores causes ultrastructural changes, including cytoplasmic vacuoles, blistering of the coccidial plasma membrane, swollen mitochondria, and pyknotic nuclei.[11,12]

In ruminants, the ionophores have been shown to improve feed efficiency (10%–20%) in feedlot and pastured cattle by altering the ruminal microflora.[13,14] This change in flora includes a shift toward bacteria that produce propionate and a decrease in the bacteria that produce acetate and butyrate volatile fatty acids. Additionally, the ionophores can decrease feed intake (approximately 10%) on grain diets, decrease (4%–31%) ruminal methane production, and reduce ruminal protein degradation with a protein-sparing effect, which all combine to increase the efficiency of production by the ruminant.[15] The ionophores may also have a potential environmental benefit due to the reduction of ammonia and methane emissions of treated cattle. The use of ionophores can reduce the production of methane by 25% to 30% and reduce feed intake by 4% without affecting animal performance.[16,17]

There are also effects of ionophores that are independent of the rumen. These effects include significantly lower serum concentrations of potassium, magnesium, and phosphorus and higher serum glucose and volatile fatty acid concentrations.[18] Additionally, in ruminants, the ionophores can reduce the incidence of bloat, decrease ruminal acidosis, and prevent tryptophan-induced atypical bovine pulmonary emphysema.

TOXICITY

The ionophores currently used in livestock production are safe and efficacious at prescribed use levels in intended species. The majority of the literature concerning the toxic effects of ionophores describes monensin, due to the earlier market entry and greater market share for this compound. Ionophore toxicosis is well documented in most domestic species, including horses, the most sensitive species[19,20]; cattle[21–23]; goats[24]; pigs[25,26]; chickens[27,28]; turkeys[29,30]; quail[31]; dogs[32,33]; and cats.[34]

Management of feeding and feedstuffs plays a major role in ionophore toxicosis. Cases of intoxication are generally due to a mixing error, ingestion of premix or concentrated products, or consumption by a nontarget species (horse).[35] In addition, intoxication has occurred in cattle and sheep after the ingestion of poultry litter.[36–38]

TOXIC DOSE

The toxic dose depends on the ionophore, the species, previous exposure to the ionophore, and nutritional background. The use of median lethal dose (LD_{50}) estimates gives a general guide for the levels of concern after exposure to potentially toxic concentrations of an ionophore. The estimated LD_{50}s (mg/kg body weight) for monensin are 2 to 3 mg/kg (horses), 11.9 mg/kg (sheep), 16.7 mg/kg (swine), 26.4 mg/kg (cattle), and 200 mg/kg (chicken).[39,40] The estimated LD_{50}s (mg/kg body weight) for lasalocid are 21.5 mg/kg (horses) and 71.5 mg/kg (chicken).[41] Lasalocid has a reported lethal dose in swine of 58 mg/kg[41] and a lethal dose in cattle of 50 to 100 mg/kg.[42] These LD_{50}s and toxic dose information are guides and veterinarians should always consider the entire clinical picture when evaluating potential ionophore toxicosis. In spite of feeding a ration with the proper concentrations of monensin, a Kansas feed yard lost 562 of 988 cattle in 8 weeks due to ionophore toxicosis potentiated by dried distillers grains that contained macrolide antibioitics.[43]

IONOPHORE TOLERANCE

After ingestion, the ionophores are rapidly absorbed and metabolized by the liver, excreted in the bile, and eliminated primarily via the feces. As a class, the ionophores do not accumulate in the tissues of cattle and poultry. The tolerances for veterinary ionophores approved in the United States are listed in **Table 1**.

In other studies, the elimination of monensin was examined under various conditions. Information in **Table 1** is based on feeding the recommended dose to each species. After feeding monensin at recommended concentrations to cattle and chickens with a zero withdrawal time, there were no detectable residues (limit of detection 0.05 ppm) in edible tissues.[44] In an experimental study, rats given elevated doses of monensin did not show accumulation or deposition in tissues.[44] Lactating dairy cows fed monensin up to 10 times the recommended dose showed no detectable residues in the milk.[45] Used at recommended concentrations, the ionophores are rapidly metabolized and eliminated.

MECHANISM OF TOXICITY

The ionophores exert their toxicologic effects by several different mechanisms. The transport of cations (sodium, potassium, and calcium) across cell membranes is one of those mechanisms resulting in pH and ionic changes across membranes and across intracellular organelles. This may disrupt cellular energetics by inhibiting or disrupting ATP generation causing decreased energy production, which may lead to cell death. The actions of the ionophores can lead to increased intracellular sodium that

Table 1
Tolerances for veterinary ionophores

Ionophore	Species	Tissue	Tolerance
Monensin	Cattle	Liver	0.10 ppm
Monensin	Cattle	Muscle and kidney	0.05 ppm
Monensin	Goat	Edible tissue	0.05 ppm
Monensin	Chicken, turkey, quail	Edible tissues	Not needed
Monensin	Cattle	Milk	Not needed
Lasalocid	Cattle	Liver	0.7 ppm
Lasalocid	Chicken	Skin with adhering fat	1.2 ppm
Lasalocid	Chicken	Liver	0.4 ppm
Lasalocid	Turkeys	Skin with adhering fat	0.4 ppm
Lasalocid	Turkeys	Liver	0.4 ppm
Lasalocid	Rabbits	Liver	0.7 ppm
Lasalocid	Sheep	Liver	1.0 ppm
Laidlomycin	Cattle	Liver	0.2 ppm
Salinomycin	Chicken	Skin with adhering fat	Not needed

Data from Refs.[4–8,10]

results in greater influx of water and swelling of intracellular organelles and cell death. Another consequence of the disruption of ionic gradients and increased intracellular sodium is triggering the release of calcium from intracellular stores. The increased free intracellular calcium can initiate a myriad calcium-mediated processes that can lead to cell death.

DRUG INTERACTIONS

Several different drugs/toxins can interact with or potentiate ionophore toxicosis. Generally the interaction is due to a competition for the enzymes or processes responsible for drug metabolism. This can lead to enhanced concentrations of the ionophore in vivo. There are reports of interaction between ionophores and dihydroquinolone antioxidants,[46–48] tiamulin,[49–53] macrolide antibiotics,[43] chloramphenicol,[54] and sulfonamides. Tiamulin and macrolide antibiotics have been shown to inhibit the cytochrome P450 activity of several species,[55,56] which may be involved in enhanced toxicity. Additionally, the interaction of tiamulin and monensin in pigs is minimized by concurrent administration of vitamin E and selenium.[57]

Several studies[44,58,59] have shown species-specific differences in the P450-mediated metabolism of several compounds. In one study, the oxidative metabolism of monensin as measured by total turnover (nmol monensin/min/nmol P450) was greatest for the chick, intermediate for cattle, and lowest for the horse.[58] Chick and cattle microsomes also showed the highest catalytic efficiency for two P450 3A-dependent substrates (erythromycin and triacetyloleandomycin). These differences may account for some of the species-specific sensitivity to the ionophores (especially monensin).

CLINICAL SIGNS

The clinical presentation of ionophore toxicosis may depend on the species, the ionophore, and the dose ingested. In cattle the clinical signs are generally referable to the cardiac and musculoskeletal systems. In some cases, there may be no initial clinical signs, only sudden deaths.[43] Anorexia is an early and common clinical signs of intoxication.[9,42,43,45,60–62] The presence of clinical signs generally occurs a few days after exposure and may include any one or more of the following: anorexia, ruminal atony, depression, muscle tremors, watery diarrhea, tachycardia, ataxia, recumbency, and decreased weight gain.[9,39,63–66]

PATHOLOGY

Depending on the toxic dose and the species affected, acute death may occur with few if any lesions noted. When they occur, lesions of ionophore toxicosis are most typically noted in the cardiac and skeletal muscles of affected animals. Lesions may also be noted in hepatic, renal, or neurologic tissues of different species. In cattle, sheep, and poultry, lesions are most often found in both the heart and skeletal muscles. In horses, gross lesions are most often noted in the heart muscle. In swine, the lesions are most commonly seen in skeletal muscles.[9,67] At necropsy it is common to note hydropericardium, hydrothorax, pulmonary congestion, pulmonary edema, hepatic congestion, and accentuated hepatic lobular pattern.

Gross lesions of ionophore-induced myonecrosis include pale myocardial tissues, yellow-tan myocardial streaks, enlarged ventricles, and flabby myocardium.[9,19,43,61,63,68] The histologic lesions of ionophore toxicosis may include focal degeneration of myocytes, vacuolation, swelling and eosinophilic staining of cardiomyocytes, swelling of mitochondria, and disrupted cristae.[69,70] After ionophore-mediated damage occurs to cardiomyocytes injured tissue is replaced by fibrosis.[9] The skeletal myopathy induced in turkeys after monensin overdose presents with ataxia, rear limb paresis, and paralysis. Histologically, birds exhibit dose-dependent, necrotizing skeletal myopathy of the leg muscles with intrafiber edema and myocardial vacuolation.[71]

With some ionophores (eg, lasalocid and salinomycin), neurotoxic clinical signs have been reported.[19,34] These syndromes reflect a peripheral neuropathy. The histologic lesions noted in these cases are typically restricted to the peripheral nervous system and are related to demyelination, including fragmentation and loss of myelin, formation of digestion chambers, and swollen Schwann cells.[19,32,34]

CLINICAL PATHOLOGY CHANGES

Clinical pathologic changes are associated with ionophore-induced toxicosis. These generally involve elevated enzyme levels of muscle origin—aspartate transaminase, creatine kinase, lactate dehydrogenase, and alkaline phosphatase[65]—or possible increased serum urea nitrogen. Serum calcium and potassium concentrations may decline to life-threatening levels in monensin-intoxicated ponies or horses.[9] In one study of lasalocid toxicosis, the findings are reflective of dehydration rather than targeted organ damage.[42] More recently, the use of cardiac troponin I as a biomarker for myocardial injury has been examined in ionophore toxicosis. In one study, horses were dosed with monensin and the cardiac troponin I concentrations were highest in the horses with the most severe cardiac disease.[60] This technology requires some additional study but may provide greater insight to specific cardiac injury in poisoned veterinary patients.

DIAGNOSIS

Diagnosis of ionophore toxicosis is initially tentative because clinical signs and lesions are not pathognomonic. Any feed-related problem that involves multiple animals exhibiting clinical signs consistent with ionophore intoxication warrants a presumptive diagnosis of ionophore toxicosis.[9] Observation of gross and histopathologic lesions suggestive of ionophore toxicity can help support the presumptive diagnosis. Confirmation requires consideration of differential diagnoses as well as necropsy findings and additional history. To make a definitive diagnosis-specific analysis of the feed or stomach/rumen, content is required to determine the specific ionophore and concentrations. One of the greatest challenges is to obtain a representative feed sample (ensure complete mixing and multiple samples). It is important to obtain samples of the complete ration and any components (premix or vitamin/mineral supplement) to find the suspect ionophore.

DIFFERENTIAL DIAGNOSIS

The differential diagnosis of ionophore toxicosis in cattle includes other causes of cardiac/skeletal muscle injury and vitamin or mineral deficiencies. Gossypol intoxication from cottonseed meal may produce a similar syndrome in cattle and sheep (especially preruminant), swine, and poultry.[72,73] Ingestion of plants that can induce a skeletal or cardiac myopathy should be considered as it can produce symptoms and signs similar to ionophore toxicosis in cattle, horses, and sheep. Some of these plants include Taxus spp (yews), oleander (*Nerium oleander*), senna (*Cassia occidentalis*), white snakeroot (*Eupatorium rugosum*), vetch, and coyotillo (*Karwinskia humboldtiana*). (See the article on southeastern plants by Nicholson elsewhere in this issue for more information.) Additionally, vitamin E or selenium deficiencies can produce a similar syndrome in cattle, sheep, and swine. In horses, the differential diagnosis should also include colic, cantharidin (blister beetle) toxicosis, and azotemia.

TREATMENT AND PROGNOSIS

There are no specific antidotes for ionophore intoxication but removal of the adulterated feedstuff from these animals is essential and central to therapy. Offering affected animals a high-quality feed and minimizing stressors or all types can also be of benefit. Gastric decontamination using activated charcoal and a saline cathartic may be beneficial for individual cases if attempted early to help reduce ionophore absorption and reduce the toxic effects. Symptomatic therapy of affected animals may include intravenous fluids and electrolytes to address dehydration.

The prognosis for animals suffering from ionophore intoxication is guarded. Animals may continue to show signs and sequelae for an extended period of time. There may be mortalities from cardiac myopathy weeks or months after exposure.[43] Some animals may collapse and die acutely after exercise or handling as a result of permanent cardiac damage. Cattle that survive the initial episode of intoxication can be fed for salvage but may exhibit poor feeding performance. Horses that are affected require an extended period (6 weeks) of stall rest and may never again attain their level of athletic performance. These horses are at greater risk of sudden cardiac arrest/death and more likely to suffer exercise intolerance and congestive heart failure. These animals also present a greater risk to owners and riders.

REFERENCES

1. Pressman BC, Harris EJ, Jagger WS, et al. Antibiotic-mediated transport of alkali ions across lipid barriers. Proc Natl Acad Sci U S A 1967;58:1949–56.
2. Westley JW. Polyether antibiotics: versatile carboxylic acid ionophores produced by Streptomyces. Adv Appl Microbiol 1977;22:177–223.

3. Pressman BC. Biological applications of ionophores. Annu Rev Biochem 1976; 45:501–30.
4. FDA-CVM. NADA 095–735. Monensin sodium. Rumensin 80. Freedom of Information Summary. 2005.
5. FDA-CVM. NADA 140–937. Monensin sodium. Coban. Freedom of Information Summary. 1994.
6. FDA-CVM. NADA 096–298. Lasalocid. Avatec. Freedom of Information Summary. 2001.
7. FDA-CVM. NADA 141–250. Lasalocid sodium. Bovatec. Freedom of Information Summary. 2006.
8. FDA-CVM. NADA 128–686. Salinomycin. Freedom of Information Summary. 2003.
9. Novilla MN. The veterinary importance of the toxic syndrome induced by ionophores. Vet Hum Toxicol 1992;34:66–70.
10. FDA-CVM. NADA 141–025. Laidlomycin proprionate. Freedom of Information Summary. 1994.
11. Augustine PC, Watkins KL, Danforth HD. Effect of monensin on ultrastructure and cellular invasion by the turkey coccidia Eimeria adenoeides and Eimeria meleagrimitis. Poult Sci 1992;71:970–8.
12. Daszak P, Ball SJ, Pittilo RM, et al. Ultrastructural studies of the effects of the ionophore lasalocid on Eimeria tenella in chickens. Parasitol Res 1991;77:224–9.
13. Bergen WG, Bates DB. Ionophores: their effect on production efficiency and mode of action. J Anim Sci 1984;58:1465–83.
14. Quigley JD 3rd, Boehms SI, Steen TM, et al. Effects of lasalocid on selected ruminal and blood metabolites in young calves. J Dairy Sci 1992;75:2235–41.
15. Schelling GT. Monensin mode of action in the rumen. J Anim Sci 1984;58: 1518–27.
16. Tedeschi LO, Fox DG, Tylutki TP. Potential environmental benefits of ionophores in ruminant diets. J Environ Qual 2003;32:1591–602.
17. Guan H, Wittenberg KM, Ominski KH, et al. Efficacy of ionophores in cattle diets for mitigation of enteric methane. J Anim Sci 2006;84:1896–906.
18. Armstrong JD, Spears JW. Intravenous administration of ionophores in ruminants: effects on metabolism independent of the rumen. J Anim Sci 1988;66:1807–17.
19. Aleman M, Magdesian KG, Peterson TS, et al. Salinomycin toxicosis in horses. J Am Vet Med Assoc 2007;230:1822–6.
20. Matsuoka T. Evaluation of monensin toxicity in the horse. J Am Vet Med Assoc 1976;169:1098–100.
21. Mathieson AO, Caldow GL, Anderson R. Acute cardiomyopathy in heifers. Vet Rec 1990;126:147–8.
22. Van Vleet JF, Ferrans VJ. Ultrastructural myocardial alterations in monensin toxicosis of cattle. Am J Vet Res 1983;44:1629–36.
23. Gabor LJ, Downing GM. Monensin toxicity in preruminant dairy heifers. Aust Vet J 2003;81:476–8.
24. Dalvi RR, Sawant SG. Studies on monensin toxicity in goats. Zentralbl Veterinarmed A 1990;37(5):352–5.
25. Van Vleet JF, Amstutz HE, Weirich WE, et al. Acute monensin toxicosis in swine: effect of graded doses of monensin and protection of swine by pretreatment with selenium-vitamin E. Am J Vet Res 1983;44:1460–8.
26. Kavanagh NT, Sparrow DS. Salinomycin toxicity in pigs. Vet Rec 1990;127(20): 507.
27. Howell J, Hanson J, Onderka D, et al. Monensin toxicity in chickens. Avian Dis 1980;24:1050–3.

28. Wagner DD, Furrow RD, Bradley BD. Subchronic toxicity of monensin in broiler chickens. Vet Pathol 1983;20:353–9.
29. Van Assen EJ. A case of salinomycin intoxication in turkeys. Can Vet J 2006;47: 256–8.
30. Ficken MD, Wages DP, Gonder E. Monensin toxicity in turkey breeder hens. Avian Dis 1989;33:186–90.
31. Sawant SG, Terse PS, Dalvi RR. Toxicity of dietary monensin in quail. Avian Dis 1990;34(3):571–4.
32. Safran N, Aizenberg I, Bark H. Paralytic syndrome attributed to lasalocid residues in a commercial ration fed to dogs. J Am Vet Med Assoc 1993;202:1273–5.
33. Wilson JS. Toxic myopathy in a dog associated with the presence of monensin in dry food. Can Vet J 1980;21:30–1.
34. van der Linde-Sipman JS, van den Ingh TS, van nes JJ, et al. Salinomycin-induced polyneuropathy in cats: morphologic and epidemiologic data. Vet Pathol 1999;36:152–6.
35. Roder JD, Stair EL. Ionophore toxicosis. Vet Hum Toxicol 1999;41:178–81.
36. Bastianello SS, McGregor HL, Penrith ML, et al. A chronic cardiomyopathy in feedlot cattle attributed to toxic levels of salinomycin in the feed. J S Afr Vet Assoc 1996;67:38–41.
37. Bastianello SS, Fourie N, Prozesky L, et al. Cardiomyopathy of ruminants induced by the litter of poultry fed on rations containing the ionophore antibiotic, maduramicin. II. Macropathology and histopathology. Onderstepoort J Vet Res 1995;62: 5–18.
38. Fourie N, Bastianello SS, Prozesky L, et al. Cardiomyopathy of ruminants induced by the litter of poultry fed on rations containing the ionophore antibiotic, maduramicin. I. Epidemiology, clinical signs and clinical pathology. Onderstepoort J Vet Res 1991;58:291–6.
39. Todd GC, Novilla MN, Howard LC. Comparative toxicology of monensin sodium in laboratory animals. J Anim Sci 1984;58:1512–7.
40. Potter EL, VanDuyn RL, Cooley CO. Monensin toxicity in cattle. J Anim Sci 1984; 58:1499–511.
41. Galitzer SJ, Oehme FW. A literature review on the toxicity of lasalocid, a polyether antibiotic. Vet Hum Toxicol 1984;26:322–6.
42. Galitzer SJ, Oehme FW, Bartley EE, et al. Lasalocid toxicity in cattle: acute clinicopathological changes. J Anim Sci 1986;62:1308–16.
43. Basaraba RJ, Oehme FW, Vorhies MW, et al. Toxicosis in cattle from concurrent feeding of monensin and dried distiller's grains contaminated with macrolide antibiotics. J Vet Diagn Invest 1999;11:79–86.
44. Donoho AL. Biochemical studies on the fate of monensin in animals and in the environment. J Anim Sci 1984;58:1528–39.
45. Bagg R, Vessie GH, Dick CP, et al. Milk residues and performance of lactating dairy cows administered high doses of monensin. Can J Vet Res 2005;69:180–5.
46. Laczay P, Varga I, Mora Z, et al. Potentiation of ionophorous anticoccidials with dihydroquinolines: reduction of adverse interactions with antimicrobials. Int J Parasitol 1994;24:421–3.
47. Varga I, Laczay P, Lehel J, et al. Potentiation of ionophorous anticoccidials with dihydroquinolines: battery trials against Eimeria tenella in chickens. Int J Parasitol 1994;24:689–94.
48. Szucs G, Bajnogel J, Varga A, et al. Studies on the toxic interaction between monensin and tiamulin in rats: toxicity and pathology. Acta Vet Hung 2000;48: 209–19.

49. Weisman Y, Herz A, Yegana Y, et al. The effect of tiamulin administered by different routes and at different ages to turkeys receiving monensin in their feed. Vet Res Commun 1983;6:189–98.
50. Ratz V, Laczay P, Mora Z, et al. Recent studies on the effects of tiamulin and monensin on hepatic cytochrome P450 activities in chickens and turkeys. J Vet Pharmacol Ther 1997;20:415–8.
51. Miller DJ, O'Connor JJ, Roberts NL. Tiamulin/salinomycin interactions in pigs. Vet Rec 1986;118:73–5.
52. Mezes M, Salyi G, Banhidi G, et al. Effect of acute salinomycin-tiamulin toxicity on the lipid peroxide and antioxidant status of broiler chicken. Acta Vet Hung 1992; 40:251–7.
53. Umemura T, Nakamura H, Goryo M, et al. Histopathology of monensin-tiamulin myopathy in broiler chicks. Avian Pathol 1984;13:459–67.
54. Broz J, Frigg M. Incompatibility between lasalocid and chloramphenicol in broiler chicks after a long-term simultaneous administration. Vet Res Commun 1987;11: 159–72.
55. Zweers-Zeilmaker WM, Van Miert AS, Horbach GJ, et al. In vitro complex formation and inhibition of hepatic cytochrome P450 activity by different macrolides and tiamulin in goats and cattle. Res Vet Sci 1999;66:51–5.
56. Carletti M, Gusson F, Zaghini A, et al. In vitro formation of metabolic-intermediate cytochrome P450 complexes in rabbit liver microsomes by tiamulin and various macrolides. Vet Res 2003;34:405–11.
57. Van Vleet JF, Runnels LJ, Cook JR Jr, et al. Monensin toxicosis in swine: potentiation by tiamulin administration and ameliorative effect of treatment with selenium and/or vitamin E. Am J Vet Res 1987;48:1520–4.
58. Nebbia C, Ceppa L, Dacasto M, et al. Oxidative monensin metabolism and cytochrome P450 3A content and functions in liver microsomes from horses, pigs, broiler chicks, cattle and rats. J Vet Pharmacol Ther 2001;24:399–403.
59. Nebbia C, Dacasto M, Rossetto Giaccherino A, et al. Comparative expression of liver cytochrome P450-dependent monooxygenases in the horse and in other agricultural and laboratory species. Vet J 2003;165:53–64.
60. Divers TJ, Kraus MS, Jesty SA, et al. Clinical findings and serum cardiac troponin I concentrations in horses after intragastric administration of sodium monensin. J Vet Diagn Invest 2009;21:338–43.
61. Jones A. Monensin toxicosis in 2 sheep flocks. Can Vet J 2001;42:135–6.
62. Gonzalez M, Barkema HW, Keefe GP. Monensin toxicosis in a dairy herd. Can Vet J 2005;46:910–2.
63. Janzen ED, Rodostits OM, Orr JP. Possible monensin poisoning in a group of bulls. Can Vet J 1981;22:92–4.
64. VanderKop PA, MacNeil JD. The effect of sodium selenite supplementation on monensin-induced growth inhibition and residue accumulation in broiler chicks. Vet Hum Toxicol 1990;32:1–5.
65. Galitzer SJ, Bartley EE, Oehme FW. Preliminary studies on lasalocid toxicosis in cattle. Vet Hum Toxicol 1982;24:406–9.
66. Oehme FW, Pickrell JA. An analysis of the chronic oral toxicity of polyether ionophore antibiotics in animals. Vet Hum Toxicol 1999;41:251–7.
67. Plumlee KH, Johnson B, Galey FD. Acute salinomycin toxicosis of pigs. J Vet Diagn Invest 1995;7:419–20.
68. Litwak KN, McMahan A, Lott KA, et al. Monensin toxicosis in the domestic bovine calf: a large animal model of cardiac dysfunction. Contemp Top Lab Anim Sci 2005;44:45–9. American Association for Laboratory Animal Science.

69. Van Vleet JF, Ferrans VJ. Ultrastructural alterations in the atrial myocardium of pigs with acute monensin toxicosis. Am J Pathol 1984;114:367–79.
70. Anderson TD, Van Alstine WG, Ficken MD, et al. Acute monensin toxicosis in sheep: light and electron microscopic changes. Am J Vet Res 1984;45:1142–7.
71. Cardona CJ, Galey FD, Bickford AA, et al. Skeletal myopathy produced with experimental dosing of turkeys with monensin. Avian Dis 1993;37:107–17.
72. Morgan S, Stair EL, Martin T, et al. Clinical, clinicopathologic, pathologic, and toxicologic alterations associated with gossypol toxicosis in feeder lambs. Am J Vet Res 1988;49:493–9.
73. Morgan SE. Gossypol as a toxicant in livestock. Vet Clin North Am Food Anim Pract 1989;5:251–62.

Ruminant Mycotoxicosis

Michelle S. Mostrom, DVM, PhD[a,*], Barry J. Jacobsen, MS, PhD[b]

KEYWORDS

• Molds • Mycotoxins • Ruminants • Toxicosis

Mycotoxins are naturally occurring compounds or secondary metabolites produced by fungi growing on plants in the field or during storage periods. The source of toxigenic fungi or mold in both cases is the field. *Fusarium* species and *Claviceps purpurea* can act as plant pathogens on cereal crops or grasses in the field. *Fusarium verticillioides* and *Aspergillus flavus* can produce mycotoxins on stressed or senescent plants, particularly corn. Fungi that occur on developing kernels in the field and later proliferate in storage, especially on ensiled cereals or baled forages, are typically the *Penicillium* and *Aspergillus* species. Additional fungi have been associated with grass endophytes such as *Neotyphodium coenophialum* in tall fescue. Numerous mycotoxins can be produced by fungi invading plant material; however, only a few mycotoxins have been recognized as toxic to animals. This article focuses on mycotoxins affecting ruminants in North America. Ruminants are often considered less sensitive to mycotoxins than are monogastrics because of rumen microflora metabolism to less toxic compounds. However, ruminants occupy wide agricultural niches from roaming range or grass pastures to housing in dairy lots or small farms with localized feed sources to confinement in feedlots using numerous commercial sources of grains or by-products, which exposes animals to diverse toxins in widely different conditions.[1] Often, the more moldy and potentially highly contaminated feeds end up at a feedlot and, in poor crop years, beef cows can be fed contaminated screenings, straw, and cereal by-products, poorly preserved silages or baled forages, or be turned onto moldy fields for crop salvage. In the United States during 2008, approximately 70% to 75% of agricultural commodities were sent into commercial channels with only 25% to 30% retained for on-farm use (Kim Koch, PhD, Fargo, ND, personal communication, September 2010). Therefore, veterinary practitioners need to be aware of the local environmental conditions and potential mycotoxins in animal feed and regional mycotoxin problems in grain that could be brought into local channels.

The authors have nothing to disclose.
[a] Veterinary Diagnostic Laboratory, Veterinary Diagnostic Services, North Dakota State University, 1523 Centennial Boulevard, Van Es Hall, Department 7691, PO Box 6050, Fargo, ND 58108-6050, USA
[b] Montana State University, Plant Pathology, 205 Plant BioSciences Building, Bozeman, MT 59717-3150, USA
* Corresponding author.
E-mail address: michelle.mostrom@ndsu.edu

Vet Clin Food Anim 27 (2011) 315–344
doi:10.1016/j.cvfa.2011.02.007 **vetfood.theclinics.com**
0749-0720/11/$ – see front matter

A critical factor in mycotoxicosis is obtaining a representative sample of suspect feed or feeds that livestock have been consuming. Analytical results and their interpretation depend on representative sampling. This review covers factors associated with mold production in feedstuffs and major mycotoxins affecting ruminants: aflatoxin, ergot alkaloids, trichothecene mycotoxins, and several mycotoxins associated with tremors, photosensitization, and silage contamination. The estrogenic mycotoxin zearalenone and the reproductive effects of ergot alkaloids and associated summer slump and fat necrosis are discussed by Tim J. Evans elsewhere in this issue.

CROP MOLDS AND POTENTIAL MYCOTOXINS

Veterinarians frequently evaluate suspect feeds associated with clinical illness in livestock. Feeds can be cultured by mycologists and plant pathologists for mold identification providing a record or biologic indicator of storage conditions and potential mycotoxins. Mold cultures can provide direction in analytical testing for mycotoxins. Stored grains and seeds can be damaged by insects and fungi if not properly conditioned and protected. Damage from field and storage molds can include reduced germination, heating, reduction in market grade and grain value, loss of feed and oil quality, mycotoxin contamination, fires, explosions, and worker health hazards associated with dust and mycotoxin inhalation and falling through crusted grain. Mold damage occurs both before and after harvest. Those fungi associated with damage before harvest are termed field molds and they grow in equilibrium with relative humidity greater than 90% to 95% (**Table 1**). Fungi associated with damage in storage can grow in equilibrium with relative humidity between 65% and 85% (**Table 2**). Grains and seeds readily absorb or lose moisture and achieve moisture in equilibrium with the moisture vapor available in the air between seeds or grains. Moisture and temperature are the primary factors determining the ability of molds to grow, as well as their rate of growth. The growth of storage fungi results in increased temperatures and increased moisture caused by the metabolism of these fungi. Thus, once molds begin growth, grains and seeds gain in moisture and allow growth of storage fungi that require higher equilibrium moistures. For example, *Aspergillus glaucus* can grow at 15% moisture in starchy grains but, as it grows, it produces heat and moisture that allow growth of *Aspergillus candidus* or even *A flavus* or *Penicillium* species that require 16% to 18% moisture. Growth of *A glaucus* and *A candidus* can be rapid and generate temperatures as high as 60°C (140°F). A good management practice is to avoid blending low-moisture and high-moisture grains; grain moisture in a blending process will progress to the high moisture levels.

Grain and seeds are at highest quality and have the lowest storage risk when they are fully mature before harvest, free of field mold damage, have no mechanical damage to the seed coat, and harvest is not delayed by weather or other factors. The intact seed coat is an effective barrier to seed infection by storage molds, and extra care in preventing mechanical damage during harvest and handling is critical to managing storage mold damage. Grain or seeds infected by field molds such as *Fusarium*, *Helminthosporium*, *Penicillium*, *Sclerotinia*, *Botrytis*, *Ascochyta*, *Alternaria*, and *Cladosporium* are at higher risk for damage by storage molds than intact seeds and will likely have lower germination rates. **Table 1** lists diseases caused by field molds that may predispose grains and seeds to damage by storage molds. **Table 3** lists selected molds and associated mycotoxicoses in ruminants. Even though toxigenic molds may grow in a given set of conditions, they do not necessarily produce mycotoxins. The mold can undergo additional stress conditions

Table 1
Field mold problems that can cause predisposition to storage mold damage and reduce germination

Crop	Disease Name/Pathogen Genus	Favored By
Cereal grains	Fusarium head blight, scab Several *Fusarium* species	Warm, wet weather at anthesis and shortly after
	Black head molds *Alternaria* and *Cladosporium* spp	Plants killed prematurely (eg, by diseases, frost)
	Head molds *Fusarium* and *Penicillium* spp	Wet weather–delayed harvest, snow cover
	Black point *Helminthosporium* spp	Wet weather during grain maturation
Corn	Ear and kernel rots *Fusarium* spp, *Gibberella*, *Diplodia*, *Helminthosporium*, *Bipolaris*	Warm, wet weather in 21 d after pollination, delayed harvest, hail, bird, or insect damage. *F verticillioides* and *F proliferatum*; droughty conditions, insect damage to ear. *Fusarium*; hail damage
	Aspergillus, *Penicillium*	*Aspergillus*; droughty conditions, insect damage to ear. *Penicillium*; hail damage milk stage or later, insect damage, cool, wet weather–delayed harvest
Soybeans	Pod and stem blight; *Phomopsis, Diaporthe* spp	Wet weather during pod-fill, weather-delayed harvest
	Anthracnose; *Colletotrichum*	Wet weather during pod-fill
Peas, Lentils, Chickpea, dry bean	Ascpchyta blight; *Ascochyta*, gray mold; *Botrytis*, Anthracnose; *Colletotrichum*	Wet weather during pod-fill
Safflower	*Alternaria* blight; *Alternaria*	Warm temperatures and high humidity from flower to seed set, wet weather–delayed harvest
Hay	*Fusarium* spp, *Cladosporium*, *Alternaria*	These fungi cannot grow at moistures <20%

leading to mycotoxin production, which can be generated fairly rapidly in field or storage conditions. More than 1000 μg/kg (ppb) of aflatoxins can be produced on corn inoculated with *A flavus* within 4 days and *Fusarium* mycotoxins (zearalenone, deoxynivalenol [DON or vomitoxin] and HT-2 toxin) can be found in mg/kg (ppm) levels within 4 to 7 days following hail damage on maturing corn. Mold culture and identification provides a direction to test for potential mycotoxins. The use of mold spore counts is limited; it provides an indication of mold presence (mold spores can deteriorate) and whether the feedstuff has gone bad, but does not equate to the presence or identification of a mycotoxin(s). Most mycotoxins can remain stable for years in feeds, and many survive ensiling and food processing. Mycotoxins can be concentrated several-fold in cereal by-products and typically concentrate threefold in distillers coproducts.

Table 2
Percentage relative humidity (%RH), equilibrium moistures for various grains and seeds and storage fungi that can grow at these moistures

%RH	Starchy Grains Corn, Wheat, Barley (%)	Soybean, Pea, Bean, Lentils (%)	Peanut, Canola, *Camelina*, Safflower (%)	Fungi
65–70	12.5	12.0	5.0	*Aspergillus halophilcus* *Aspergillus restrictus*
70–75	14.0	13.0	6.0	*A glaucus*
75–80	15.0	14.0	7.0	*A candidus*
80–85	16.0	15.0	8.0	*A flavus* *Penicillium* sp
85–90	18.0	18.0	10.0	As above + *Penicillium*
>95	22.0	20.0	13.0	Yeasts/bacteria/most field molds

AFLATOXINS

Sources and Production

Aflatoxins are an important group of structurally related difuranocoumarin compounds produced primarily by *A flavus*, *Aspergillus parasiticus*, and *Aspergillus nomius*. These mycotoxins are found worldwide, but more commonly are produced in warm, subtropical, and tropical climates. Aflatoxins can occur before harvest on starchy cereal crops, cottonseeds, and peanuts or after harvest on stored commodities (see **Table 3**). Aflatoxins are potent hepatotoxins, immunosuppressants, carcinogens, and mutagens, and can be important public health problems. Clinical signs of aflatoxicosis include poor weight gains and feed conversion, liver disease with increased hepatic enzymes and bilirubin, prolonged clotting times, and reduced immune competence (ie, vaccine failure or poor antibiotic response). Aflatoxins affect cell-mediated immunity, cytokine production, and nonspecific humoral factors such as complement, interferon, and some bactericidal serum components.[2] Numerous governments regulate the allowable concentrations of aflatoxins in animal feeds, human foods, and fluid milk (**Table 4**).

Strains of *A flavus* typically invade damaged or senescent plant tissue and mainly produce aflatoxin B_1. Aflatoxin B_1 is generally found in the highest concentration and considered the most toxic and carcinogenic of the aflatoxins. Strains of *A parasiticus* can produce aflatoxins B_1 and B_2, and G_1 and G_2 that fluoresce blue or green, respectively, under ultraviolet light. Aflatoxins M_1 and M_2 are 4-hydroxylated metabolites of aflatoxin B_1 and B_2, respectively, and can occur in feed contaminated with aflatoxin and in tissues, milk, and dairy products. Aflatoxin B_1 has been associated with hepatocellular carcinoma in humans and is included in group 1 as a human carcinogen by the International Agency for Research on Cancer (IARC). Aflatoxin M_1 is acutely toxic with lower carcinogenic activity. Sterigmatocystin, a mycotoxin produced by *Aspergillus versicolor* and other molds, is a precursor in the synthesis of aflatoxins, a hepatotoxin and carcinogen, and capable of toxicosis similar to, but less toxic than, aflatoxins.

Chemistry and Metabolism

Aflatoxins are low molecular weight, lipophilic compounds that are passively absorbed from the gastrointestinal tract. Absorption of aflatoxin may occur in the mouth or esophagus before entering the rumen, based on detection of aflatoxin M_1 in the plasma within 5 minutes after dosing dairy cows.[3] Aflatoxins are absorbed from the intestinal tract into the hepatic portal system. Young animals absorb aflatoxins more efficiently than older animals. Rumen microbial degradation of aflatoxins has been studied and findings are inconsistent. Aflatoxins can be degraded slightly in the rumen, but type of ration, feeding time, animal species, individual animal, and incubation time in rumen influence degradation of aflatoxins.[4–6] Aflatoxin B_1 can bind reversibly to albumin, with unbound aflatoxin B_1 passing from the circulation into tissues. Aflatoxins do not readily accumulate in tissues, although repeated exposures can generate toxic effects in tissues. Aflatoxins may cross the placenta and damage fetal tissue; however, little work has focused on reproductive effects. Aflatoxin elimination is through the bile, feces, urine, and into milk and eggs. Most species eliminate the toxin within 24 hours after exposure.[7]

The liver and, to a lesser extent, kidney, intestinal tract, and other organs biotransform aflatoxin B_1 into several products, with the most important toxic product being aflatoxin B_1-8,9-epoxide. The covalent binding of aflatoxin 8,9-epoxide to DNA, RNA, and proteins results in tissue adducts and reduced synthesis of these products, and disruption of cellular processes and organ function. The outcome results in cellular necrosis, immune suppression (both humoral and cell-mediated immunity), mutagenesis, and neoplasms. Additional biotransformation products (eg, aflatoxin M_1, aflatoxin M_2, aflatoxin Q_1, aflatoxicol) are less toxic; conjugation of these products with glucuronide and sulfate are detoxification reactions. The metabolite aflatoxicol, which is a carcinogen to animals and possibly a carcinogen to humans, can be oxidized back to aflatoxin B_1 and serve as a source for aflatoxin B_1 in the body. Aflatoxicol has been detected in milk, eggs, fermented dairy products, and tissues. Pasteurization and ultrapasteurization of milk with various levels of fat content did not destroy aflatoxicol.[8] Aflatoxin M_1 is the major excretion product in urine and milk and can be monitored for exposure. Aflatoxin M_1 appears quickly in milk; goats in midlactation given a single oral dose of 0.8 mg aflatoxin B_1/head had detectable concentrations of aflatoxin M_1 in milk 1 hour after administration, maximum concentrations in milk 3 to 6 hours after administration, and concentrations less than 50 ng/L (0.05 ppb, the European Union maximum allowed level) 36 hours after aflatoxin B_1 administration.[9] Excretion of M_1 in milk varies with animal species, individual, lactation status, and milkings after exposure. Aflatoxin M_1 excretion in milk approaches a steady-state condition about 3 to 6 days after daily ingestion of aflatoxins.[7] The dietary threshold for cows to excrete aflatoxin in milk is about 15 μg aflatoxins/kg ration (ppb); lactating cows consuming a diet with 20 μg aflatoxins/kg (ppb) or less excrete less than 0.1 μg aflatoxin M_1/kg (ppb) in milk (US Food and Drug Administration [FDA] action limit is 0.5 ppb in milk). The ratio of aflatoxin M_1 excreted in milk to the amount of aflatoxin B_1 ingested is generally between nondetectable and 4% in cows, between 1% and 3% in dairy ewes,[10] and approximately 0.26% in dairy goats.[9] After removal from the contaminated ration, aflatoxin M_1 becomes undetectable in milk after 2 to 4 days.

Toxic Effects

All animals are susceptible to aflatoxins, but the sensitivity varies between species. Young animals and monogastrics are more at risk for toxicosis. The major impact in dairy herds is reduced milk production and potential milk residue violations, with recent questions focused on possible immune suppression. Aflatoxins in the total ration of immature ruminants and dairy cows should not exceed 20 ppb. **Table 4** lists the FDA action levels set for aflatoxins in animal feeds. Ruminants fed rations with more than several hundred ppb aflatoxins may exhibit some decreased feed intake

Table 3
Molds and environmental conditions favoring growth, their mycotoxins, and clinical disease in ruminants

Toxicant	Mold	Feeds Affected	Environmental Conditions	Clinical Signs	Lesions	References
Aflatoxins B1, B2, G1, G2	*Aspergillus flavus*, *Aspergillus parasiticus*	Cereal grains Peanuts Cottonseed Soybeans Others	13–42°C (54–108°F) Optimum: 25–30°C (81–86°F), 75% relative humidity, grain moisture >18%; peanut moisture >8%–9%; oxygen>0.5%	Hepatotoxic, reduced feed conversion and weight gains, immunosuppression, hemorrhage, abortions, death, increased liver enzymes (especially γ-glutamyltransferase), increased bilirubin, increased prothrombin time	Hepatic fatty degeneration, megalocytosis and necrosis, fibrosis, biliary hyperplasia, possible veno-occlusive lesions, hemorrhages	1,16,62
Sterigmatocystin	*A glaucus*, *Aspergillus nidulellus*, *Aspergillus versicolor*	Wheat Cereals	Stored cereals at 14%–15% moisture	Hepatotoxin Carcinogen Bloody diarrhea Lower milk production		62,69
Ergot alkaloids	*C purpurea* *Claviceps africana* *Claviceps cyperi*	Rye Triticale Grains Grasses Sorghum Nut sedges	Cool, damp spring weather delaying pollination increases infection, and warm weather favors growth of the sclerotia	Vasoconstriction with loss of extremities (ears, feet, tail) Skin necrosis, Agalactia (abortions) Summer slump Hyperthermia Decreased milk production Open-mouth breathing, shade seeking	Thickening of blood vessel walls, tissue necrosis and sloughing	23,24,63

Ergot alkaloids (ergovaline)	*Neotyphodium coenophialum*	Tall fescue (*Festuca arundinacea* syn. *Lolium arundinaceum*)	Drought and rainy conditions, highest in summer and late fall	Reduced weight gain Ill thrift Fescue foot Summer slump Fat necrosis	Tissue necrosis and sloughing	25
Deoxynivalenol	*Fusarium graminearum* *Fusarium culmorum*	Cereal grains Straws Silages Hay	Optimum growth at temp of ~21–28°C at a water activity (a_W) greater than 0 87	Lower feed intake Lower milk production Diarrhea Immune alterations		1,64
Trichothecenes (T-2 toxin, HT-2 toxin, diacetoxyscirpenol)	*Fusarium poae* *F acuminatum* *F sporotrichioides* *F equiseti*	Cereal grains (overwintered) Straws Hay	Moderate to low temperatures, sharp fluctuations in temperature may increase mycotoxin production, high humidity	Cytotoxicity, Anorexia Inflammation of GIT Hemorrhage Hematotoxicity Diarrhea, ill thrift, Poor growth, abortions, Immunosuppression, death	Hemorrhage Dermonecrosis	1,34,64
Zearalenone, zearalenol	*Fusarium graminearum* *F culmorum* *F equiseti*	Cereal grains Ear corn Hay	High oxygen, moist Moderate temperatures (cooler at night, warmer in the day)	Hyperestrogenism Infertility	Enlarged genitalia	1
Fumonisin B1 and B2 (B3)	*F verticillioides* *F proliferatum*	Corn in the field	Drought followed by cool, wet weather during pollination	Decreased feed intake Decreased milk production Increase serum hepatic enzymes Increased serum urea nitrogen and creatinine (lambs)	Mild hepatopathy Tubular nephrosis	18,29,37,40

(*continued on next page*)

Table 3
(continued)

Toxicant	Mold	Feeds Affected	Environmental Conditions	Clinical Signs	Lesions	References
Ochratoxin A	*Aspergillus alutaceus* var. *alutaceus* (*ochraceus*), *Penicillium viridicatum*	Wheat Cereal grains	Grain moisture of 16%–18% and equilibrium relative humidity >85%, Temperatures 12–25°C (54–77°F)	Hepatotoxic and nephrotoxic Poor feed conversion and weight gains, Ill thrift, Polyuria/polydipsia Immunosuppressive	Enlarged kidneys Interstitial fibrosis Dilated renal tubules Thickened basement membranes Glomerular sclerosis	18,41,42
Citrinin	*Penicillium citrinum* *Penicillium viridicatum* *Monascus ruber*	Wheat Barley Oats Rye	Grain moisture of 16%–18% and equilibrium relative humidity >85%, Temperatures 12–25°C (54–77°F)	Uremia	Degeneration and necrosis of proximal convoluted tubules	2,42,62
Roridin E, satratoxins G and H, Verrucarin J	*Stachybotrys alternans* (syn. *Stachybotrys atra* and *Stachybotrys chatarum*)	Wet, mildewed forages Cereal grains	Temperatures 0–40°C Relative humidity ~90% Moisture content of 15% in substrate	Anorexia, fever Salivation, oral necrosis Bloody diarrhea Skin necrosis Abortions, sudden death	Hemorrhage and necrosis of gastrointestinal tract	64,65
(neurotoxin?) Cases in South Africa and South America	*Diplodia maydis* (syn. *Stenocarpella maydis*)	Corn, close to 50% of plants in silk	Wet weather, moderate temperatures	Neuromuscular syndrome; High-stepping gait, ataxia, incoordination, constipation, salivation, paresis, and paralysis Stillborn/nonviable fetuses	Rare	58,59

…amine	*Rhizoctonia legumicola*	Clover (*Trifolium* sp) Other legumes Black patch disease	Wet weather and cool temperatures during regrowth of forages (mid to late summer)	Excessive salivation Lacrimation Watery diarrhea Bloat Dyspnea	Severe cases: dilated, fluid-filled intestines	18
Tremorgenic toxins Paspalitrem A and B Lolitrem B	*Claviceps paspali* *Neothyphodium lolii*	Dallis grass (*Paspalum dilatatum*) Bahia grass Perennial ryegrass (*Lolium perenne*)		Staggers Tremors Convulsions		1,2,44
Sporidesmin	*Pithomyces chartarum*	Dead plant material and pasture litter	Warm, humid weather during late summer and fall	Photosensitization Skin edema and necrosis Sheep hepatic lesions and urinary cystitis		1,56
Roquefortine C Mycophenolic acid Marcfortine A and B Andrastin A PR toxin Other toxins?	*Penicillium roqueforti* (*P paneum* Frisvad, *P carneum* Frisvad)	Corn and grass silage	Low oxygen High levels of organic acids	Ill thrift Poor milk production Poor reproduction Immunosuppression Inappetance, ketosis		51,52,54
Unknown toxicant? (Patulin?)	*Aspergillus clavatus*	Hydroponically grown sprouted barley or wheat Sprouted grains Beer residues (malting by-products)		Posterior ataxia Knuckling of fetlocks Tremors, recumbency Salivation Good appetite Paralysis Death	Degenerative and necrotic neuronal changes of nuclei of brainstem and neurons of ventral horns of spinal cord. Vacuolation and myelin depletion in spinal cord	45–50

(*continued on next page*)

Table 3
(continued)

Toxicant	Mold	Feeds Affected	Environmental Conditions	Clinical Signs	Lesions	References
Patulin	*Penicillium* *Aspergillus* *Byssochlamys*	Silages Apple juice	0–25°C	Impairs cellulose digestion Decreased feed intake Decreased milk production Neurotoxicosis?		1,30,50,70
Dicoumarol	*Penicillium* *Mucor* *Humicolor*	Sweet clover hay (*Melilotus* sp) Sweet vernal grass (*Anthoxanthum odoratum*)	Damp weather	Hemorrhages Prolonged clotting time	Hemorrhages	18
Gliotoxin	*Aspergillus fumigatus* *Candida albicans*	Grains Hay Animal tissues; bovine udder		Immunosuppression Diarrhea (Case in camels)	Edema and hemorrhage in abomasum and intestines	1,66
Luteoskyrin Islanditoxin Skyrin Rubroskyrin Cyclochlorotine	*Penicillium islandicum*	Stored corn Rice	High relative humidity, moderate weather (10–45°C)	Reduced milk production Anorexia Depression Abdominal pain Fever Polyuria Death	Hepatomegaly, Periportal to midzonal necrosis and fibrosis, binucleated hepatocytes Biliary hyperplasia Necrosis proximal renal tubules	67,68

and growth. Chronic aflatoxicosis in cattle is associated with clinical signs of reduced appetite, feed efficiency, milk production, and icterus. Hepatic enzymes are typically increased and prothrombin time can be prolonged. The sensitive indicator of aflatoxicosis is decreased performance, the cause of which is multifactorial, involving nutritional interactions, anorexia, altered hepatic protein and lipid metabolism, and disruptions of hormonal metabolism.[1] **Table 5** lists several subacute to chronic experimental studies with aflatoxin B_1 in ruminants. In a study of young, crossbred steers fed between 0 and 1000 ppb aflatoxin B_1 in a ration for 133 days (4.5 months) no toxic effects were observed in the animals fed 300 ppb or less of aflatoxin B_1.[11] Aflatoxins B_1 and M_1 can be detected in livers of animals fed aflatoxins, with increasing aflatoxins in liver reflecting increasing aflatoxin dietary concentrations. No clinical signs of toxicity were observed in young steers (183 kg) fed naturally contaminated aflatoxin corn incorporated into rations containing between 350 and 455 ng aflatoxin/g (ppb) for 15 and 17.5 weeks.[12] The calves did not have adverse effects in weight gain, feed conversion, or antibody production to *Brucella abortus* strain 19 vaccination, but the cutaneous hypersensitivity to johnin protein (*Mycobacterium paratuberculosis*) tended to decrease after 12 weeks. Aflatoxin B_1 and M_1 were detected in urine and pooled blood during the feeding trial, with aflatoxin M_1 detected up to 14 days in urine of calves after the contaminated feed was eliminated in the diet. Sheep are considered the most resistant domesticated species to toxic effects of aflatoxins.[13] Lambs fed increased concentrations of aflatoxins (1.0–1.75 ppm) in concentrate for 5 years were slower to grow, had reduced fertility, and developed hepatic cell carcinoma and nasal tumors, but did not develop liver disorders consistent with aflatoxicosis.[14]

High concentrations of aflatoxins can occur in field crops with insect damage and hot weather, such as a case of moldy, unharvested sweet corn containing more than 2300 ng aflatoxin/g (ppb) of corn that caused death in a cow grazing the field[15]; sweet corn is considered more hazardous than field corn because of higher sugar content. Veterinarians need to consider multiple sources of aflatoxins in rations and commodity storage conditions on a farm. In one field case, young calves of 140 to 200 kg fed corn, whole cottonseed, gin trash, molasses, and mineral for 60 to 120 days started to show clinical signs of depression, lethargy, ataxia, poor performance, respiratory disease with poor treatment response, and death.[16] Aflatoxin B_1 was detected in multiple samples of cottonseed between 96 and 1700 ng/g (ppb), in 2 samples of gin trash at 110 and 857 ng/g, and corn at 14 ng/g. The commodities had been stored on the farm outside on the ground and in heavy rains for several months, with mold visible in the cottonseed. The concern in this investigation, and in many field cases, is that the feed consumed by the animals before the farm visit or investigation may not be available for chemical testing and mycotoxin determination. Neurologic signs of proprioceptive hindlimb deficits, circling, ataxia, depression, absence of response to stimuli, and lateral recumbency were observed in beef calves between 6 and 15- months old fed a home-produced cornmeal contaminated with 1400 ppb aflatoxin B_1 (1670 ppb total aflatoxins) and 15 ppm fumonisins.[17] Calves deteriorated and died within 48 hours of clinical examinations. Postmortem results included severe hepatopathy, moderate to severe edema of the brain white matter, and lesions in the cerebral and cerebellar cortices. The fumonisin concentration in cornmeal was not considered toxic for cattle.

Diagnosis

A diagnosis of aflatoxicosis is based on typical clinical signs, lesions, and showing toxic (not trace) concentrations in the ration. Positive fluorescence of grain under a black light (blue-green color at 365 nm) suggests *Aspergillus* metabolites, but not

Table 4
Guidelines for maximum mycotoxins in final rations (mg/kg = ppm; μg/kg = ppb)

Mycotoxin	Dairy Cows		Beef Cattle		Other		Ref
DON	5 ppm[a]	>4 mo of age	10 ppm[a]	>4 mo of age	2 ppm[b]		FDA 2010[71]
	Complementary and complete feedstuffs: 5 ppm				2 ppm	Calves (<4 mo), lambs and kids	EC[72]
	1 ppm	Young calves & lactating dairy	5 ppm				CFIA fact sheet[73]
Aflatoxins	20 ppb	Corn, peanut products, cottonseed meal, and other animal feeds and feed ingredients	300 ppb	Feedlot beef using corn, peanut products	20 ppb	Corn, peanut products, cottonseed meal, and other animal feeds for other ruminants	FDA action levels CPG 683.100[74]
			300 ppb	Beef regardless of age or breeding status using cottonseed meal			
			100 ppb	Breeding beef using corn, peanut products			
			20 ppb	Immature animal using corn, peanut products and other feed ingredients (excluding cottonseed meal)			
Aflatoxin M1					0.5 ppb	Fluid milk	FDA[75]
					0.05 ppb	Raw milk, heat-treated milk	EC[76]

Fumonisins (B1+B2+B3)	30 ppm (≤50% of diet)	Lactating dairy cows	60 ppm (≤ 50% of diet)	Ruminants more than 3 mo old and fed for slaughter	FDA 2001[77]
			30 ppm (≤ 50% of diet)	Breeding ruminants	
			10 ppm (≤ 50% of diet)	Ruminants less than 3 mo of age	
Zearalenone	0.5 ppm		0.5 ppm	Calves, sheep, lambs, goats, kids	EC[72]
	<2–4 ppm (lower with phytoestrogens, pregnancy, early postnatal period)		<5–10 ppm (lower with phytoestrogens, pregnancy, early postnatal period)		MO[d] ND[e]
	Cow diets 10 ppm (1.5 if other toxins present) recommended tolerance				CFIA[73]
HT-2 toxin	0.025 ppm		0.1 ppm		CFIA[73]
T-2 toxin + HT-2 toxin	<2 ppm		<5 ppm feeder cattle		ND[e]
Ergot alkaloids[c]	<100–200 ppb based on species, physiologic state, environmental conditions, dose, and duration of exposure				MO[d]
Ochratoxin A	0.25 ppm in feed materials fed to animals in a daily ration				EC[72]

Abbreviations: CFIA, Canadian Food Inspection Agency-Fact Sheet; CPG, Compliance Policy Guide; EC, European Community; FDA, US Food and Drug Administration.

[a] FDA guidelines: 10 ppm DON on grains and grain by-products (12% moisture basis) and 30 ppm in distillers' grains, brewers' grains, and gluten feed and gluten meals derived from grains destined for ruminating beef and feedlot cattle and dairy cattle older than 4 months, with the added recommendation for the total ration (all grains, all grain by-products, hay, silage, and roughage) given in the table.

[b] FDA guidelines: 5 ppm DON on grains and grain by-products, with the added recommendation that these ingredients not exceed 40% of their diet.

[c] CFR Title 7 - Agriculture, Part 810, Official US Standards for Grain: ergoty grain products are: wheat >0.05% ergot sclerotia; barley, oats, triticale >0.1% ergot sclerotia; rye >0.3% ergot sclerotia; mixed grain predominately wheat or rye >0.3% ergot sclerotia; and other mixed grains >0.1% ergot sclerotia.

[d] Guidelines provided by University of Missouri Columbia, Veterinary Medicine Diagnostic Laboratory.

[e] Guidelines provided by North Dakota State University, Veterinary Diagnostic Laboratory.

Table 5
Aflatoxin dose, duration, and clinical effects in ruminants

Initial Weight (kg)	Feed Aflatoxin B1 μg/kg (ppb)	Days Fed	Comments	References
189 steers	300	133	Altered liver enzymes	11
184 steers	700		Lower weight gains and feed efficiency; enlarged, fibrous livers	
197 steers	1000		Lower weight gains and feed efficiency, deaths at 59 and 137 d; enlarged, fibrous livers	
225 steers	60	155	Aflatoxins B_1 and M_1 (<1 ppb, wet tissue) in liver during feeding trial	78
236 steers	300		Aflatoxins B_1 and M_1 (<2 ppb, wet tissue) in liver during feeding trial	
228 steers	600		Decrease in growth rate and rate of gain; slight increase in liver enzymes; mild fibrosis and disruption of liver structure. Aflatoxins B_1 and M_1 (<3 ppb, wet tissue) in liver during feeding trial	
183 steers	<456	123	No effect on weight gain and immune effects (lymphoblastogenesis and antibody production) with a trend toward reduction in delayed cutaneous hypersensitivity. Aflatoxins B_1 and M_1 detected periodically in urine and blood and in liver, kidney, muscle, and other tissues at necropsy	12
183 steers	<456 (followed by 18 d on noncontaminated diet)	105	No adverse effects. Aflatoxins B_1 and M_1 detected in urine and blood. Aflatoxins B_1 (0.09 ng/g) detected only in rumen contents at necropsy	
27 lambs	2000 (followed by35 days on noncontaminated diet)	37	Decrease in average daily gain and bacteriostatic activity of serum; increase in neutrophil phagocytosis and immunoglobulin G levels; no difference in white blood cell and differential leukocyte counts	79
15 lambs	2500	21	Decrease in body weight, relative liver weight, and average daily gains; increase in relative kidney weights. No mortality or gross lesions; moderate fatty vacuolation in liver. Increased γ-glutamyltransferase and decreased serum urea and alkaline phosphatase activities	80
3-mo-old lambs, initially	1750 in concentrate for 3.5 y 1000 in concentrate for 1.5 y	~1280	Grew slightly slower for 18 mo, lower fertility, no typical liver symptoms of aflatoxicosis. Neoplasms in liver and nasal cavity	14

aflatoxins. Various analytical methods can be used to determine aflatoxins in feedstuffs; the most important aspect of analysis is to acquire a representative sample of the suspect feed or feeds. When sampling for aflatoxins in feed, the larger and more random the sampling, the better the chances to detect aflatoxins. In a small sample, even 1 contaminated kernel can dramatically alter analytical results. Uneven distribution of mold and mycotoxins in a storage facility requires multiple samples at both the perimeter and center of the bin.[18,19] A more representative sample is obtained by periodic sampling from a flowing or moving stream of suspect feed to generate a large sample volume (5–10 kg), mixing the sample, and subsampling for analysis. To avoid inadequate or insufficient sampling, retain a minimum of 5 kg from each batch of feed or grain purchased or used.[19]

Treatment and Prevention

No specific treatment is available for aflatoxicosis beyond quickly removing the contaminated ration and replacing with an uncontaminated feed. Providing optimum dietary protein, vitamins, and trace elements may aid recovery, although some affected animals may not recover. To prevent aflatoxin production after harvest, storage moisture of less than 12% is recommended for cereals grains and less than 8% to 9% moisture for oilseeds within a wide range of temperatures. Store grains and oilseeds in clean, weatherproof structures; cleaning grain to remove lightweight or broken grain can reduce mycotoxins. Several measures have been taken to reduce aflatoxin contamination of feeds, including mold inhibitors, fermentation, physical separation, thermal treatment (roasting), irradiation, ammoniation, ozonation, and using mycotoxin adsorbents. No method is without drawbacks, including cost, large-scale application, and only partial success. Treating grain with anhydrous ammonia may reduce aflatoxin concentrations by about 30%. Numerous products are marketed to sequester or bind mycotoxins and reduce absorption from an animal's gastrointestinal tract, although in the United States these agents are typically sold as anticaking or free-flow agents. Agents tested include sodium calcium aluminosilicates, activated charcoal, bentonite and various clays, yeast cultures, and esterified glucomannan. Several of these compounds show potential in partially binding aflatoxin B_1 and reducing aflatoxin M_1 contamination in milk.[20–22] Positive responses in reducing aflatoxin M_1 in milk are not consistent for all of these binders; refereed publications indicate that several clay products only partially bind aflatoxins in ruminants (unknown rumen compounds compete for binding sites on clay) and may reduce aflatoxin M_1 residue by 20% to 40% (G. Rottinghaus, PhD, Columbia, MO, personal communication, October 2010). Incorporating sodium calcium aluminosilicates or clay products at low concentrations in the diet is a reasonable investment to partially sequester aflatoxin, reducing potential toxicosis and milk residues in lactating cows. The use of yeast products may stimulate some immune responses and partially offset some adverse effects, but do not seem to substantially reduce toxicosis or milk residues. The FDA has not licensed any product for use as a mycotoxin binder in animal feeds.

ERGOT

Ergot can refer to the disease caused by *Claviceps* spp invading the developing ovary of certain grasses and to the visible sclerotium or ergot body of *C purpurea* growing on rye. It may be questionable whether the condition called nervous or convulsive ergotism is a real syndrome, because it could be confused with tremorgens and the mycotoxins produced by *Claviceps paspali*.[23] Ergot alkaloids can be produced in both ergotism and tall fescue toxicosis, and aspects of these conditions are similar.

Historically, ergot has been associated with gangrene and reproductive effects of abortion and agalactia. Ergot bodies are *C purpurea* mycelia and hardened exudates of honeydew with fungal conidia that replace a grass or cereal grain ovary with the hardened, dark sclerotium. The ergot bodies drop to the ground and overwinter until the spring when sclerotia germinate and produce filamentous ascospores that infect the stigma of grass or cereal grain flowers. Within a few days, conidia (asexual spores) are produced on the plant ovary and extrude a sweet matrix (honeydew) attracting insects to spread conidia to other flowers or susceptible grasses. Rye, triticale, wheat, barley, oats, and various grasses can be infected by *C purpurea*. The US Standards for Grain define ergoty wheat and barley at more than 0.05% and more than 0.3% ergot sclerotia, respectively (see **Table 4**). Endophyte-infected and endophyte-free fescue grasses can also be infected by *C purpurea*. In the spring, cool damp weather delays pollination and allows *C purpurea* germination and development. No-till farming, shallow cultivation, and failure to rotate crops increase the potential for ergot germination. Sporadic cases of cutaneous and gangrenous ergotism occur when livestock are turned out into pasture grasses with infected seed heads. Ergot alkaloids are composed of primary toxicants or ergopeptine alkaloids (ergotamine, ergocristine, ergosine, ergocryptine, ergocornine, and ergovaline) and ergoline alkaloids (ergonovine, lysergic acid, lysergol, and lysergic acid amide). Following ingestion of the ergopeptine alkaloids, the compounds are rapidly cleared from the blood by the liver, undergo primarily biliary excretion, and are not excreted in the milk of cows. Ergopeptine alkaloids cause vasoconstriction through inhibition of the D_1 dopaminergic receptor and partial agonism of the α_1-adrenergic and serotonin receptors. Constriction of small arteries can lead to ischemia and necrosis of the distal portions of the limbs, tail, and ears; uterine contractions in late pregnancy are associated with stimulation of α_1-adrenergic receptors, but evidence for abortion is vague. Decreased prolactin secretion by lactotropes in the anterior pituitary is associated with ergopeptine alkaloid stimulation of D_2-dopamine receptors.

Susceptibility of livestock to ergotism seems to vary with species, breed, age, gender, and physiologic state. Ruminants are considered susceptible because of the types of diets (both grains and grasses) and ruminal pH that can favor fermentation and enhanced extraction of ergot alkaloids from sclerotia. Numerous risk factors influence the development of clinical signs, including extremes in environmental temperatures (too cold or hot), physiologic state (eg, lactating, late gestation), and ergot alkaloid dose. The concentration of ergot alkaloids in *C purpurea* sclerotia is highly variable, between 0 and almost 10,000 mg/kg (ppm), and the relative concentrations of individual ergopeptine alkaloids vary. The threshold concentrations of total ergot alkaloids or ergopeptine alkaloids capable of causing ergotism in animals have not been established; however, the threshold ergovaline concentrations that produce clinical fescue toxicosis are approximately 200 to 800 μg/kg (ppb) in a total ration and likely approximate the threshold concentrations of ergopeptine alkaloids that produce ergotism in livestock.[23] Cattle consuming sclerotia with total ergot alkaloid concentrations from 1300 mg/kg (ppm) to 3100 mg/kg for several weeks developed ergotism. Broken ergot sclerotia can concentrate in screenings; therefore, avoid feeding grain screenings to animals unless tested for mycotoxins. Dietary concentrations of 0.3% to 1% sclerotia have been associated with clinical signs of ergotism in cattle. Initial clinical signs of ergotism can appear as pain and lameness (eg, stamping the feet), with affected areas feeling cool to the touch. With disease progression, a sharp line of demarcation appears between healthy and nonviable tissue, which can be followed by necrosis and sloughing of tissue. Additional clinical signs may affect the gastrointestinal tract (eg, constipation, diarrhea, or internal bleeding). During hot, humid weather, clinical signs of ergotism in lactating cattle include hyperthermia and lower milk production and feed intake. Hyperthermia is related to poor heat dissipation from the body surface, and reduced milk production is associated with hypoprolactinemia. A summer syndrome involving a 30% decrease in milk production, open-mouth breathing, need to seek shade or wade into water even at night, and lower fertility developed in lactating dairy cattle in South Africa.[24] Field investigations determined that a common weed, nut sedge (*Cyperus esculentus*), was infected with the ergot *Claviceps cyperi* and heavily contaminated maize silage and teff (*Eragrostis curvula*) hay on several farms. The ergot alkaloid content in contaminated maize silages was 115 to 975 ppb on one farm and 875 ppb on a second affected farm, with the predominant alkaloid ergocryptine. Treatment of ruminants for ergotism includes removal of ergot source from the ration, providing good bedding for lame animals, and reducing stress in the environment (providing shade and water holes). Antibiotics may be necessary to control secondary bacterial infections. Livestock with severe gangrene of the extremities may require euthanasia. To avoid adverse effects of ergot on livestock performance, the total dietary concentrations of ergot alkaloids should be less than 100 to 200 ppb (see **Table 4**).

FESCUE

Fescue toxicosis is a descriptive term for several syndromes (fescue foot, summer slump, and fat necrosis) associated with ingestion of tall fescue grass (*Lolium arundinacea*). This article focuses on fescue foot. For a discussion of fescue effects on reproduction, see the article by Tim J. Evans elsewhere in this issue.

Tall fescue grass is a popular cool-season, perennial grass that naturally contains alkaloids (eg, loline, perloline, and perlolidine alkaloids) and can be infected with an endophyte, *N coenophialum*, which grows within the intercellular spaces of the leaf sheaths, stems, and seeds. The symbiotic relationship between tall fescue and the endophyte can result in production of ergot alkaloids, including ergoline alkaloids (lysergic acid, lysergol, lysergic acid amide, ergonovine) and ergopeptine alkaloids (eg, ergovaline, ergosine, ergotamine, ergocryptine, ergocristine, and ergocornine).[25] Although the exact roles of these toxins are debated, most clinical signs of fescue toxicosis are attributed to the ergopeptine alkaloids, of which ergovaline predominates. The mechanisms of action of ergot alkaloids are described earlier. Fescue foot is similar to the condition of dry gangrene of the extremities observed with exposure to ergot alkaloids in cold weather. Fescue foot generally occurs in late fall or winter with cooler environmental temperatures. The ergovaline concentration in the feed is usually greater than 400 ppb. Vasoconstriction generally affects the hind limbs first. The condition appears initially as swelling and reddening at the coronary band, and progresses to knuckling at the pastern joint, shifting hind leg lameness, unthriftiness, and ischemic necrosis of the hooves. Tips of ears and the tail can become ischemic. Sheep may develop clinical signs of fescue toxicosis similar to cattle; dietary ergovaline concentrations greater than 500 ppb and cooler temperatures are associated with fescue foot in sheep. Sheep can also develop tongue necrosis.

Ergovaline concentrations in fescue grass can range between 200 and 600 μg/kg (ppb), and seed head concentrations can exceed 1000 ppb. Ergovaline concentrations of 150 μg/kg diet (ppb) or 6.8 μg/kg body weight have reduced growth rate and lowered blood prolactin concentrations in lambs.[25] Summer fescue toxicosis in heat-stressed steers has been reported at low concentrations of ergovaline in the total ration, about 200 ppb. Fescue foot has been reproduced in cattle and sheep with concentrations of ergovaline in the diet at 400 to 750 ppb in cattle and at 500 to 800 ppb in sheep. Diagnostic testing for fescue toxicosis can involve analysis for ergot alkaloids or ergovaline in forage or hay and detection of the endophyte in the leaf sheaths, stems, or seed of tall fescue. Contact agronomists or testing laboratories for protocols to collect samples of forages or seeds before testing.

TRICHOTHECENES

Fusarium molds are the most economically important source of trichothecene mycotoxins. Trichothecenes are sesquiterpenoid compounds with an epoxy group at C12 to C13 that is considered essential for toxicity. Although more than 100 trichothecene mycotoxins have been identified, veterinary medicine is focused on a few trichothecenes. Type A trichothecenes include some of the most toxic trichothecenes (eg, T-2 toxin, its deacetylated metabolite HT-2 toxin, and diacetoxyscirpenol [DAS or anguidine]). Type B trichothecenes are common field contaminants of grains and include DON and its acetylated derivatives 15-acetyl DON and 3-acetyl DON, nivalenol, and fusarenone-X (4-acetylnivalenol). In North American, *Fusarium graminearum* characteristically produces DON and 15-AcDON; during cooler, wet conditions production of 3-AcDON and nivalenol can be detected in cereals. The relative cytotoxicity of the type B trichothecenes has been evaluated in vitro using bioassays. In summary, the toxicity of DON, 15-AcDON, nivalenol, and fusarenone-X are similar, and 3-AcDON is considered slightly less toxic.[26] Trichothecenes are stable compounds and can remain present at toxic concentrations in feed for years. Field reports of trichothecene toxicity in livestock in North America typically involve DON contamination. Most trichothecene exposures are of a chronic to subchronic nature with low dietary DON concentrations associated with nutritional impairment, reduced production, and possible diminished immune responses. Swine and monogastrics are more sensitive to trichothecenes than are ruminants.

Fusarium is most common in temperate climates, but contamination of grains is reported worldwide. Although not a trichothecene, the estrogenic mycotoxin zearalenone is produced by several *Fusarium* species and often found together with DON in North America (**Table 6**). *Fusarium* infection of immature corn generally results in higher trichothecene and zearalenone concentrations in the cob, compared with kernel mycotoxin concentrations. In unusually wet, cool periods, *Fusarium* mycotoxins not only occur in the grain but also in the vegetative part of the plant (hay and straw). *Fusarium* contamination can occur in hay baled wet or stored in higher moisture

Table 6
***Fusarium* species and related mycotoxins produced by the molds**

Fusarium	Mycotoxins
F graminearum	DON, 15-ADON, 3-ADON, nivalenol, zearalenone
F culmorum	DON, 3-ADON, nivalenol, zearalenone
F equiseti	Nivalenol, zearalenone, diacetoxyscirpenol
F poae	Nivalenol, diacetoxyscirpenol, T-2, HT-2
F acuminatum	Diacetoxyscirpenol, T-2, HT-2
F sporotrichioides	Diacetoxyscirpenol, T-2, HT-2
F verticillioides (moniliforme) *F proliferatum*	Fumonisins

conditions (>20%) and in silage inadequately packed or where aerobic conditions exist. Wheat straw contamination with DON in scabby years may be as high as 50 to 100 mg DON/kg (ppm, dry weight basis).[27] These extremely high levels of contamination are medically relevant when contaminated forages are used for fiber in dairy feeds or bedding for swine (with potential ingestion).

Trichothecenes have multiple effects on eukaryotic cells, including inhibition of protein, RNA and DNA synthesis, alteration of membrane structure and mitochondrial function, stimulation of lipid peroxidation, induction of programmed cell death or apoptosis, and activation of cytokines and chemokines.[2] The hallmark clinical sign of trichothecene toxicosis in animals is feed refusal, which has led to speculation that animals may not voluntarily consume enough contaminated ration to cause marked poisoning. However, when the only available feedstuffs are contaminated with trichothecenes, poisoning can result. Diarrhea is fairly common following trichothecene ingestion. Altered intestinal absorption of compounds and impaired permeability are caused by morphologic and functional damage to intestinal mucosa.[28] Significant metabolism of trichothecenes can occur in the rumen and gastrointestinal tract before absorption. The rumen metabolite of oral DON is de-epoxy deoxynivalenol (DOM-1). De-epoxidation of DON to DOM-1 is considered a deactivation step resulting in a much less toxic compound. Rumen microbes, in particular protozoa, seem to be active in the deacetylation of the trichothecenes.[4]

Low concentrations of DON do not seem to adversely affect ruminating beef growth or reproduction. In one study, crossbred steers fed up to 9.2 mg DON/kg diet (ppm) for 84 days during the growing period and up to 12.6 mg DON/kg diet (ppm) for 100 days during the finishing period had no significant differences in beef performance including feed intake, feed efficiency, rate of gain, or carcass quality.[29] The FDA advisory level for DON in the final ration for beef cattle more than 4 months of age is 10 mg/kg or ppm (see **Table 4**). Pregnant yearling heifers consumed DON-contaminated barley at 10.2 mg DON/kg diet or 13 mg DON/kg diet from midgestation through the first 45 days of lactation.[29] No significant changes were noted in feed intake, heifer weight gain, or calf body weights; calf weight gains were higher for calves nursing heifers fed the DON-contaminated barley during calving and lactation. Ovine responses to trichothecene exposure are similar to beef cattle. In general, beef cattle and sheep are more tolerant of higher DON concentrations in their rations than are dairy cattle. The different susceptibilities could be associated with greater stress for dairy cows and increased dry-matter intake, faster rumen turnover, and decreased rumen microbial degradation time for dairy cows.[30] When feeding dairy cows, questions arise about the possible impact of DON on milk production and milk residues; data from several controlled studies are available. Primiparous Holstein cows fed DON-contaminated grains up to 12.09 mg DON/kg of dry-matter concentrate (maximum daily intake 104 mg DON) for 10 weeks in a lactation study had no changes in total milk output or feed intake, and no detectable residues (<1 ng/mL or ppb) of DON or DOM-1 in milk.[31] High-producing dairy cows provided DON-contaminated barley diets up to 14.6 mg DON/kg concentrate (~8.5 ppm in diet, 0.31 mg DON/kg body weight) for 3 weeks showed no significant changes in milk production or feed intake.[32] The FDA advisory level for DON in the final ration for dairy cattle more than 4 months of age is 5 mg/kg or ppm (see **Table 4**). Lactating cows dosed orally with 920 mg of DON had only trace DON levels in serum (<2 ng DON/mL) detected 24 hours after administration.[33] Free and conjugated DON were detected in cow's milk at low levels (<4 ng/mL) with an estimated 0.0001% of the administered dose excreted in milk (**Table 7**).

Clinical signs of the more toxic type A trichothecenes include emesis, feed refusal and weight loss, diarrhea, immunomodulation, coagulopathy and hemorrhage, and

Table 7
Mycotoxins and milk carryover

Mycotoxins	Exposure	Carryover Rates to Milk	Biologic Metabolism	References
Aflatoxin B_1	>30 ppb Aflatoxin B_1 in feed (dry matter) may exceed 0.5 ppb in milk; >3 ppb in feed exceeds 0.05 ppb M_1 in milk	1%–3% (up to 6.2%)	Aflatoxin M_1	30
Ergot alkaloids	~16 μg/kg body weight	None detected	Unchanged	83
DON		DOM<0.0024	De-epoxy DON	82
	920 mg orally	DON<0.0001%	Free and conjugated	33
		DON none detected DOM-1<0.0011		84
Ochratoxin A		<1% (sheep)	Ochratoxin α	85
T-2 toxin		0.05%–2%	various	81,86
Zearalenone		0.008%–0.06%	α-zearalenol, β-zearalenol	81
Fumonisin B_1		0%–0.05%	Unchanged	81

Data from Yiannikouris A, Jouany JP. Mycotoxins in feeds and their fate in animals: a review. Anim Res 2002;51:92–3; and Fink-Gremmels J. Mycotoxins in cattle feeds and carry-over to dairy milk: a review. Food Addit Contam 2008;25:175–6.

cellular necrosis of mitotically active tissues such as intestinal mucosa, skin, bone marrow, spleen, testis, and ovary.[2] T-2 and HT-2 toxin, often found together in plants, are some of the most toxic trichothecenes detected in feeds. Ruminants can rapidly deacetylate T-2 toxin to HT-2 toxin. It is often difficult to distinguish the effects of T-2 toxin from HT-2 in vivo; therefore, it is reasonable to sum the concentrations of these toxins to evaluate clinical effects. Decreased feed consumption was reported in beef calves (85–200 kg) orally dosed with T-2 toxin at 0.3 mg/kg (~10 mg T-2/kg diet or ppm) for 6 weeks.[34] Calves dosed with 0.6 mg/kg (~20 mg T-2/kg diet) developed marked anorexia, weight loss, rough hair coats, and intermittent diarrhea. In a field case, clinical signs of anorexia, periodic increased temperatures, abortions in midgestation, and a 20% death loss were associated with feeding moldy, high-moisture corn to lactating Holstein dairy cows during a 5 month period in late winter.[35] Among the fungi cultured from corn were *Fusarium tricinctum*, *Fusarium roseum*, and *Fusarium moniliforme*, and various *Penicillium* spp. A sample of feed from this field investigation contained 2 mg T-2 toxin/kg, which was considered a low value because of analytical methodology (low recovery). Additional mycotoxins could have been present in the feed and contributed to clinical toxicity in the dairy cows, but were not analyzed. Potential infectious causes, particularly viruses, may not have been ruled out as the cause. Wet, cooler conditions in the northern United States and in Canada during the fall have been associated with significant concentrations of T-2 and HT-2 toxins in grass hay bales (~9 ppm) and in corn (4.5–5 ppm) (M. Mostrom, Fargo, ND, unpublished data, 2006). Feeder calves have been fed contaminated corn silage in a ration with almost 5 ppm T-2 plus HT-2 toxins with no adverse effects, supporting earlier research. However, higher concentrations of type A trichothecenes in rations should be avoided in pregnant animals and dairy. T-2 toxin can cross the placenta. Multiple abortions were reported in beef cows fed primarily grass hay contaminated with 7.5 ppm (T-2+HT-2 toxins), however, necropsies were not performed on the fetuses to rule out infectious or nutritional causes (M. Mostrom, Fargo, ND, unpublished data, 2006). Dramatic weather patterns have created wet, cooler conditions in central and southern United States leading to *Fusarium* growth on wet pasture grasses and production of T-2 toxin, HT-2 toxin, and other mycotoxins in pastures used for livestock grazing. This is not a common occurrence.

Because of the vague nature of toxic effects attributed to low concentrations of trichothecenes, a solid link between low-level exposure and a specific trichothecene(s) is difficult to establish. Mycotoxins may play a role in some subtle animal diseases, but diagnostic consideration needs to move beyond just testing the feed for toxins and evaluate nutrition, disease, management, and environment conditions. Storage of grains at less than 13% to 14% moisture (<0.70 α_w) and hay/straw at less than 20% moisture are important in preventing trichothecene production. After the contaminated feed is removed from the diet and exposure stopped, animals generally have a good prognosis for recovery. The use of mycotoxin adsorbents (smectite clays, humic substances, and yeast wall products) to bind trichothecenes in dietary rations reducing clinical effects in ruminants is generally discouraging (G. Rottinghaus, PhD, Columbia, MO, personal communication, October 2010). A potential cost-effective process to reduce DON contamination of wet, stored cereal grains (15%–20% moisture) is through incorporation of sodium metabisulfite, with or without propionic acid, into grain.[36] A decrease in DON concentrations was paralleled by an increase in DON sulfonate, which was considered biologically less active in pigs. The stability of DON sulfonate in the rumen is unknown.

FUMONISINS

Fumonisins are a group of heat-stable, water-soluble mycotoxins generally produced in white and yellow corn in the field by *F verticillioides* (syn. *F moniliforme*) and *Fusarium proliferatum*. A period of drought during the growing season followed by wet, cooler conditions during pollination of corn favors development of fumonisins. Toxicity is associated with fumonisins B_1 and B_2, with fumonisin B_2 usually occurring at about 30% of fumonisin B_1. These toxins can be concentrated in corn screenings; horses are the most sensitive species. Fumonisins are chemically characterized as an aliphatic hydrocarbon with a terminal amine group and tricarboxylic acid side chains, and are structurally similar to sphingolipids in cellular membranes.[18] Fumonisins inhibit enzymes involved with the conversion of sphinganine to sphingosine, which can interfere with cellular growth, differentiation, and cell communication resulting in toxicity and carcinogenicity. Ruminants are fairly resistant to fumonisins; feed containing 148 μg fumonisins/g (ppm) was less palatable to feeder calves (~230 kg) that developed increased liver enzymes and mild liver lesions (see **Table 3**).[37] In a chronic study of feeder steers (86–127 kg) fed *F moniliforme* culture material with 417 ppm fumonisins B_1 and B_2 in the final corn mixture, a few days of feed refusal were observed in the calves.[38] The liver sphinganine/sphingosine ratios in the calves fed fumonisin were greater than 1; normal ratios are considered to be less than 0.5. Renal and hepatic damage were reported in lambs fed high concentrations of fumonisins (~470 ppm).[39] Dairy cows seem to be more susceptible to fumonisins and FDA guidelines recommend lower fumonisin concentration in their rations, compared with ruminants fed for slaughter (see **Table 4**). Dairy cows provided a naturally contaminated ration with 100 μg fumonisin/g (ppm) for 7 days before parturition and 70 days after parturition developed reduced feed intake and milk production.[40]

OCRHRATOXIN A AND CITRININ

Ochratoxins are phenylalanine-dihydroisocoumarin compounds produced primarily by *Aspergillus alutaceus* var. *alutaceus* (*Aspergillus ochraceus*) and *Penicillium viridicatum.* Ochratoxins are potent nephrotoxins, immunosuppressants, and possible human carcinogens. They inhibit protein synthesis and deplete humoral factors, especially immunoglobulins, and decrease natural killer cell activity.[2] The most toxic of the ochratoxins is ochratoxin A. Another nephrotoxic mycotoxin often found with ochratoxins is citrinin. Citrinin is produced by *Penicillium* molds in similar conditions as ochratoxins (see **Table 3**). Ruminants are more resistant to ochratoxin, compared with monogastrics, because rumen protozoal metabolism quickly converts ochratoxin A to the less toxic ochratoxin α. The elimination half-life in ruminants is short, about 17.3 hours, compared with 100 hours in pigs.[30] However, rapid changes in rations and an increased percentage of concentrates can decrease ruminant metabolism of ochratoxin A to less toxic compounds. Regulatory concerns for ochratoxin A in ruminants are chronic exposure and potential for accumulation in tissues or milk residues (see **Table 7**).

Ochratoxin A and citrinin target the renal proximal tubule. Adult cattle given a single oral dose of ochratoxin A at 13 mg/kg body weight developed anorexia, reduced milk production, diarrhea, and incoordination, with eventually recovery.[41] Ochratoxin (up to 6 ppm) and citrinin (up to 4 ppm) were detected in feeds of several cases of suspect field toxicosis in which cattle had clinical signs of uremia (eg, depression, anorexia, profuse diarrhea, dehydration, hypothermia) and died.[42] Histologic lesions included nephrosis with hyaline casts, dilated tubules and fibrosis in the kidneys, and fatty changes in the liver.

TREMORGENS

The term staggers refers to a group of nervous disorders, of different fungal origins, that are characterized by similar clinical signs, including muscle tremors, incoordination, and generalized weakness exacerbated by stress.[1] Perennial ryegrass (*Lolium perenne*) is a common pasture grass in New Zealand, Australia, Europe, and northwestern United States. Cases of staggers predominately occur on intensively grazed pastures. Disease outbreaks generally appear in the summer and fall and are characterized by high morbidity, low mortality, and no lesions or biochemical changes in recovered animals. A group of indole terpenoids, including lolitrem A and B, paxilline, and related compounds are produced by an endophyte, *Neothyphodium lolii*, and are believed to act on γ-aminobutyric acid receptors disrupting neuromuscular control. Lolitrem B is the predominant tremorgen responsible for clinical signs, which start as head tremors and muscle fasciculations of the neck and shoulders and later involve extremities. With disease progression, animals tend to sway, lie down, and convulse when stressed. The maximum tolerable dose is about 2 mg toxin (lolitrem B)/kg dry matter in sheep and cattle.[43] Deaths rarely occur and animals can recover completely within 7 days when removed from infected grasses and kept in a quiet, secure location.

Paspalum staggers or Dallis grass staggers are associated with infection of Dallis and Bahia (*Paspalum* spp) grasses by *C paspali* and formation of indole-diterpene tremorgens or paspalitrems, such as paspalinine and paspalitrem A and B. Animals can be at risk with ingestion of sclerotia and perhaps honeydew formed in the grasses. Paspalitrem B is the most abundant mycotoxin associated with tremors in cattle and sheep. Sporadic outbreaks of tremors in cattle, similar to paspalum staggers, have been associated with grazing Bermuda grass (*Cynodon dactylon*) infected with

Claviceps cynodontis.[44] Infected seedheads of Bermuda grass contained sclerotia and paspalitrems and paspalinelike indole-diterpenes and low concentrations of ergonovine and ergine.

Aspergillus clavatus has been associated with numerous field outbreaks of tremors, posterior ataxia with knuckling of fetlocks, paresis, recumbence, and death reported in sheep, beef, and dairy cattle.[45–47] The animals generally maintain a good appetite. A common denominator is feeding sprouted cereals, hydroponically grown sprouts, or malted by-products contaminated with *A clavatus*. Symptoms include degeneration of large neurons in the brain stem and neuronal chromatolysis in the spinal cord gray matter.[48,49] Although *A clavatus* can produce patulin, no specific mycotoxin was associated with these outbreaks. Several field outbreaks of neurotoxicosis in Belgium cattle, accompanied by lesions involving neuronal degeneration in the central nervous system and axonal degeneration in the peripheral nervous system, were associated with malting residues contaminated with *A clavatus* and traces of patulin in the compacted fodder.[50]

SILAGE AND FORAGE MOLDS

Ruminant diets contain a significant amount of fiber, usually grass, hay, straw, and silages. These feedstuffs can be contaminated in the field with *Fusarium*, *Alternaria*, *Claviceps*, and *Cladosporium* molds. With poor growth, production, or storage conditions, additional fungal spoilage and mycotoxin contamination continue in forages. Generally, when oxygen is excluded from acidic silages or tight forage bales, further mold growth and mycotoxin production is unlikely; however, if air gains access to these feedstuffs they are at risk for storage molds. Corn and grass silages are often contaminated with molds, including *Aspergillus*, *Penicillium*, *Mucor*, *Geotrichium*, and *Monascus*.[43,51,52] *Fusarium* spp require oxygen for growth, are pH sensitive, and generally vanish in days following routine silage methods. However, significant concentrations of *Fusarium* mycotoxins (DON, 15-acDON, zearaleneone) can routinely be detected in corn silages, and occasionally lower (<3 ppm) concentrations of T-2 and HT-2 toxins can be found in hays and straws in the Midwest. (M. Mostrom, unpublished data, 2009).

Geotrichum candidum occurs in silages and gives off a rancid odor that tends to repel animals, reducing feed consumption.[53] In Europe, *Penicillium* molds, particularly *Penicillium roqueforti*, contaminate corn silage, grass, and sugar beet products and can produce numerous mycotoxins, including: roquefortine, andrastin A, mucophenolic acid, and PR toxin (see **Table 4**). In a field case, *P roqueforti* was identified on barley kernels stored in a bunk silo for 1.5 months before feeding dairy cows.[54] Adverse effects noted in the cows were inappetance, ketosis, mastitis, paralysis, and abortions; roquefortine C, an indole alkaloid, was identified at approximately 25.6 mg/kg (ppm) in feed grain. No additional *Penicillium* mycotoxins (ie, patulin, PR toxin, and penicillic acid) were found and clinical signs disappeared after feeding the moldy grain stopped. The toxicity of roquefortine in ruminants has not been established. Oral administration of roquefortine to ewes by stomach tube of equivalent amounts of 0 to 25 mg roquefortine/kg silage through 1 estrous cycle (16–18 days) resulted in no clinical illness or changes in serum chemistry or hematology parameters.[55] The only apparent effect was a decrease in rumen pH by 0.5 units, perhaps caused by a shift to gram-positive bacteria.

Stored straw and hay can be invaded by *Stachybotrys atra*, a mold that prefers growing on cellulose in cool, damp conditions. Stachybotryotoxicosis, a historical disease in the 1930s and 1940s, has been reported in ruminants and horses in Eastern

Europe (see **Table 3**). Sporadic cases in animals have been reported elsewhere. There is also intense interest in *Stachybotrys* because this black mold grows on drywalls in flooded buildings or wet, poorly ventilated areas and has been associated with pulmonary hemorrhage and respiratory difficulties in humans. *Stachybotrys* can be occasionally cultured from silages, although methodology to test for *Stachybotrys* toxins in forages is not available (no pure reagent standards).

PHOTOSENSITIZATION

Photosensitization is clinically characterized as skin (without protection of hair, wool, or pigmentation) hyperreactivity to sunlight because of photodynamic compounds circulating in peripheral blood. The condition may be primary or secondary. Primary photosensitization occurs when photodynamic compounds are absorbed through the skin or gastrointestinal tract and reach the skin to interact with light. Secondary photosensitization is the most common form of photosensitization and occurs when a breakdown product of chlorophyll in the gut (phylloerythrin) accumulates in the plasma and skin because of hepatic injury. Phylloerythrin can absorb and release energy, creating a phytotoxic reaction in skin. Facial eczema or pithomycotoxicosis is reported in ruminants grazing intensive pasture systems containing dead plant material contaminated with *Pithomyces chartarum*. Toxicoses generally occur in late summer and fall when hot, dry weather and occasional rain and high humidity promote the growth and sporulation of *P chatarum* and production of sporidesmin mycotoxins. The predominant mycotoxin is sporidesmin A.[56] Clinical signs usually occur 10 to 14 days after ingestion of sporidesmin and reflect cholestatic liver disease and dermal photosensitization. Edema and erythema of the ears, eyelids, face, and lips are visible in sheep. Animals can develop secondary bacterial infection and become icteric. Dairy cows may develop a sudden decrease in milk production and ill thrift followed by dermal photosensitization several weeks later.

The term lupinosis applies to a hepatic disease in sheep and cattle resulting from ingestion of phomopsins produced by *Diaporthe toxica* and *Diaporthe wooddii* on dead lupin plants. The hepatotoxicosis is prevalent in Western Australia where dead lupin plants are used for fodder in the summer and autumn.[57] Phomopsins are cytotoxic and antimitotic agents. The course of the disease may be acute, subacute, or chronic depending on the dose and exposure time. Clinical signs are severe liver damage, inappetance, lethargy, icterus, and death. Abortions occur in late pregnant sheep and cattle. Photosensitization is seen in cattle, but rarely in sheep.

DIPLODIA

Another fungus contaminating corn or maize worldwide is *Stenocarpella maydis* (syn. *Diplodia maydis*). Ear corn is most susceptible to *Diplodia* infection within a week or two of midsilk (50% of plants with silks), with wet weather and moderate temperatures allowing spores to splash onto the plant and infect the stalk or ear. The *Diplodia* spores germinate and penetrate the ear shank, starting at the base of the ear and growing toward the tip; ear rot appears as white-gray-brownish mycelia. *Diploidia* is not considered a mycotoxin producer in the United States; however, in southern Africa, diplodiosis is an important mycotoxicosis in harvested maize fields used for winter forage. *Diplodia* can cause a neuromuscular paretic syndrome, (eg, high-stepping gait, ataxia, incoordination, constipation, salivation, paresis, and paralysis) in sheep or cattle.[58] Lesions in the central nervous system are rare and most animals recover. A report of diplodiosis in Argentina involved beef heifers grazing a harvested maize field for about 2 weeks and developing incoordination of hindquarters, stiffness, ataxia, recumbency, and paralysis.[59]

SUMMARY

Mycotoxins occurring on grains and in grasses can adversely affect ruminants. Detection and characterization of mycotoxins occurring in silages, forages, and some of the cereal by-products that are routinely fed to dairy and beef has been limited. In general, ruminants tend to be less susceptible to mycotoxins compared with monogastrics and young animals. Dose-response relationships often have not been established for reproductive or immune effects of mycotoxins in ruminants. Our analytical capabilities to detect very low concentrations of several mycotoxins in feedstuffs can be far lower than feed concentrations associated with clinical effects in livestock. Just detecting mycotoxins at trace levels can lead to interpretations that mycotoxins explain a variety of adverse effects, without a scientific basis. Testing feed for mycotoxins is not the easy answer to often complex problems involving nutrition, environment, animal physiology, genetics, other toxins, and disease.

Often, several mycotoxins can be detected in moldy feed (eg, aflatoxins, fumonisins, DON in cereal by-products) and knowledge of interaction(s) of effects in ruminants is limited. Some mycotoxins can exist in conjugated form, either soluble (masked mycotoxins) or incorporated into, associated with, or attached to macromolecules in plants (insoluble or bound mycotoxins).[60] Food and animal feed tested for recognized mycotoxins may not necessarily be safe, because they might contain mycotoxins in disguise. Plants can convert mycotoxins into more polar metabolites and store them in vacuoles or conjugated to cell wall components. The significance of conjugated mycotoxins is an unknown; no data are available on the toxicity or bioavailability of these mycotoxins. A lack of pure standards for conjugated mycotoxins and adequate clean-up before detection constrains analysis for conjugated mycotoxins by liquid chromatography-mass spectrometry (LC/MS). Validated analysis for DON and zearalenone are being developed for LC/MS/MS. Government regulations for maximum mycotoxins in commodities are typically established to protect the consumer from harmful effects of these compounds, and regulations for mycotoxins in food and feed will probably expand with better analytical methods and more standardized sampling methods.[61] Much of the current research has focused on carryover in tissues and milk, reflecting public health concern and consumer demand for safety in the food chain. More research is needed for effective, cost-efficient inactivation of mycotoxins (especially trichothecenes).

No feed sample submitted for mycotoxin analysis can ever be labeled as safe to feed to animals because laboratories do not have the analytical capability or mycotoxin standards to test for all possible mycotoxins produced by molds and there is lack of toxicity data in ruminants for many mycotoxins, particularly for *Penicillium* mycotoxins. Based on mold cultures, analytical findings, and knowledge of mycotoxin concentrations associated with clinical effects, feed can be channeled for use in various animals in specified conditions. Often, the moldy and more contaminated feeds are used in feedlots, where the physiologic demands of pregnancy and lactation are avoided and a more frequent turnover in sources or batches of feed reduce duration of exposure. However, this is not a foolproof approach to avoiding mycotoxicosis. The golden rule is not to feed moldy feed; a practical approach is to test suspect feeds in a ration, avoid moldy feed if possible, and dilute with clean feed to minimize effects.

REFERENCES

1. Raisbeck MF, Rottinghaus GE, Kendall JD. Effects of naturally occurring mycotoxins on ruminants. In: Smith JE, Henderson RS, editors. Mycotoxins and animal foods. Boca Raton (FL): CRC Press; 1991. p. 647–77.
2. Mycotoxins: risks in plant, animal and human systems. Task Force Report No. 139. Ames (IA): CAST (Council for Agricultural Science and Technology); 2003.
3. Gallo A, Moschini M, Masoero F. Aflatoxins absorption in the gastro-intestinal tract and in the vaginal mucosa in lactating dairy cows. Ital J Anim Sci 2008;7:53–63.
4. Kiessling K-H, Pettersson H, Sandholm K, et al. Metabolism of aflatoxin, ochratoxin, zearalenone and three trichothecenes by intact rumen fluid, rumen protozoa and rumen bacteria. Appl Environ Microbiol 1984;47:1070–3.
5. Westlake K, Mackie RI, Dutton MF. *In vitro* metabolism of mycotoxins by bacterial, protozoal and ovine ruminal fluid preparations. Anim Feed Sci Technol 1989;25:169–78.
6. Upadhaya SD, Sung HG, Lee CH, et al. Comparative study on the aflatoxin B1 degradation ability of rumen fluid from Holstein steers and Korean native goats. J Vet Sci 2009;10:29–34.
7. Meerdink GL. Aflatoxins. In: Plumlee KH, editor. Clinical veterinary toxicology. St Louis (MO): Mosby; 2004. p. 231–5.
8. Carvajal M, Rojo F, Méndez I, et al. Aflatoxin B_1 and its interconverting metabolite aflatoxicol in milk: the situation in Mexico. Food Addit Contam 2003;20:1077–86.
9. Mazzette A, Decandia M, Acciaro M, et al. Excretion of aflatoxin M_1 in milk of goats fed diets contaminated by aflatoxin B_1. Ital J Anim Sci 2009;8(Suppl 2):631–3.
10. Battacone G, Nudda A, Cannas A, et al. Excretion of aflatoxin M_1 in milk of dairy ewes treated with different doses of aflatoxin B_1. J Dairy Sci 2003;86:2667–75.
11. Keyl AC, Booth AN. Aflatoxin effects in livestock. J Am Oil Chem Soc 1971;48:599–604.
12. Richard JL, Pier AC, Stubblefield RD, et al. Effect of feeding corn naturally contaminated with aflatoxin on feed efficiency, on physiologic, immunologic, and pathologic changes, and on tissue residues in steers. Am J Vet Res 1983;44:1294–9.
13. Newberne PM. Chronic aflatoxicosis. J Am Vet Med Assoc 1973;163:1262–7.
14. Lewis F, Markson LM, Allcroft R. The effect of feeding toxic groundnut meal to sheep over a period of five years. Vet Rec 1967;80:312–4.
15. Hall RF, Harrison LR, Colvin BM. Aflatoxicosis in cattle pastured in a field of sweet corn. J Am Vet Med Assoc 1989;194:938.
16. Osweiler GD, Trampel DW. Aflatoxicosis in feedlot cattle. J Am Vet Med Assoc 1985;187:636–7.
17. D'Angelo A, Bellino C, Alborali GL, et al. Neurological signs associated with aflatoxicosis in Piedmontese calves. Vet Rec 2007;160:698–700.
18. Osweiler GD. Mycotoxins. In: Toxicology (The National Veterinary Medical Series). Philadelphia: Williams & Wilkins; 1996. p. 409–36.
19. Osweiler GD. Mycotoxins. Contemporary issues of food animal health and productivity. Vet Clin North Am Food Anim Pract 2000;16:511–30.
20. Smith EE, Phillips TD, Ellis JA, et al. Dietary hydrated sodium calcium aluminosilicate reduction of aflatoxin M1 residue in dairy goat milk and effects on milk production and components. J Anim Sci 1994;72:677–82.

21. Diaz DE, Hagler WM, Blackwelder JT, et al. Aflatoxin binders II: reduction of aflatoxin M1 in milk by sequestering agents of cows consuming aflatoxin in feed. Mycopathologia 2004;157:233–41.
22. Kutz RE, Sampson JD, Pompeu LB, et al. Efficacy of Solis, NovasilPlus and MTB-100 to reduce aflatoxin M1 levels in milk of early to mid lactation dairy cows fed aflatoxin B1. J Dairy Sci 2009;92:3959–63.
23. Evans TJ, Rottinghaus GE, Casteel SW. Ergot. In: Plumlee KH, editor. Clinical veterinary toxicology. St Louis (MO): Mosby; 2004. p. 239–43.
24. Naudé TW, Botha CJ, Vorster JH, et al. *Claviceps cyperi*, a new cause of severe ergotism in dairy cattle consuming maize silage and teff hay contaminated with ergotised *Cyperus esculentus* (nut sedge) on the Highveld of South Africa. Onderstepoort J Vet Res 2005;72:23–37.
25. Evans TJ, Rottinghaus GE, Casteel SW. Fescue. In: Plumlee KH, editor. Clinical veterinary toxicology. St Louis (MO): Mosby; 2004. p. 243–50.
26. Sundstøl Eriksen G, Pettersson H, Lundh T. Comparative cytotoxicity of deoxynivalenol, nivalenol, their acetylated derivatives and de-epoxy metabolites. Feed Chem Toxicol 2004;42:619–24.
27. Mostrom M, Tacke B, Lardy G. Field corn, hail, and mycotoxins. In: Proceedings, North Central Conference of the American Association of Veterinary Laboratory Diagnosticians. Fargo (ND): NDSU Veterinary Diagnostic Laboratory; 2005.
28. Ueno Y. General toxicology. In: Ueno I, editor. Trichothecenes - chemical, biological, and toxicological aspects. New York: Elsevier; 1983. p. 135–46.
29. Anderson VL, Boland EW, Casper HH. Effects of vomitoxin (deoxynivalenol) from scab infested barley on performance of feedlot and breeding cattle. J Anim Sci 1966;74:208.
30. Jouany J-P, Diaz DE. Effects of mycotoxins in ruminants. In: Diaz DE, editor. The mycotoxin blue book. Nottingham (UK): Nottingham University Press; 2005. p. 295–321.
31. Charmley E, Trenholm HL, Thompson BK, et al. Influence of level of deoxynivalenol in the diet of dairy cows on feed intake, milk production, and its composition. J Dairy Sci 1993;76:3580–7.
32. Ingalls JR. Influence of deoxynivalenol on feed consumption by dairy cows. Anim Feed Sci Technol 1996;60:297–300.
33. Prelusky DB, Trenholm HL, Lawrence GA, et al. Nontransmission of deoxynivalenol (vomitoxin) to milk following oral administration to dairy cows. J Environ Sci Health B 1984;19:593–609.
34. Osweiler GD, Hook BS, Mann DD, et al. Effects of T-2 toxin in cattle. Proceedings United States Animal Health Association, 85th Annual Meeting. St Louis (MO): US Animal Health Association; 1981. p 214–31.
35. Hsu IC, Smalley EB, Strong FM, et al. Identification of T-2 toxin in moldy corn associated with a lethal toxicosis in dairy cattle. Appl Microbiol 1972;24:684–90.
36. Dänicke S, Pahlow G, Beyer M, et al. Investigations on the kinetics of the concentration of deoxynivalenol (DON) and on spoilage by moulds and yeasts of wheat grain preserved with sodium metabisulfite (Na2S2O5, SBS) and propionic acid at various moisture contents. Arch Anim Nutr 2010;64:190–203.
37. Osweiler GD, Kehrli ME, Stabel JR, et al. Effects of fumonisin-contaminated corn screenings on growth and health of feeder calves. J Anim Sci 1993;71:459–66.
38. Baker DC, Rottinghaus GE. Chronic experimental fumonisin intoxication of calves. J Vet Diagn Invest 1999;11:289–92.

39. Edrington TS, Kamps-Holtzapple CA, Harvey RB, et al. Acute hepatic and renal toxicity in lambs dosed with fumonisin-containing culture material. J Anim Sci 1995;73:508–15.
40. Diaz DE, Hopkins BA, Leonard LM, et al. Effect of fumonisin on lactating dairy cattle. J Dairy Sci 2000;83:1171 [abstract].
41. Meerdink GL. Citrinin and ochratoxin. In: Plumlee KH, editor. Clinical veterinary toxicology. St Louis (MO): Mosby; 2004. p. 235–9.
42. Lloyd WE, Stahr HM. Ochratoxin toxicosis in cattle. In: 22nd Annual Proceedings, American Association Veterinary Laboratory Diagnosticians. San Diego (CA): AAVLD; 1979. p. 223–38.
43. Fink-Gremmels J. Mycotoxins in forages. In: Diaz DE, editor. The mycotoxin blue book. Nottingham (UK): Nottingham University Press; 2005. p. 249–68.
44. Uhlig S, Botha CJ, Vrålstad T, et al. Indole-diterpenes and ergot alkaloids in *Cynodon dactylon* (Bermuda grass) infected with *Claviceps cynodontis* from an outbreak of tremors in cattle. J Agric Food Chem 2009;57:1112–9.
45. Shlosberg A, Zadikov I, Perl S, et al. *Aspergillus clavatus* as the probable cause of a lethal mass neurotoxicosis in sheep. Mycopathologia 1991;114:35–9.
46. Kellerman TS, Newsholme SJ, Coetzer JA, et al. A tremorgenic mycotoxicosis of cattle caused by maize sprouts infested with *Aspergillus clavatus*. Onderstepoort J Vet Res 1984;51:271–4.
47. McKenzie RA, Kelly MA, Shivas RG, et al. *Aspergillus clavatus* tremorgenic neurotoxicosis in cattle fed sprouted grains. Aust Vet J 2004;82:635–8.
48. Van Der Lugt JJ, Kellerman TS, Van Vollenhoven A, et al. Spinal cord degeneration in adult dairy cows associated with the feeding of sorghum beer residues. J S Afr Vet Assoc 1994;65:184–8.
49. Loretti AP, Colodel EM, Driemeier D, et al. Neurological disorder in dairy cattle associated with consumption of beer residues contaminated with *Aspergillus clavatus*. J Vet Diagn Invest 2003;15:123–32.
50. Sabater-Vilar M, Maas RFM, Bosschere HD, et al. Patulin produced by an *Aspergillus clavatus* isolated from feed containing malting residues associated with a lethal neurotoxicosis in cattle. Mycopathologia 2004;158:419–26.
51. O'Brien M, Nielsen KF, O'Kiely P, et al. Mycotoxins and other secondary metabolites produced *in vitro* by *Penicillium paneum* Frisvad and *Penicillium roqueforti* Thom isolated from baled grass silage in Ireland. J Agric Food Chem 2006;54:9268–76.
52. Sumarah MW, Miller JD, Blackwell BA. Isolation and metabolite production by *Penicillium roqueforti*, *P. paneum* and *P. crustosum* isolated in Canada. Mycopathologia 2005;159:571–7.
53. Scudamor K, Livesey C. Occurrence and significance of mycotoxins in forage crops and silage: a review. J Sci Food Agric 1998;77:1–17.
54. Häggblom P. Isolation of roquefortine C from feed grain. Appl Environ Microbiol 1990;56:2924–6.
55. Tüller G, Armbruster G, Widenmann S, et al. Occurrence of roquefortine in silage – toxicological relevance to sheep. J Anim Physiol Anim Nutr 1998;80:246–9.
56. Dalefield R. Sporidesmin. In: Plumlee KH, editor. Clinical veterinary toxicology. St Louis (MO): Mosby; 2004. p. 264–8.
57. Allen J. Phomopsins. Ergot. In: Plumlee KH, editor. Clinical veterinary toxicology. St Louis (MO): Mosby; 2004. p. 259–62.
58. Kellerman TS, Coetzer JA, Naudé TW, et al. Neurological disorders without notable pathological lesions. In: Kellerman TS, Coetzer JA, Naude TW, et al, editors. Plant

poisonings and mycotoxicoses of livestock in Southern Africa. 2nd edition. Cape Town (South Africa): Oxford University Press Southern Africa; 2005. p. 63–86.
59. Odriozola E, Odeón A, Canton G, et al. *Diplodia maydis*: a cause of death of cattle in Argentina. N Z Vet J 2005;53:160–1.
60. Berthiller F, Schuhmacher R, Adam G, et al. Formation, determination and significance of masked and other conjugated mycotoxins. Anal Bioanal Chem 2009; 395:1243–52.
61. van Egmond HP, Schothorst RC, Jonker MA. Regulations relating to mycotoxins in food. Anal Bioanal Chem 2007;389:147–57.
62. Jacobsen BJ, Coppock RW, Mostrom M. Mycotoxins and Mycotoxicoses. Bozeman (MT): Montana State University Extension; 2007. Pub. EB0174.
63. Blaney BJ, Ryley MJ, Boucher BD. Early harvest and ensilage of forage sorghum infected with ergot (*Claviceps africana*) reduced the risk of livestock poisoning. Aust Vet J 2010;88:311–2.
64. Mostrom MS, Raisbeck. Trichothecenes. In: Gupta R, editor. Veterinary toxicology, basic and clinical principles. New York: Academic Press; 2007. p. 951–76.
65. Hintikka EL. Stachybotryotoxicosis in horses. In: Wyllie TD, Morehouse LG, editors, Mycotoxic fungi, mycotoxins, mycotoxicoses. mycotoxicoses of domestic and laboratory animals, poultry, and aquatic invertebrates and vertebrates, vol. 2. New York: Marcel Dekker; 1978. p. 181–5.
66. Gareis M, Wernery U. Determination of gliotoxin in samples associated with cases of intoxication in camels. Mycotoxin Res 1994;10:2 8.
67. Coppock RW, Mostrom MS, Ferns, et al. Luteoskyrin induced hepatotoxicity in a dairy herd. Toxicologist 1993;13:233 [abstract].
68. Enomoto M, Ueno I. *Penicillium islandicum* (toxic yellowed rice)–luteoskyrin–islanditoxin–cyclorchlorotine. In: Purchase IF, editor. Mycotoxins. New York: Elsevier; 1974. p. 303–25.
69. Vesonder RF, Horn BW. Sterigmatocystin in dairy cattle feed contaminated with *Aspergillus versicolor*. Appl Environ Micro 1985;49:234–5.
70. Tapia MO, Stern MD, Koski RL, et al. Effects of patulin on rumen microbial fermentation in continuous culture fermenters. Anim Feed Sci Technol 2002;97: 239–46.
71. FDA (US Food and Drug Administration). Available at: http://www.fda.gov/downloads/Food/GuidaneComplianceRegulatoryInformation/GuidanceDocuments/NaturalToxins/UCM217558.pdf. Accessed July 7, 2010.
72. Anon. Commission recommendation on the presence of deoxynivalenol, zearalenone, ochratoxin A, T-2 and HT-2 and fumonisins in products intended for animal feeding. 17 August 2006. 2006/576/EC. Official Journal of the European Union 2006;49,Part 229:7–9.
73. CFIA (Canadian Food Inspection Agency), Charmley LL, Trenholm HL. Fact sheet – Mycotoxins. Available at: http://www.inspection.gc.ca/english/anima/feebet/pol/mycoe.shtml. Accessed April 23, 2009.
74. FDA. CPG Sec. 683.100 Action levels for aflatoxins in animal feeds. Available at: http://www.fda.gov/ICECI/ComplianceManuals/CompliancePolicyGuidanceManual/ucm074703.htm. Accessed August 28, 1994.
75. FDA. CPG Sec. 527.400 Whole milk, lowfat milk, skim milk - Aflatoxin M1. Available at: http://www.fda.gov/ICECI/ComplianceManuals/CompliancePolicyGuidanceManual/ucm074482.htm. Accessed November 29, 2005.
76. Anon. Commission regulation (EC) no. 1881/2006 of 19 December 2006 setting maximum levels for certain contaminants in foodstuffs. 01.07.2010. p. 17. Official Journal of the Europen Union L364/5–24.

77. FDA. Available at: http://www.fda.gov/Food/GuidanceComplianceRegulatoryInformation/GuidanceDocuments/ChemicalContaminantsandPesticides/ucm109231.htm. Accessed November 9, 2001.
78. Helferich WG, Garrett WN, Hsieh DP, et al. Feedlot performance and tissue residues of cattle consuming diets containing aflatoxins. J Anim Sci 1986;62:691–6.
79. Fernández A, Hernández H, Verde MT, et al. Effect of aflatoxin on performance, hematology, and clinical immunology in lambs. Can J Vet Res 2000;64:53–8.
80. Fernández A, Ramos JJ, Sanz M, et al. Alterations in the performance, haematology and clinical biochemistry of growing lambs fed with aflatoxin in the diet. J Appl Toxicol 1996;16:85–91.
81. Yiannikouris A, Jouany JP. Mycotoxins in feeds and their fate in animals: a review. Anim Res 2002;51:81–99.
82. Fink-Gremmels J. Mycotoxins in cattle feeds and carry-over to dairy milk: a review. Food Addit Contam 2008;25:172–80.
83. Schumann B, Lebzien P, Uebershär K-H, et al. Effects of the level of feed intake and ergot contaminated concentrate on ergot alkaloid metabolism and carry over into milk. Mol Nutr Food Res 2009;53:931–8.
84. Kreese C, Meyer U, Valenta H, et al. No carry over of unmetabolised deoxynivalenol in milk of dairy cows fed high concentrate proportions. Mol Nutr Food Res 2008;52:1514–29.
85. Boudra H, Barouin J, Dragacci S, et al. Aflatoxin M1 and ochratoxin A in raw bulk milk from French dairy herds. J Dairy Sci 2007;90:3197–201.
86. Yoshizawa T, Mirocha CJ, Swanson SP. Metabolic fate of T-2 toxin in a lactating cow. Food Cosmet Toxicol 1981;19:31–9.

Diminished Reproductive Performance and Selected Toxicants in Forages and Grains

Tim J. Evans, DVM, MS, PhD

KEYWORDS

- Toxicants • Reproductive performance
- Enzootic toxic stressors

Reproduction is a critical biologic process in all living systems and is required for species survival.[1] Reproduction is also essential for the production of such important agricultural commodities as milk and meat for human and companion animal consumption. Several other articles of this book cover in great detail the potential adverse reproductive effects of several phytotoxins and mycotoxins. This article takes a novel, integrated approach to discuss the possible roles of reproductive toxicants, especially those associated with common forages and grains, in diminished reproductive performance in ruminant species. Toxicants are discussed not only as the potential primary causes of observed reproductive abnormalities but also in the context of contributing to the adverse effects of other factors that can affect ruminant reproduction. Although impaired reproductive function can have a single, diagnosable, toxic cause, the causes of diminished reproductive efficiency in ruminants can be difficult to distinguish and may be multifactorial, involving various predisposing factors and/or stressors, including toxicants.

PRECAUTIONARY NOTE

This article's treatment of multifactorial causes of negative reproductive outcomes should not be misconstrued as an attempt to indict trace amounts of some potential toxicants, particularly mycotoxins, or subtle alterations in micronutrient content, for playing major roles in observed reproductive problems in ruminants. Rather, on the contrary, this approach to investigating subfertility is a holistic (ie, looking at the whole) effort to understand how negative reproductive outcomes might occur in ruminants when there is no smoking gun or obvious

---

Veterinary Medical Diagnostic Laboratory, Department of Veterinary Pathobiology, College of Veterinary Medicine, University of Missouri, 1600 East Rollins Street, Columbia, MO 65211, USA
E-mail address: evanst@missouri.edu

Vet Clin Food Anim 27 (2011) 345–371
doi:10.1016/j.cvfa.2011.03.001 vetfood.theclinics.com

single cause. When no clear, single cause of diminished reproductive performance is evident, it is important to take an integrated approach and objectively evaluate the relative contributions of a wide variety of variables to the reproductive problems that are apparent. Multiple predisposing factors and stressors, including toxicants, plus possible contributions of interactions involving these variables and management, can all have adverse effects on fertility. This is the whole, which should be considered when attempting to explain and remediate herd reductions in reproductive efficiency.

The predisposing factors and stressors discussed in this article are enzootic in nature because they are common under normal ruminant husbandry conditions. The adverse effects of these predispositions and stressors, which negatively affect animal production systems, can generally be prevented or greatly ameliorated with sound management practices. However, conversely, suboptimal management can have the opposite effect and exacerbate the adverse reproductive effects of these ubiquitous predisposing and stress-related factors. This article discusses potential reproductive problems, related to the ingestion of various toxic compounds found in forages or grain crops of agronomic importance. The emphasis of these discussions is on possible adverse reproductive effects associated with toxicants in common pasture grasses and legumes (eg, fescue, bromes, clovers) frequently grazed by ruminants, as well as grains routinely used in ruminant rations, such as corn, oats, barley, wheat, and triticale. These potential reproductive toxicants, especially nitrate, ergot alkaloids, and xenoestrogens, can all play primary or important contributory roles in various types of diminished reproductive efficiency in ruminant species. The recognition and, most importantly, the prevention of the adverse effects of these enzootic toxic stressors are essential for optimal ruminant reproductive performance.

REPRODUCTION

Before going into greater detail about variables that can adversely affect reproductive function in ruminants, it is appropriate to briefly review normal reproduction. Reproduction is a critical biologic process, which is required for species but not individual animal survival.[1] Reproduction is also essential for the production of such important agricultural commodities as milk and meat consumed by humans and their pets. The success or failure of a producer is often determined by the ability of their livestock to reproduce in an efficient manner. Reproduction in ruminants, as in most other mammalian species, encompasses the wide range of physiologic processes and the associated behaviors and anatomic structures necessary for the birth of the next generation of a given species.[2] As shown in **Fig. 1**, reproduction is a dynamic continuum of physiologic processes involving precise coordination and integration of the functions of multiple organs, within both male and female animals, as well as the conceptus.[1,2] The efficient production of viable and functional gametes and their transport and union to form a zygote that develops into a healthy and fertile individual require that stringent physiologic and metabolic needs be met.[1] A thorough understanding of normal reproductive processes is essential to recognize, treat, and/or prevent abnormal reproductive function, as well as subtle changes in reproductive efficiency in domestic ruminants.[1,2] Although most readers have a more than adequate understanding of normal reproductive physiology and anatomy to appreciate the major take-home points of this article, some individuals might need or seek additional background information. Although further, detailed discussion of reproductive

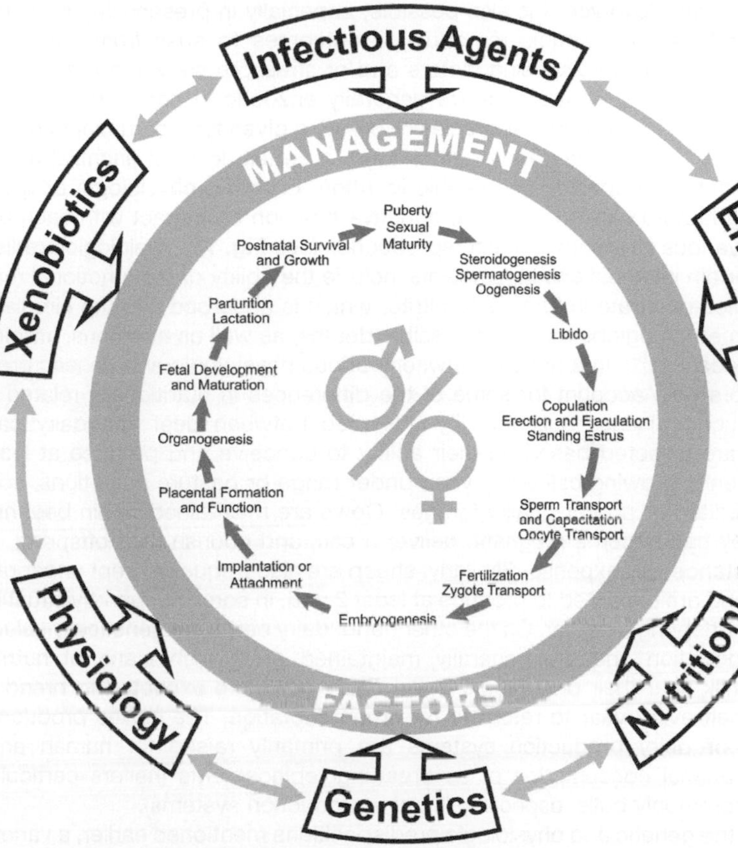

Fig. 1. The continuum of developmental stages and reproductive functions taking place in males and/or females, as well as the embryo and fetus, illustrates the complexity of reproduction in ruminant species. The possible influences of genetic and physiologic predispositions, as well as nutritional, environmental, infectious, and, especially, toxic stressors on decreased reproductive performance are also shown, along with the role management can play in modulating those influences on reproductive function. (*Adapted from* Evans TJ. Reproductive toxicity and endocrine disruption. In: Gupta RC, editor. Reproductive and developmental toxicology. New York: Academic Press/Elsevier Inc; 2011. p. 8; with permission; *modifications and artwork courtesy of* Don Connor and Howard Wilson.)

physiology and anatomy is beyond the scope of this article, there are several publications that provide a comprehensive overview of animal reproduction.[1–5]

NEGATIVE REPRODUCTIVE OUTCOMES AND ENZOOTIC PREDISPOSITIONS AND STRESSORS

Delayed puberty, estrous cycle abnormalities, conception failure, embryonic death, teratogenesis, abortions, stillbirths, and diminished lactation leading to suboptimal postnatal growth and development are all negative reproductive outcomes that can have devastating effects on livestock production and the livelihood of producers.[1] Each of these abnormalities can be associated with the adverse reproductive effects of a single cause. However, it is also possible, especially in present-day production systems, for these undesirable reproductive outcomes to arise from interactions between the multiple predisposing factors and/or stressors shown in **Fig. 1**. These predisposing factors and stressors are generally enzootic in nature because they are inherent to a particular animal species or breed, a given type of ruminant production system (eg, dairy, meat, and/or wool/fiber), a certain level of financial or labor investment, and/or a specific geographic location. Enzootic physiologic or genetic predisposing factors can influence reproductive function or interact with each other and/or with various stressors to affect reproduction (see **Fig. 1**). Physiologic predispositions to certain intoxications in ruminants include the ability of the functional rumen to convert dietary nitrate in forages to nitrite, which is absorbed into the circulation, resulting in methemoglobinemia and possible deaths, as well as abortions, stillbirths, and/or weak calves.[6–8] Interactions between various physiologic and genetic predisposing factors help account for some of the differences in nutritionally related and toxicant-induced disease susceptibility observed between beef and dairy cattle. Beef cattle are selected based on their ability to conceive and produce at least 1 viable, efficiently growing calf every year, under range or pasture conditions, sometimes with limited or poorer-quality forages. Cows are maintained within beef herds because they can become pregnant, deliver a calf, and nourish their offspring, with limited assistance and expense. Similarly, sheep are also frequently kept under range conditions and are expected to produce at least 2 and, in some husbandry situations, more than 2 offspring per year. On the other hand, dairy cattle are genetically selected for milk production and are generally maintained on a high plane of nutrition, producing milk near their physiologic limits. Dairy cows are expected to breed and produce a calf every year to return to maximum lactation. The calves produced in either beef or dairy production systems are primarily raised for human and/or companion animal consumption or as breeding replacements (heifers particularly; much less commonly bulls, especially in dairy production systems).

Similar to the genetic and physiologic predispositions mentioned earlier, a variety of nutritional, environmental, infectious, and/or toxic stressors can also, either alone or through multifactorial interactions, influence reproductive performance. Inadequate nutrition can delay puberty, cause irregular estrous cycles, and/or adversely affect pregnancy rates.[2–5] Nutritional deficiencies can also impair immune function, making animals more susceptible to infections which can affect reproduction. Suboptimal environmental conditions (eg, weather factors, geographic location, topography, adequacy and hygiene of facilities) can affect reproductive function in multiple ways, such as by limiting estrus detection by male animals or by exacerbating the heat stress-related adverse effects of fescue toxicosis and ergotism.[4,5,8–10] There are many examples of how various infectious agents (ie, viruses, bacteria, protozoa, fungi, and internal and external parasites) can negatively affect ruminant reproduction.[4,5] These infectious agents, some of which can cause endometritis and early return to estrus, teratogenesis, and birth defects or, even, abortions, can be associated with isolated cases of impaired reproduction or widespread herd outbreaks of contagious reproductive disease. Conditions that affect some animals and not others might be addressed by simple changes in management practices or individual animal treatment. Conversely, infectious diseases that can be spread rapidly from animal to animal might require herd/flock prophylaxis and/or long-term disease management strategies to boost immunity and prevent disease transmission.

Various enzootic forage-related or grain-related toxicants also have the potential to diminish reproductive performance.[4,5] Xenobiotics, meaning any chemicals foreign to the body (ie, drugs or toxicants), particularly those that are associated with forages and grains common within a given climate, can have deleterious effects on reproductive efficiency, either by acting alone or by interacting with other predisposing factors and stressors to contribute to multifactorial causes of impaired reproductive function (see **Fig. 1**). The relative role of these enzootic toxicants in decreased reproductive efficiency is often determined, in large part, by the size of the dose. Exposure to a high dose of a given xenobiotic suggests that the xenobiotic might represent the potential primary cause of the observed adverse reproductive effect. On the contrary, an exposure involving a lesser but still potentially relevant dose of the xenobiotic, which is outside the normal background levels of exposure for that chemical, suggests that that specific xenobiotic played a contributory role in the negative reproductive outcome.

THE IMPORTANCE OF MANAGEMENT FACTORS TO OPTIMAL REPRODUCTIVE EFFICIENCY

In addition to the multiple steps involved in successful mammalian reproduction and the various factors that can adversely affect ruminant reproductive function, **Fig. 1** also shows how management constitutes an important interface between enzootic predisposing factors and/or stressors and the ultimate goal of optimal reproductive performance. Management can maximize reproductive efficiency or, conversely, augment the adverse reproductive effects of the predisposing factors and stressors inherent to a given situation. Management factors can determine whether reproductive performance and/or specific production outcomes (ie, milk, offspring for breeding or meat, and/or wool or fiber) are optimized and profitable or, just the opposite, suboptimal and financially draining on a production system. As management systems become more intensive, the level of skill required for success increases, and the room for error or shortcuts decreases proportionately. Management systems can amplify the adverse effects of some enzootic stressors if there is less than adequate attention to important details or insufficient resources available to sustain an optimal level of production. Artificial insemination (AI) of cryopreserved semen and timed-AI ovulation synchronization protocols involve low numbers of sperm already stressed by cryopreservation methods and packaged into a single insemination dose. In this instance, the thresholds for tolerable errors on the part of the technician and the potentially harmful effects of enzootic stressors, which can have a negative effect on reproductive efficiency, have been lowered. Likewise, economic pressures and/or adverse weather conditions could force managers of intensive production systems to use less than optimal feedstuffs, although still demanding the same high levels of production to maintain financial stability.

Some of the management factors that have the greatest influence on reproductive performance in livestock (the first 5 of which are critical determinants of the others) are as follows:

1. Size/type of production system, including animal species/breed and products marketed
2. Knowledge of ruminant husbandry, health care, and reproductive management
3. Understanding of the causes of suboptimal reproductive performance in ruminants
4. Expectations for levels of reproductive performance and livestock production
5. Capital available for investment and financial solvency of principal parties
6. Quality of nutrition relative to physiologic demands
7. Animal supervision/labor intensity and skill level
8. Structure and hygiene of facilities

9. Veterinary involvement in health and reproductive management
10. Prebreeding examinations of males, including semen evaluations
11. Adequate male/female ratios and heat detection during breeding season
12. Appropriately timed breeding/insemination
13. Estrus/ovulation synchronization protocols suitable for production system
14. Pregnancy examinations of females
15. Prophylactic measures for common infectious agents/contagious diseases/parasites
16. Records pertaining to individual animal health and reproductive activity/function
17. Surveillance of herd reproductive performance and production outcomes.

There is a tendency to think that bigger and more modern always equates to improved reproductive function and greater profitability. Intensive livestock production systems and state-of-the-art facilities allow for higher levels of production and future expansion in response to market demands. These types of production systems and facilities can incorporate emerging technologies and new marketing strategies and, therefore, have the potential to be extremely productive and profitable. However, there is no substitute in animal agriculture for adequate nutrition, appropriately skilled employees, and suitable health and reproductive management.

Within reason and practicality, it can be argued that the reproductive efficiency and ultimate financial stability or success of ruminant production systems is not so dependent on the specific levels of management factors 6 to 17 as on whether those levels are appropriate for management factors 1 to 5. The levels of knowledge and practical husbandry skills, investment capabilities, and the expectations of management must be adequate for and consistent with the specific animal production system involved. Depending on market demands livestock-based commodities, complex systems for producing animal-related commodities, such as might be observed in modern, large, high-producing dairy herds using timed-AI and ovulation synchronization programs, likely require a higher level of management and greater financial outlay to initially have as healthy and productive animals and the same level of profitability, as a similarly sized, established cow-calf operation, using natural mating systems. Experienced and informed management of livestock production systems can facilitate reproductive efficiency and financial success without a lot of "bells and whistles," as long as there is suitable hygiene, nutrition, health care, and reproductive management, all of which need to take into account enzootic predisposing factors and stressors, including toxicants, and the limitations for expansion of such a system. Likewise, financial hardship and poor reproductive performance are all but guaranteed when novice livestock producers, with a large capital investment and high reproductive performance and production expectations, attempt to develop an intensive livestock production system without skilled labor, a basic knowledge of animal husbandry, an understanding of ruminant reproductive management, and an awareness of the enzootic factors, including toxic xenobiotics, that can impair reproductive function.

BASIC PATHOPHYSIOLOGY OF NEGATIVE REPRODUCTIVE OUTCOMES IN RUMINANTS

Delayed puberty and estrous cycle abnormalities, conception failure, embryonic death, teratogenesis, abortions and stillbirths, and agalactia are all negative reproductive outcomes that can have devastating effects on ruminant production systems.[1,3–5] The pathophysiology of these negative reproductive outcomes can be simple (ie, poor estrus detection preventing copulation and the appearance of conception failure) or complex (ie, fetal stress initiating the endocrine cascade leading to abortion).

An attempt to understand the basic "how?" of these abnormal reproductive events can be extremely useful in improving reproductive management and, ultimately, reproductive performance within a herd.

Although reproduction is essential for the survival of ruminant species, it is not necessary for individual animal survival, other than preventing a particular animal from being culled. Stress, implying excessive stimulation of the hypothalamic-pituitary-adrenal (HPA) axis and the release of large amounts endogenous glucocorticoid (ie, cortisol in sheep, goats, and cattle) can adversely affect several reproductive processes. The amplitude of the pulsatile release of luteinizing hormone (LH) can be greatly reduced by glucocorticoids. If prolonged, this effect has the potential to affect the release of gonadal steroids (ie, estrogens and androgens) in sexually mature animals. In addition, maturation of the fetal HPA axis and the appropriately timed release of cortisol by the fetus initiate the cascade of events leading to parturition, under normal, physiologic circumstances.[1,2] However, maternal or fetal stress occurring at a susceptible stage of pregnancy can lead to premature parturition.[1] Nutrition and body condition also play important roles in regulating reproductive function. Puberty, characterized by normal estrous cycles in females and spermatogenesis in males, generally takes place at some time point within a species-specific range of ages but is dependent on adequate nutrition and body condition.[2] Likewise, normal estrous cycles also require that females be adequately fed and have sufficient energy stores.[4,5] Poor body condition, which can be associated with greater energy output than input, nutritional deficiencies, parasitism, or, even, viral or bacterial disease, which is most likely associated with a stress component, can interfere with reproductive cyclicity and diminish pregnancy rates. Sexual reproduction requires copulation at the appropriate time and the union of a normal ovum of female origin with a functionally mature sperm cell produced by the male. In natural breeding situations, male animals must be able to detect sexually receptive females in estrus and successfully introduce adequate numbers of spermatozoa into the female reproductive tract, generally before ovulation. These accomplishments, on the part of the male, are necessary to ensure that enough, normal, motile sperm cells are transported to the female's uterine tubes in order for 1 healthy spermatozoa to be available and able to fertilize each viable ovum, which is transported to the site of fertilization. Standing estrus in females, estrus detection by the male, and copulation not only require adequate nutritional status and energy but also sensory and physical access and structural soundness on the parts of both the male and female. Circumstances that interfere with these processes (eg, rough terrain, high environmental temperatures, competition with other, less fertile bulls, lame females, or males that cannot engage in coitus) can result in what appears as a failure of conception. Impaired sperm transport within the female reproductive tract, which has been associated with exposure to xenoestrogens in sheep, or other factors that interfere with sperm capacitation or movement of the ovum within the uterine tubes can also prevent conception and decrease pregnancy rates.[1,11]

Many of the same nutritional, environmental, and toxic stressors that can adversely affect pregnancy rates can also impair embryonic development. Inadequate nutrition and high environmental temperatures, especially in conjunction with exposure to ergot alkaloids, can negatively affect oocyte and sperm quality, thereby interfering with conception, as well as normal embryonic development. Recent studies have suggested that exposure of females or, even, males to ergot alkaloids of tall fescue endophyte or ergot origin can also affect embryo quality and subsequent development.[9,10,12,13] Likewise, cow comfort issues can also adversely affect reproductive function. Teratogenesis can be characterized by embryonic or fetal mortality, structural or functional abnormalities, and/or alterations in birth weight, with the phenotypic effects being dependent on genetic predispositions and critically timed exposures to teratogens at specific stages of development.[1]

A special mention should be made of the inadvertent, potential contributory role of more intensive reproductive management protocols to the pathophysiology of diminished reproductive performance. Appropriately supervised and executed use of cryopreserved semen, timed AI, and/or ovulation synchronization protocols, as well as other assisted reproductive techniques, can be successful under certain management conditions. Effective ovulation synchronization can eliminate the need for heat detection, which is a limiting factor in many ruminant production systems, especially those involving dairy cattle. However, as mentioned earlier, the negative effect of enzootic predispositions and/or stressors can be amplified in reproductive management situations, in which the immense surplus of spermatozoa in the male ejaculate is removed and sperm numbers are reduced to an insemination dose or in which ovarian function is completely dependent on appropriate responses to pharmacologic manipulations.

THE ADVERSE REPRODUCTIVE EFFECTS OF PHYTOTOXINS AND MYCOTOXINS IN RUMINANTS

Although the primary and integrated, contributory adverse effects of specific forage-related and grain-related reproductive toxicants are reviewed in greater detail later, it is appropriate to make note of the negative impacts of other phytotoxins and mycotoxins, which are discussed elsewhere in this issue: plant toxins, particularly those in the western United States, that cause adverse reproductive effects in ruminants, including teratogens and abortifacients, are carefully reviewed in the article by Panter and Stegelmeier (however, although many of the plants discussed in that article are enzootic in various geographic locations, especially the western states, they are typically plant species that, although having some nutritional value, are primarily eaten when other, safer pasture forages are unavailable or less prevalent); other plant toxins without primary reproductive effects that are enzootic to the northeastern and southern United States are reviewed in the articles by Bischoff and Nicholson; the nonreproductive effects of selected mycotoxins are reviewed in the article by Mostrom.

However, regardless of primary toxic effects of a given phytotoxin or mycotoxin, whether they are reproductive or nonreproductive in nature, xenobiotics, either alone or in conjunction with nutritional, environmental, or infectious stressors, can cause acute or chronic stress conditions associated with glucocorticoid release, which can be detrimental to ruminant reproductive performance. Excessive stimulation of the maternal and/or fetal HPA, resulting in dramatic increases in glucocorticoid secretion related to acute maternal and/or fetal stress, can initiate the cascade of endocrine events that leads to premature parturition, as shown by abortion, stillbirth, or neonatal weakness and death. This situation is especially true in systemic intoxications interpreted as life threatening by homeostatic mechanisms within the dam and/or fetus. Maternal and/or fetal hypoxia is a particularly strong, stressful stimulus for the release of glucocorticoid hormones, such as cortisol. High maternal dietary concentrations of nitrate, as well as toxic xenobiotics associated with pulmonary disease, or cardiotoxins (eg, cardiac glycosides, grayanotoxins, and taxine alkaloids) can result in inappropriately timed parturition. Although the observance of clinical disease or death of the dam or other animals is expected in most of the aforementioned circumstances, there are clinical situations, especially in the case of dietary nitrate, in which maternal illness or clinical signs in herd mates might not be evident without forced activity or careful examination.

Toxicants, especially mycotoxins, as well as interactions involving various predisposing factors, other stressors, such as nutritional deficiencies, parasitism, or even viral or bacterial disease, can cause chronic stress, resulting in diminished reproductive performance of both male and female animals. Cow discomfort related to ergot alkaloid-associated hyperthermia or lameness can adversely affect herd reproductive efficiency. Similarly, aflatoxin-induced, impaired hepatic function or decreased immunity associated with exposure to several common mycotoxins can interfere with an animal's optimal reproductive function. However, the adverse reproductive effects of these toxins should be considered secondary to their primary effects (ie, impaired hepatic function in the case of aflatoxins). The level of exposure to mycotoxins is still critical in these instances. Based on current, evidence-based knowledge, dietary exposures to aflatoxins associated with minimal violative residues in milk and, especially, those aflatoxin concentrations in which no violative residues of aflatoxin M_1 are anticipated in milk, should not be expected, under normal husbandry and management conditions, to adversely affect ruminant reproductive function.[13] Although it might not be possible or practical to eliminate all measurable mycotoxins from livestock feeds, especially under certain agronomic conditions, there is not a nutritional requirement for mycotoxins, including aflatoxins and vomitoxin (deoxynivalenol [DON]), in ruminant rations. It is probably not advisable to consider ruminants intended for breeding purposes as the ultimate destination for forages and/or grains deemed unsatisfactory for consumption by other livestock species or humans. First, any observed, negative reproductive outcomes are most likely incorrectly or disproportionately blamed on the lesser-quality, contaminated feedstuffs. Second, breeding animals or those animals eventually intended for breeding, especially those currently producing at their physiologic limits (eg, lactating dairy cows) or those females that are already in the later stages of pregnancy, require higher levels of nutrition. Feedstuffs containing mycotoxins, depending on the measured concentrations of the contaminants and the results of nutritional analyses, might not be unsatisfactory for ruminant consumption because of their mycotoxin content but, rather, because of their nutritional inferiority. Studies involving the inclusion of binders in rations with low mycotoxin concentrations sometimes seem to minimize this possibility and attribute most of the observed adverse outcomes directly to the toxic effects of mycotoxins. This experimental approach, although helpful in showing value of secondary fungal metabolites as biomarkers for lesser-quality feeds, tends to discount the contributions of enzootic predisposing factors and nonxenobiotic stressors, as well as the role of management, when reproductive performance and production outcomes are less than anticipated. Several books, National Research Council publications, and government Web sites discuss some of the nutritional aspects of ruminant reproduction (some with references to mycotoxin contamination) and are worthy of review.[4,5,14–18] Taking into consideration the measured concentrations of mycotoxins detected (particularly if more than one is found) and the nutritional quality of selected feedstuffs, it is advisable to keep dietary mycotoxin concentrations as low as is practical, given the specific type of production system and market factors, as well as crop growth, harvest, and storage conditions. It is especially critical to keep mycotoxin concentrations less than regulatory action levels and/or recommendations for a given species and stage of production. A reasonable management approach to possible mycotoxin contamination in rations fed to potential and current breeding animals (ie, both males and females) includes (1) producer education by careful review of the current, producer-oriented literature and consultations with veterinarians, extension specialists, toxicologists, and nutritionists; (2) when indicated by growth, harvest, storage conditions, feed appearance, and/or diminished reproductive performance, analyses for concentrations of relevant mycotoxins and evaluation of the nutritional quality of representative samples of feedstuffs incorporated in the diet; (3) consideration of other predisposing factors and stressors pertinent to a particular type of production system and geographic location; and (4) to compensate for differences in individual animal susceptibility, sampling techniques, or potential mycotoxin hot spots, a target concentration for a specific mycotoxin, at least no more than approximately half of what is the current action or guidance level for the dietary concentration of that particular mycotoxin for a certain species and type of production (ie, calculated out to 50 ppb of aflatoxin for breeding cattle; 10 ppb of aflatoxin for dairy animals; 7.5 ppm of fumonisins for breeding ruminants; 2.5 ppm of fumonisins for dairy animals; 2 ppm of vomitoxin for breeding cattle; and 1 ppm of vomitoxin for dairy cattle and other ruminants intended for breeding).[19] If multiple mycotoxins are present in contaminated feedstuffs, the possibility of additive, adverse effects should be taken into consideration.

SPECIFIC FORAGE-RELATED AND GRAIN-RELATED REPRODUCTIVE TOXICANTS

Common forages, including grasses and legumes, and typical grain crops used in ruminant rations can contain concentrations of xenobiotics, which can adversely affect reproductive performance in ruminants. These enzootic xenobiotics can be the major cause of impaired reproductive function, or, as mentioned earlier, they can often be an integral part of multifactorial causes of diminished reproductive efficiency (see **Fig. 1**). Of greatest interest are the potential adverse reproductive effects of nitrate, ergot alkaloids (particularly ergopeptine alkaloids), and xenoestrogens (ie phytoestrogens and zearalenone), at least one of which is present in the forages and grains listed in **Table 1**. Each of these xenobiotics is reviewed individually, concentrating on sources, mechanisms of action, adverse reproductive effects, interactions with predisposing factors and other stressors, diagnosis, and management.

NITRATE

Sources

Ruminants and, in particular, cattle are commonly at increased risk, especially under adverse weather conditions, for excessive consumption of nitrate-accumulating forages. Ingestion of large amounts of these forages can predispose these animals to illness and even death, as well as diminished reproductive performance. Nitrate in the soil are assimilated into plants and undergo reduction in the process of nitrogen being incorporated into plant proteins and other nitrogen-containing compounds.[6] Nitrate reductase activity is highest in the leaves, where photosynthesis takes place, so that nitrate concentrations are lowest in the leaves and seeds or grains and highest in the roots and lower portions of the stems or stalks, which are in closer proximity to the soil.[6,8] Decreased photosynthesis-dependent nitrate-reductase activity in several agronomically important grains, grasses, and/or legumes (see **Table 1**) commonly results in nitrate accumulation within the roots, stems, and/or stalks of these plants.[6–8] Various other plant genera, including pigweed (*Amaranthus* spp), lambsquarters (*Chenopodium* spp), fireweed (*Kochia* spp), nightshades (*Solanum* spp), and docks (*Rumex* spp) are also prone to sufficiently decreased nitrate-reductase activity to have the potential to accumulate excessive concentrations of nitrate.[6,8] Nitrate reductase activity decreases in response to several plant-related and environment-related stress factors, such as herbicide application, drought, frost, and hail.[6] Being water soluble, plant nitrates in rain-soaked stacked hay bales can leach into the bales below, resulting in nitrate concentrations that are higher than those present in the uppermost bales. These lower hay bales are typically the last ones to be fed. The ingestion of these nitrate-concentrated bales frequently occurs during the winter, when

Table 1
Toxicants commonly associated with agronomically important crops and forages[a]

Plant Name	Ergot Alkaloids (Ergopeptine Alkaloids)	Excessive Nitrates	Xenoestrogens
Oats and wild oats *Avena* spp	**Yes**[b] Ergot	**Yes**	Yes Zearalenone
Brome grasses *Bromus* spp	Yes Ergot	No	No
Orchard grasses *Dactylis* spp	Yes Ergot	No	No
Wild ryes *Elymus* spp	Yes Ergot	No	No
Soybeans *Glycine max*	No	Yes	Yes Isoflavones
Barley *Hordeum* spp	**Yes** Ergot	Yes	Yes Zearalenone
Tall fescue *Lolium arundinaceum*	**Yes** Endophyte and ergot	Yes	No
Rye grasses Other *Lolium* spp	**Yes** Endophyte and ergot	No	No
Alfalfa *Medicago sativa*	No	Yes	**Yes** Coumestans
Pearl millet *Pennisum typhoides*	No	**Yes**	No
Timothy grasses *Phleum* spp	Yes Ergot	No	No
Rye *Secale cereale*	**Yes** Ergot	Yes	No
Johnson grass *Sorghum halepense*	No	**Yes**	No
Sorghum sudan *Sorghum vulgare*	No	**Yes**	No
Clovers[c] *Trifolium* spp	No	No	**Yes** Primarily isoflavones
Wheat *Triticum aestivum*	**Yes** Ergot	Yes	**Yes** Zearalenone
Corn *Zea mays*	No	**Yes**	**Yes** Zearalenone

[a] Although many of the small grains, grasses, and legumes listed can occasionally accumulate nitrate or be infected by *Fusarium* molds under specific circumstances, the "No" for a given toxicant means that a toxicant is associated with that plant species only sporadically, if at all.
[b] A "Yes" in bold font indicates that a particular plant species has commonly been associated with clinical cases of a given intoxication.
[c] Other clovers can be involved, but *Trifolium subterraneum* and *pratense* (ie, subterranean and red clover) are the species of clover most often associated with xenoestrogenic exposures.

late-gestational cattle are likely to tank up on such forages, especially just before the onset of inclement weather.

Mechanisms of Action

Dietary nitrate is not particularly toxic to livestock. Nitrate is usually converted primarily into nitrite and, then, into ammonia (ammonium ion under slightly acidic conditions) by microbial organisms within the reticulorumen. The nitrogen from the ammonium cation is eventually incorporated into microbial protein and other nitrogenous compounds. When excessive dietary nitrates are available to ruminants, microbes in the reticulorumen rapidly convert nitrate into nitrite, which is slowly metabolized to ammonia.[6] Both nitrates and nitrites, when present in concentrations that exceed microbial metabolic reduction capabilities, can be rapidly absorbed into the systemic circulation. Nitrite facilitates the oxidation of the ferrous iron in heme molecules of hemoglobin to the ferric state (ie, methemoglobin), which cannot combine with oxygen and transport it to the brain and/or peripheral tissues.[6–8] Nitrates and nitrites are also vasoactive compounds and can cause vasodilation and hypotension.[6] Methemoglobinemia, with or without hypotension, can lead to anxiety, hypoxia, dyspnea, exercise intolerance, and possibly death in affected animals, as well as fetal stress and subsequent abortions, stillbirths, and/or delivery of weak neonates.[1,6–8]

Adverse Reproductive Effects

Experimental results indicate that nitrite can easily cross the placenta and induce methemoglobinemia in fetal erythrocytes.[6] Abortions, stillbirths, and/or weak neonates, which might not be able to stand and suckle, are the major negative reproductive outcomes generally associated with nitrate/nitrite intoxication in pregnant cattle and occur 3 to 7 days or later after toxic maternal exposures.[6–8] In 1 survey of the possible causes of bovine abortion, nitrate/nitrite-induced abortions accounted for approximately 5% of the confirmed causes (approximately 29% of the total observed abortions).[20] In addition, hypoxic and/or hypotensive animals are certainly stressed and should not be expected to perform optimally with regards to reproductive function. In 1 study, prolonged exposure of bulls to nonlethal doses of potassium nitrate resulted in methemoglobinemia, increased plasma cortisol concentrations, impaired hepatic steroid metabolism, and a greater percentage of sperm abnormalities, in addition to degenerative changes within the testes.[21] Similarly, decreased pregnancy rates, defective embryos, and an increased incidence of congenital defects have been reported in several animal species after exposure of bred animals to excessive dietary nitrate.[22]

Interactions with Predisposing Factors and Other Stressors

There continues to be considerable debate about whether excessive dietary nitrate can induce premature parturition in the absence of maternal, nitrate-related/nitrite-related disease in ruminants. In instances in which there is controversy regarding the adverse effects of a particular toxicant, it is likely that interactions involving predispositions and other stressors might contribute to the occurrence of certain xenobiotic-induced negative reproductive outcomes. There are several fetus-related, predisposing factors that suggest that clinically obvious maternal disease is not a prerequisite for nitrate-induced/nitrite-induced fetal disease. Fetal bovine hemoglobin is susceptible to conversion to methemoglobinemia by nitrite. The elimination half-life of nitrate in the bovine fetus is longer than that in adult cattle (24 hours vs 9 hours), and the fetus is sensitive to hypoxic conditions, particularly in the later stages of gestation. In addition, maternal methemoglobinemia can be difficult to recognize if animals are not being handled on a regular basis. It is therefore not surprising if the pathophysiologic requirements for induction of premature parturition associated with fetal stress can be met and the fetus aborted, under circumstances in which subclinical maternal methemoglobinemia is present but not necessarily recognized.[6] Conversely, there is experimental evidence in support of the belief that nitrate-induced/nitrite-induced parturition is not common, unless the dam is clinically ill and her life is at serious risk. Experimental administration of nitrite to pregnant cattle, which consistently resulted in diagnosed maternal methemoglobinemia (methemoglobin does not cross the placenta), did not induce premature parturition in the treated cattle. These seemingly contradictory results have been interpreted by some as evidence that nitrate-associated/nitrite-associated abortions are overdiagnosed and are a rare occurrence in cattle. On the other hand, it seems just as likely that other dam-related and/or fetus-related predisposing factors or stressors, not accounted for in an experimental setting, could play a role in exacerbating nitrate-associated/nitrite-associated maternal and/or fetal stress under certain conditions, thereby precipitating the cascade of events leading to premature parturition.[6,22]

Rumen metabolism, variations in microbial populations, and rapid feed intake, especially by aggressive and/or dominant individuals, can all predispose cattle to nitrate/nitrite intoxication. Inclement weather leading to tanking up on available feedstuffs, low-concentrate diets, rapid introduction to and ingestion of forages with high stem/leaf ratios and/or specific types of grasses, grains, and/or legumes (see **Table 1**), as well as other nitrate-accumulating plants, are environmental and nutritional stressors that commonly contribute to the incidence of nitrate/nitrite intoxication.[6–8] Similarly, nitrate fertilizers and nitrate-contaminated, nitrite-contaminated, or *N*-nitroso-contaminated water, as well as chlorate herbicides, represent other well-known, additional sources of dietary nitrate or other compounds that can cause the formation of methemoglobinemia.

In contrast to some of the predispositions and stressors mentioned earlier, which are frequently discussed in conjunction with nitrate/nitrite intoxication, there are several nutritional, infectious, and toxic stressors that also deserve discussion, with respect to their possible contributory roles in nitrate-associated/nitrite-associated adverse reproductive effects. Any nutritional deficiency, infectious agent, or toxicant that can induce anemia or limit the delivery of oxygen to the brain and peripheral tissues has the potential to lower the threshold of dietary nitrate necessary to induce methemoglobinemia and impair reproductive function or even cause adult mortality. Copper deficiency (possibly associated with ingestion of endophyte-infected fescue), infection by *Anaplasma marginale* or other parasitic organisms, and ingestion of some species of *Allium* (ie, onion-related plants), *Brassica* (ie, mustards and similar plants), or *Pteridium aquilinum* (ie, bracken fern) are examples of potential causes of acute and/or chronic anemia in cattle. Bacterial pneumonia and other diseases of the respiratory tract (eg, acute bovine pulmonary edema and emphysema or atypical interstitial pneumonia), sublethal exposures to carbon monoxide, plants containing 3-nitro-containing or sublethal concentrations of cyanogenic glycosides, as well as other cardiac or pulmonary toxicants, can all impede maximum tissue oxygen delivery and/or uptake.

Diagnosis and Management

The usual way to determine whether an abortion, stillbirth, or unthrifty neonate might be associated with nitrate/nitrite intoxication is a full postmortem examination, including appropriate samples collected and examined for histopathologic changes, bacterial growth, the presence of abortifacient protozoa or viruses, and, specifically, for nitrate/nitrite exposure, the concentration of nitrate (longer half-life than nitrite) in the aqueous humor (some laboratories suggest amniotic fluid or fetal stomach contents as alternatives).[6,7] Some laboratories use the diphenylamine colorimetric method to measure nitrates in ocular fluid, but this method is prone to false-positive results. Laboratories frequently differ in what is considered an increased fetal ocular fluid nitrate concentration. It is not uncommon for deceased, normal calves, within 2 weeks of their due date, to have ocular fluid concentrations approaching 20 ppm.[6] If sufficient sample is available, aqueous fluid nitrate concentrations should be at least 30 ppm or greater to be highly suggestive of nitrate-associated/nitrite-associated abortion, stillbirth, and/or neonatal weakness and death, especially if there is a compatible history and confirmed source of excessive maternal dietary nitrate.[6,7] Potential dietary sources of nitrate should be also be analyzed for their nitrate content, either qualitatively/semiquantitatively by the diphenylamine spot test or, ideally, quantitatively using one of several different methods. When interpreting the results of forage nitrate analyses, it is important to take into consideration how the nitrate content is expressed (ie, percentage or ppm of nitrate, nitrate-N, or potassium nitrate) and convert the results into units for which reference ranges are available. Forages containing greater than 0.5% nitrate (5000 ppm on a dry-matter basis) can be associated with premature parturition (ie, abortions, stillbirths, or weak neonates).[6] Some caution should be exercised before assigning a definitive diagnosis of nitrate-induced/nitrite-induced abortion, when a maternal dietary source of nitrate has yet to be identified and no other clinical disease or premature parturition has been observed within a herd or flock.

Nitrate-associated/nitrite-associated disease in live, adult ruminants is diagnosed based on clinical signs, especially chocolate brown or chocolate-colored mucous membranes and blood, and a history of exposure to nitrate-accumulating forage.[6] Some laboratories routinely measure nitrate concentrations in serum or plasma (generally at least 35% higher than ocular fluid nitrate concentrations); but chemical determination of methemoglobinemia is not performed at many veterinary diagnostic laboratories because it requires rapid collection and special preservation methods. In cases in which there is not a history of recent consumption of pigweed, sorghums, cornstalks, or other notorious nitrate-accumulating forages, identification of a specific source of excessive dietary nitrate helps to confirm nitrate/nitrite toxicosis. Forages containing greater than 0.6 to 1.0% nitrates (6000–10,000 ppm on a dry-matter basis) can be associated with adult methemoglobinemia and even acute death, depending on the circumstances.[6,7] Postmortem diagnosis of nitrate/nitrite intoxication in an adult ruminant is based on the characteristic brownish cast to all tissues and ocular fluid nitrate concentrations of at least 10 ppm (suggestive of high dietary nitrate concentrations) and, often, greater than 20 ppm (diagnostic, depending on the laboratory).[6]

In light of the prohibition of the antidotal use of methylene blue in food animals, the best way to manage the adverse reproductive effects of nitrate/nitrite intoxication is prevention. The key steps to successfully preventing and managing excessive nitrate exposure in ruminants include the following: (1) recognition of the potential for enzootic exposures, as well as predisposing factors and stressors; (2) avoidance of forages containing greater than 5000 ppm (0.5%) nitrate on a dry-matter basis in the diets of pregnant ruminants or valuable breeding stock, especially cattle[6,7]; (3) maintenance of forage nitrate concentrations less than 2000 ppm on a dry-matter basis (0.2%), when feeding pregnant animals under predisposing environmental and nutritional conditions, to compensate for variations in sampling and temporal changes in plant nitrate reductase activity; (4) ensilage of high nitrate-containing forages to reduce the nitrate content; (5) gradual introduction of animals to feedstuffs containing higher concentrations of nitrate, over at least a week and at times when the cattle are not hungry or starved; and (6) provision of diets containing adequate amounts of concentrate to maintain adequate body condition and prevent overconsumption of high-nitrate forages by pregnant ruminants.

ERGOT ALKALOIDS

Sources

Unlike nitrate, which is commonly recognized as a widespread risk to ruminant well-being, ergot alkaloids are still often viewed as a historical concern or a problem strictly in certain geographic locations. Ergot alkaloids include more than 80 indole compounds and are associated with 2 mycotoxicoses in livestock species (fescue toxicosis and ergotism), both of which are more widespread geographically than many producers realize. The potentially misleading descriptive term fescue toxicosis is derived from the temporal relationship between the development of the clinical signs of this endophytic ergot alkaloid-induced disease and the ingestion of tall fescue grass, *Lolium arundinaceum* (Schreb.), previously known as *Festuca arundinacea* (Shreber) growing in pastures or contained within hay.[9] The fungal endophyte, *Neotyphodium coenophialum* (formerly known as *Acremonium coenophialum* and *Epichlöe typhina*), has a symbiotic relationship with tall fescue grass and grows entirely within the intercellular spaces of the leaf sheaths, stems, and caryopses/seeds (highest concentrations) of this grass species.[8,9] Tall fescue endophyte produces a variety of ergot alkaloids, of which ergovaline is the primary ergopeptine alkaloid.[9] Ergotism involves the ingestion of ergot alkaloids, including several ergopeptine alkaloids to which most of the clinical signs are ascribed. These ergopeptine alkaloids are produced within the fungal sclerotia or ergot bodies of *Claviceps purpurea*, which, unlike the tall fescue endophyte, are externally visible and replace the ovarian tissue of the infected cereal grain or grass.[8,10] Cereal grains, including rye, triticale barley, and barley, as well as a variety of grasses, including both endophyte-free and endophyte-infected tall fescue, are commonly ergotized (see **Table 1**).[8–10]

The clinical signs attributed to fescue toxicosis and ergotism can both be produced experimentally by the administration of ergopeptine alkaloids.[9,10] Therefore, for the purposes of this article, unless stated otherwise, the assumption is made that ergopeptine alkaloids are the primary or, at least, the most representative type of ergot alkaloids responsible for most of the adverse reproductive effects associated with fescue toxicosis and/or ergotism.[9,10] The ergopeptine alkaloids found in ergot include ergotamine, ergocristine, ergosine, ergocornine, and ergocryptine, and their toxic effects and mechanisms of action are essentially identical to those of ergovaline.[9] Although fescue toxicosis and ergotism are frequently discussed as distinct intoxications, both of these diseases involve the adverse effects of ergopeptine alkaloids and are often clinically indistinguishable from one another.[9,10] In addition, although these 2 diseases can occur independently of one another because of differences in fungal sources and the species of animals most likely to consume those sources, there are certain geographic areas where animals can be exposed simultaneously to both ergovaline of endophytic origin and the ergopeptine alkaloids, including some ergovaline, commonly found in ergot.[8–10] It is logical to suspect that any observed clinical differences between fescue toxicosis and ergotism can probably be explained by the higher ergopeptine alkaloid concentrations in ergot than in fescue endophyte and the tendency for fescue toxicosis to involve generally longer durations of exposure.

Mechanisms of Action

Ergotism is classically divided into 4, relatively distinct disease syndromes, which, historically, have been referred to in animals as the gangrenous, hyperthermic, reproductive, and convulsive forms of ergotism.[10] However, there is some controversy regarding the nomenclature and cause of the convulsive form and its relationship to the other syndromes caused by *Claviceps purpurea*-produced ergot alkaloids. What is referred to as convulsive ergotism more closely resembles the tremorgenic syndrome associated with γ-aminobutyric acid inhibition by mycotoxins produced by *Claviceps paspali* than the other forms of *Claviceps purpurea*-related disease caused by ergopeptine alkaloids. For this reason, convulsive ergotism is not discussed further in this article, with respect to ergopeptine alkaloid-induced effects on ruminant reproductive performance. Because fescue toxicosis and ergotism are clinically indistinguishable from one another in species predisposed to both diseases, they are referred to collectively as ergopeptine alkaloid intoxication or, if a general term is deemed more appropriate in instances in which another type of ergot alkaloid (eg, ergonovine) might play a role in reproductive disease, as ergot alkaloid intoxication. The gangrenous, hyperthermic, and reproductive forms of ergopeptine alkaloid intoxication are discussed in terms of the mechanisms of action of ergopeptine alkaloids that most likely correspond to a given syndrome.

The primary mechanisms of action of the ergopeptine alkaloids, whether of tall fescue endophytic or ergot origin, involve vasoconstriction and/or hypoprolactinemia. Ergopeptine alkaloid-induced vasoconstriction is associated with D_1-dopaminergic receptor inhibition and partial agonism of α_1-adrenergic and serotonin receptors. Hypoprolactinemia is caused by the ability of ergopeptine alkaloids to stimulate lactotropic D_2-dopamine receptors in the anterior pituitary gland (ie, D_2-dopamine receptor agonism) and inhibit probating secretion.[8–10]

In ruminants, the vasoconstrictive effects of ergopeptine alkaloids, whether of endophytic or ergot origin, generally predominate and cause what can be referred to as the gangrenous and hyperthermic forms of ergopeptine alkaloid intoxication. The gangrenous syndrome generally occurs at low environmental temperatures and is characterized by diminished blood flow to the extremities, lameness, and, eventually, dry gangrene. Conversely, the hyperthermic syndrome is usually observed under heat stress conditions and develops because an animal's abilities to thermoregulate and dissipate heat are impaired.[9,10] The gangrenous or cutaneous syndrome associated with ergopeptine alkaloids is identical to what is commonly referred to as fescue foot in areas where endophyte-infected tall fescue is enzootic.[9] In these instances, the ergopeptine alkaloids are likely of endophytic origin or, when the syndrome seems less temperature dependent, probably of both endophytic and ergot origin. Ergopeptine alkaloid-induced hyperthermia associated with ingestion of fescue endophytic toxins is referred to as summer slump, the clinical signs of which can be greatly exacerbated by the ingestion of tall fescue or other grasses which have been ergotized.[9,10] In both the gangrenous and hyperthermic forms of ergopeptine alkaloid intoxication, animal comfort, lameness, and stress, as well as interactions involving environmental temperatures and reduced caloric intake, probably play major roles in the pathogenesis of any observed adverse reproductive effects. Fat necrosis or lipomatosis has been observed with chronic fescue toxicosis in a variety of ruminant species and is associated with masses of necrotic fat in the abdominal and/or pelvic cavities.[8,9] Fat necrosis most likely also arises from the vasoconstrictive effects of ergopeptine alkaloids and can be obstructive, putting extramural pressure on the birth canal and contributing to the incidence of dystocias in areas where endophyte-infected fescue is common.

The literature is somewhat confusing with respect to what exactly constitutes reproductive ergot alkaloid/ergopeptine alkaloid intoxication, but it is generally agreed that the clinical signs typically attributed to this ergopeptine alkaloid-associated syndrome are observed more commonly and more dramatically in horses than in ruminants. It is currently believed, especially in horses, that D_1-dopaminergic receptor antagonist and α_1-adrenergic and serotonergic receptor-mediated vasoconstriction does n play a major role in causing the adverse reproductive effects generally attributed this form of ergopeptine alkaloid intoxication. With the possible exception of the adverse reproductive effects of ergonovine, which is an ergoline alkaloid, the primary mechanism of action responsible for the pathogenesis of reproductive ergot alkaloid intoxication is D_2-dopamine receptor agonist-induced suppression of prolactin secretion by the anterior pituitary and the resulting hypoprolactinemia. This ability of the ergopeptine alkaloids in tall fescue endophyte (*Neotyphodium coenophialum*) and ergot (*Claviceps purpurea*) to inhibit prolactin secretion is an example of endocrine disruption (ie, a xenobiotic interfering with normal hormonal function) and can occur at low levels of ergopeptine alkaloid exposure.[1,23] Because of the diverse roles of prolactin in lactogenesis, steroidogenesis, and various reproductive pathways, as well as other homeostatic mechanisms, the reproductive form of ergopeptine alkaloid intoxication is characterized, particularly in horses eating tall fescue endophyte-infected pasture or hay, by decreased milk production, abnormal progestagen metabolism, delayed parturition, and other reproductive abnormalities, including subfertility. Although large enough doses of ergopeptine alkaloids can affect ruminant reproduction,, ruminants, unlike horses, produce a placental lactogen during pregnancy and are, therefore, not as completely dependent on prolactin for lactogenesis and, most likely, other prolactin-mediated physiologic processes as horses are.

Although vasoconstriction and/or hypoprolactinemia are probably either the direct or indirect causes of many of the reproductive abnormalities associated with ergopeptine alkaloid intoxication (ie, fescue toxicosis and/or ergotism), other ergot alkaloids might also diminish ruminant reproductive performance. The stimulation of α_1-adrenergic receptors and the resulting myometrial contractions associated with some ergot alkaloids, especially the ergoline alkaloid ergonovine (also called ergometrine), most likely play a role in the induction of abortions occasionally attributed to ingestion of ergot alkaloids.[10] The decreased feed consumption and growth, as well as disrupted copper homeostasis, frequently observed when ergopeptine alkaloids are ingested by livestock can also have a profound negative influence on reproductive function, especially when those effects are augmented by thermal stress.

Adverse Reproductive Effects

The negative reproductive outcomes associated with ergopeptine alkaloids can be subtle and characterized by slight depressions in reproductive efficiency or dramatic, involving significant reductions in pregnancy rates and increased incidence of abortions and dystocias. Ergot alkaloids can adversely affect both male and female reproductive function. Bulls grazing endophyte-infected pastures during the summer were observed to have altered sperm motility parameters, compared with bulls grazing noninfected pastures.[24] Ovarian follicular dynamics can be adversely affected by tall fescue endophytic toxins, in particular by interactions involving the hyperthermic and/or prolactin-inhibiting actions of these toxins and thermal stress.[25] Recent studies have suggested that exposure of females, as well as males, to the ergopeptine alkaloids produced by the tall fescue endophyte or ergot sclerotia can affect embryo quality and subsequent embryonic development.[9,10,12,13]

nteractions with Predisposing Factors and Other Stressors

rgopeptine alkaloids can certainly be the primary cause of reproductive problems in ıerd or flock, but, more often than not, these mycotoxins interact with enzootic pre- oosing factors, other stressors, and management to play a contributory role in the ıogenesis of impaired reproductive function. Ruminants seem to be predisposed he gangrenous and hyperthermic forms of ergopeptine alkaloid exposure.

Similarly, the species and physiologic state of the exposed ruminant can also influence the severity of the ergopeptine alkaloid-related effects on reproductive function. Because of their grazing habits, sheep generally seem to be less susceptible to ergopeptine alkaloid intoxication than cattle. On the other hand, ergopeptine alkaloid-exposed sheep with full fleeces are predisposed to hyperthermia when ambient temperatures begin to increase during the summer, and unshorn rams and recently bred ewes are both expected to be prone to ergopeptine alkaloid-associated declines in reproductive efficiency.

Although in a state of flux because of the adaptability of tall fescue grass infected with *Neotyphodium coenophialum* to a wide variety of different growing conditions and plant stressors, certain geographic areas (eg, southern midwestern states and the southeastern United States) have, traditionally, been more likely to have pastures containing endophyte-infected tall fescue than some other parts of the country. Weather conditions, such as cool, damp conditions in the spring, facilitate the life cycle of *Claviceps purpurea*. In addition, it is not uncommon for endophyte-infected fescue or other grasses growing in geographic areas, where fescue toxicosis is considered enzootic, to be ergotized. Depending on the level of ergopeptine alkaloid exposure, fescue toxicosis and ergotism can be associated with either low to high morbidity. The most severe clinical signs of ergopeptine alkaloid exposure, including reported deaths, are most likely to be related to sporadic exposures to the high concentrations of ergopeptine alkaloids (possibly as high as 10,000 ppm) that can be found in ergot sclerotia.[10] On the other hand, fescue toxicosis generally represents the effects of subacute to chronic exposures to 0.2-ppm to 0.6-ppm (200–600 ppb) concentrations of ergovaline commonly found in fescue grass pastures infected with endophyte.[9] However, the effects of ergovaline can be acutely amplified and less seasonal in nature (eg, gangrenous lesions in spring or early summer or summer slump in the spring) when endophyte-infected fescue is also contaminated with ergot.

In addition to weather conditions that favor endophyte-infected tall fescue growth and the life cycle of *Claviceps purpurea*, various other enzootic stressors have been reported to interact with ergopeptine alkaloids to adversely affect animal health. Copper homeostasis is adversely affected by ingestion of ergopeptine alkaloids, and diets low in copper or heavy internal parasite loads are likely to exacerbate ergopeptine alkaloid-related impaired reproductive function.[8,9,11] Reduced caloric intake can adversely affect reproduction in several different ways. Likewise, several studies have reported impaired immunity in animals grazing endophyte-infected pasture, suggesting that these animals might be more susceptible to infectious agents than animals not exposed to ergopeptine alkaloids.[9] In addition, severe wound infections and sepsis are further complications to the gangrenous form of ergopeptine alkaloid intoxication. As has already been suggested, perhaps the most important stressor interactions involving ergot alkaloids, specifically ergopeptine alkaloids, are those involving environmental temperature. The gangrenous form of ergopeptine alkaloid intoxication is more severe and debilitating when environmental temperatures become cooler and, particularly, as they approach freezing. Animals exhibiting lameness are less likely to graze normally, and heat detection by males, as well as standing estrus in females, is negatively affected in lame animals. In particular, heat stress can diminish reproductive performance in both male and female animals, and these adverse stressor effects are greatly amplified by exposure to the additional stress of ergopeptine alkaloids.[1,3,9,10,12,13,24,25] Animals already compromised by gangrenous or hyperthermic ergopeptine alkaloid intoxications are often unthrifty and are likel to be more severely affected by what might otherwise be a sublethal toxicant expo sure, than a healthier animal. Animals frequently recover quickly from the early stag of ergopeptine alkaloid intoxication, once they are removed from the sources of the ergopeptine alkaloids. However, it is probably not unreasonable to consider whether chronic exposures to moderate concentrations of ergopeptine alkaloids have the potential to result in chronic vascular alterations, which might predispose older animals to the gangrenous or hyperthermic forms of ergopeptine alkaloid intoxication.

Diagnosis and Management

The diagnosis of ergopeptine alkaloid-related health problems is based on clinical signs and an awareness of the geographic areas, weather conditions, and forages and grains likely to play a role in fescue toxicosis and/or ergotism (see **Table 1**). Fat necrosis can frequently be diagnosed by rectal palpation (need to to differentiate from bovine lymphosarcoma) or on postmortem examination. Ergotism should be suspected any time signs of fescue toxicosis are severe or seem to be independent of environmental temperature. Diagnostic testing for fescue toxicosis and ergotism involves detection of endophyte (less common), observation of *Claviceps purpurea* sclerotia (might require feed microscopy), and, most importantly, the determination, in enzootic areas or under suspect circumstances, of forage, hay, or processed feed concentrations of ergovaline and ergotomine, ergocristine, ergosine, ergocornine, ergocryptine, by high-performance liquid chromatography. Adverse effects on livestock performance are generally observed when the total dietary concentration of ergopeptine alkaloids exceeds 100 to 200 ppb. The clinical signs observed with excessive exposure to ergopeptine alkaloids can be variable and are dependent on the species and physiologic state of exposed animals, the environmental conditions during the period of exposure, the activities of and the interactions between the individual ergopeptine alkaloids, and the level and duration of ergopeptine alkaloid exposure.[9,10]

The early signs of ergopeptine alkaloid intoxication, whether it be fescue toxicosis or even ergotism, are often reversible, with the cutaneous vascular effects of the ergopeptine alkaloids usually subsiding shortly after removal from ergopeptine alkaloid-contaminated pastures, hay, grains, or processed feeds. Because of the challenges and costs associated with gaining regulatory approval for drug-based therapies in food animals, ergot alkaloids, like nitrate, represent a management problem that can often be addressed before serious health problems develop and reproductive function is adversely affected. The key steps to successfully preventing and managing excessive ergopeptine alkaloid exposure in ruminants include the following: (1) recognition of the potential for enzootic exposures, as well as predisposing factors and stressors; (2) the avoidance, if at all possible, of inexpensive feedstuffs containing ergot-contaminated grain screenings (fines) or, possibly, grass seed; (3) when indicated by weather conditions or clinical circumstances, determination of the total dietary concentration of ergopeptine alkaloids; (4) the early detection of the clinical signs and the removal of animals from the source of ergopeptine alkaloids by pasture rotation and/or mowing of forages to remove seed heads and possible ergot bodies[9,10]; (5) pasture/forage management, such as overseeding with legumes, limited application of nitrogen-based fertilizers, replacement of toxigenic endophyte-infected fescue with friendly endophyte, and ammoniation of lesser-quality fescue hay[9]; (6) provision of diets supplemented as necessary with trace elements and high-quality feedstuffs to compensate for decreased feed intake and alterations in copper homeostasis; (7) amelioration of the effects of temperature-related stressors by providing access to adequate housing for warmth and shade, as well as sources of potable water and ponds to aid animals in their hydration and thermoregulatory efforts, and by facilitating the removal of excessive hair, wool, or fiber from susceptible breeds and species, as warm weather approaches; (8) semen evaluations, pregnancy examinations, and record keeping to detect diminished reproductive performance; (9) selection of breeds or strains of animals capable of adapting to anticipated environmental conditions[26]; and (10) further research to identify pharmacologic or feed additive approaches that are economically feasible and capable of gaining regulatory approval for use in food animals.[27,28]

XENOESTROGENS

Sources

Instances of naturally occurring endocrine disruption involving exposures to xenoestrogens in domestic animals are often viewed as historical or sporadic and generally receive cursory treatment in the current scientific literature and popular press, compared with xenoestrogenic exposures involving wildlife, humans, or laboratory species. The term xenoestrogens (ie, estrogenic xenobiotics) classically refers to exogenous endocrine-disrupting chemicals with the ability to mimic endogenous estrogens through interactions with estrogen receptors within the exposed individual, thereby inducing estrogenic effects.[1,23] Although it is now clear that estrogenic effects can also be manifested by any mechanisms of action that increase or enhance the effects of endogenous estrogens (eg, increased half-life or production of endogenous estrogens) the discussion in this article is limited to xenobiotics capable of estrogen receptor-mediated actions.[1]

There is an information explosion of textbooks, articles, Web sites, and blogs hypothesizing and, in many instances, documenting estrogenic effects of agriculturally and industrially important synthetic chemicals and environmental contaminants in rodent and in vitro experimental models, as well as in wildlife and even human populations.[1,23] However, domestic animals are also potential targets for xenoestrogens. Several agronomically important leguminous plants, including soybeans, several clovers, and alfalfa (see **Table 1**), as well as other plants, such as hops (*Humulus lupulus*), produce naturally occurring xenoestrogenic chemicals referred to as phytoestrogens, which have the potential to adversely affect reproductive performance in domestic animals.[1,8,11,23,29] Similarly, the estrogenic mycotoxin zearalenone is also a naturally occurring xenoestrogen of clinical relevance to optimal reproductive function in livestock species and is produced by primarily by *Fusarium graminearum* (formerly *Fusarium roseum)*, under certain environmental and storage conditions, in corn, wheat, barley, and oats.[1,11,23]

The phytoestrogens of most interest to livestock producers are polyphenolic compounds generally classified as isoflavones or coumestans.[29] The isoflavones include daidzein, genistein, formononetin, biochanin A, and glycitein, which are commonly found in soybeans and clovers (see **Table 1**).[8,11,29] On the other hand, coumestrol, which is found in alfalfa and, potentially, white clover (see **Table 1**), is classified as a coumestan.[8,11] Zearalenone and its metabolites, the α- and β-zearalenols and zearalenols, are resorcyclic acid lactones produced as secondary fungal metabolites of *Fusarium graminearum* and several other *Fusarium* species found in a variety of cereal crops and, even, some grasses.[1,11]

Mechanisms of Action

For the purposes of this article, the primary mechanisms of action for the xenoestrogens of interest (ie, phytoestrogens and zearalenone) involve interactions with the estrogen receptors, whether those receptors are classic nuclear receptors, receptors located within the cytosol, or even membrane receptors. The major types of estrogen receptors are ERα and ERβ. Although most phytoestrogens have a greater affinity for ERβ than ERα, there is much variation in receptor-binding affinities between th various phytoestrogens. Phytoestrogens are frequently conjugated, and it is the nonconjugated form that interacts with endogenous estrogen receptors. There is some thought that, although coumestrol, which has an estrogenic potential similar to that of zearalenone, binds to both ERα and ERβ, its mechanism of estrogenic activity might be more dependent on its ability to enhance the sensitivity of the tissues to endogenous 17β-estradiol, than on its own ability to stimulate estrogen receptors.[11,29] Zearalenone is generally considered to have a greater affinity for ERα than ERβ, and most references suggest that α-zearalenol (predominant metabolite in most species) or β-zearalenol (predominant metabolite in cattle) has greater estrogenic activity than β-zearalenol.[30] However, there are some differences of opinion in the literature, and in vitro determinations of estrogenic activity are dependent on the type of in vitro system used to make such determinations.[11,30,31]

These naturally occurring xenoestrogens are generally considered weak estrogens, but, particularly with respect to the common phytoestrogens, their concentrations in the body can be 100-fold higher than that of endogenous estrogens.[29] Depending on the circumstances, especially the amounts of unbound endogenous estrogens available to interact with estrogen receptors and the possible bioactivation of some isoflavones from a relatively inactive form, such as formononetin, to a more active form, like equol, phytoestrogens can act as estrogen receptor agonists, partial agonists, or antagonists.[1,23,29] In some instances, phytoestrogens act like selective estrogen receptor modulators, which have different actions as estrogen receptor agonists or antagonists, depending on the tissue type or reproductive organ.[29] Like synthetic xenoestrogens, phytoestrogens and zearalenone can function as antiestrogens when high concentrations of these xenoestrogens compete with endogenous estrogens to bind with the estrogen receptor, thereby preventing the actions of endogenous estrogens and resulting in antiestrogenic effects, like the inhibition of LH release from the anterior pituitary.[1,29]

Adverse Reproductive Effects

In some of the older literature, there is a pervasive opinion that phytoestrogens and particularly zearalenone have little or no adverse effects on cattle reproduction.[8,11,32] It is likely that these observations are correct, from the perspective that adverse effects on reproductive function in cattle, associated with naturally occurring xenoestrogens, are observed only sporadically and the reproductive effects tend to be subtle. However, subtle changes in reproductive efficiency can have a dramatic financial effect on livestock producers. The adverse reproductive effects observed in ruminants exposed to xenoestrogens depend on the specific estrogenic xenobiotic, its concentration in feedstuffs, and whether that xenoestrogen is acting as an estrogen receptor agonist or antagonist. The estrogenic or antiestrogenic effects of a xenoestrogen can vary between animal species and even tissue types and reproductive organs within the same animal, as well as the sex, stage of development (eg, early prenatal, late gestational, neonatal, prepubertal, peripubertal, and/or postpubertal exposures), and, in the case of exposed females, day of the estrous cycle at the time of exposure.[1,29] Xenoestrogen exposures, especially in younger, sexually immature animals, can result in hyperestrogenism in females characterized by the following dramatic observations: precocious mammary gland development (**Fig. 2**); vulvar, vaginal, and uterine enlargement; changes in the vaginal and/or uterine epithelium (eg, squamous metaplasia, hyperplasia); alterations in uterine glandular development and architecture; ovarian atrophy; and abnormal sexual behavior.[1,8,11,29] In sexually immature males, hyperestrogenism can cause preputial swelling and testicular atrophy.[1,8,11] Other effects associated with xenoestrogenic exposures, particularly

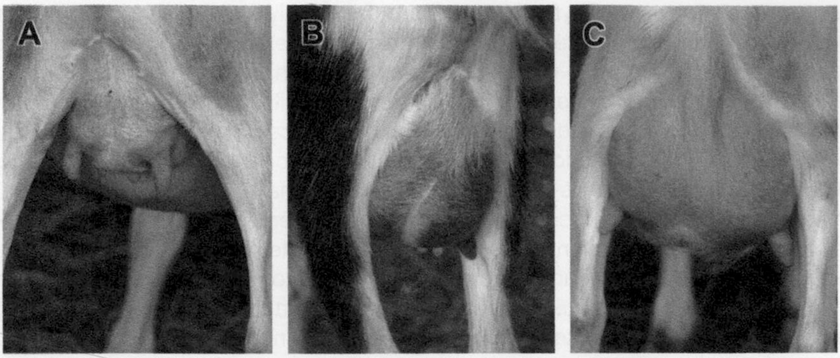

Fig. 2. A–C show the range in precocious mammary gland development and lactation, from mild (*A*) to moderate (*B*) to severe (*C*), observed in nonpregnant, 6-month-old to 8-month-old dairy goats, which were accidentally exposed to formononetin-contaminated, mixed grass-clover hay. (*Photographic assistance and modifications courtesy of* Howard Wilson and Don Connor.)

in cyclic and bred females and, to a lesser extent, mature males, are generally less dramatic than those observed in younger animals and include: reduced frequency of the gondadotropin releasing hormone pulses; inhibited LH release from the pituitary; irregular estrous cycles; cystic ovaries; possible abnormal sexual behavior; changes in cervical structure that can affect sperm transport and fertility (ie, clover disease in sheep); an abnormal environment within the uterine tubes, which can adversely affect successful fertilization; alterations in spermatogenesis and epididymal sperm maturation and transport, resulting in less than optimal sperm function; and, potentially, abnormal embryonic or fetal development, with possible fetal death, abortion, and even dystocia.[1,8,11,23,29,30]

Interactions with Predisposing Factors and Other Stressors

With respect to xenoestrogens, there are many intrinsic, toxicant-related factors, as well as genetic and physiologic predispositions pertaining to exposed animals, which influence the occurrence of xenoestrogen-associated, negative reproductive outcomes. These toxicant and predisposing factors include the metabolism and estrogenic receptor-binding affinity of a specific xenoestrogen, as well as the species, stage of development, and sex of the exposed animal, all of which determine the severity of the observed abnormalities in reproductive function. Although zearalenone is a potent xenoestrogen in swine, some studies report that the effects of this xenoestrogen are minimal in cattle.[33] However, the older literature, from which many current studies derived their conclusions, did not always appreciate the clinical significance of subtle changes in reproductive function, such as altered oocyte quality and slightly decreased pregnancy rates, which can dramatically affect overall herd reproductive performance and profitability.[32,34] Certain species, such as sheep and possibly goats, seem to be more predisposed to the adverse effects of certain phytoestrogens and even zearalenone than cattle. Formononetin in subterranean clover (2% to 4% dry weight of plant) and red clover (1% to 2% dry weight of plant) has almost no estrogenic activity but is converted in the rumen to a relatively potent phytoestrogen, equol, which binds both ERα and ERβ. Although the excretion of equol is slower in sheep than in cattle, it is believed that the primary reason sheep are more susceptible to the effects of phytoestrogens and, probably, other xenoestrogens than cattle is the greater sensitivity of ovine estrogen receptors compared those of bovine.[8,11] The unborn fetus, in particul and sexually immature, prepubertal animals are generally more susceptible to the most obvious detrimental effects of xenoestrogens, probably, in large part, because sexual differentiation and other important aspects of prenatal and postnatal sexual development are occurring at these stages of life (see **Fig. 1**).[1,23] In addition, there are lower concentrations of endogenous estrogens circulating in prepubertal animals, so there is not much competition for estrogen receptor binding between xenoestrogens and endogenous 17β-estradiol. Virgin dairy heifers also seem to be more susceptible to the adverse reproductive effects of xenoestrogens than mature dairy cows.[32,34] There is a natural tendency to discount the possibility of adverse effects of xenoestrogens on male animals. Although it is true that males are probably, depending on their stage of development at the time of exposure, less sensitive to long-term, deleterious effects of xenoestrogens, there are potentially subtle changes in male reproductive function that can be attributed to xenoestrogens.[1,23,30]

As has been emphasized throughout this article, enzootic nutritional, environmental, infectious, and toxic stressors all have the potential to lower the threshold dose at which a given reproductive toxicant, including a xenoestrogen, can have a negative effect on ruminant reproductive performance (see **Fig. 1**). In addition, there might not be a smoking-gun cause of reproductive inefficiency. Several different enzootic stressors and interactions with predisposing factors and management can all contribute to a multifactorial cause of subfertility. Some types of forages and grains (see **Table 1**) are predisposed to phytoestrogen production and infection by *Fusarium graminearum*. Diseased and stressed legumes (eg, infected by viruses or fungi or drought stressed), as well as phosphorus deficiency favor higher phytoestrogen concentrations in these predisposed plants.[8] Moldy feedstuffs are likely to be of less nutritional value, which might contribute to some subtle adverse reproductive effects. Certain environmental conditions (ie, 20–25°C; >23% to optimal 45% moisture) favor initial fungal growth in the field or during storage and subsequent zearalenone production (drop in temperature to 15°C; >23% moisture).[11] Infectious diseases, particularly those accompanied by fever and malaise, have the potential to affect physiologic processes also susceptible to the adverse effects of xenoestrogens, such as normal spermatogenesis and epididymal sperm maturation and transport, the occurrence of standing estrus in the female, heat coitus with a male, fertilization, and early embryonic development. Interactions with other toxic stressors can also exacerbate the effects of xenoestrogens. Simultaneous exposures to multiple xenoestrogens, such as might happen with ingestion of more than 1 phytoestrogen or ingestion of both phytoestrogens and zearalenone, are more likely to result in decreased reproductive efficiency than exposure to a single toxic stressor. Zearalenone is metabolized to more estrogenic metabolites, and species variations in its metabolism and toxicokinetics can result in differences in susceptibility.[11,30,31] The conditions that favor *Fusarium* fungal growth and zearalenone production frequently lead to simultaneous production of zearalenone and vomitoxin (DON) by *Fusarium graminearum* or other *Fusarium* species.[11] Although the adverse effects of vomitoxin are likely to be less severe in ruminants than in swine, concerns have been raised, especially in dairy cattle, about the adverse effects of low concentrations of this trichothecene mycotoxin. It is possible that these concerns might have more of a nutritional than a toxicologic basis.

Diagnosis and Management

As with the other intoxications reviewed in this article, the diagnosis of xenoestrogen-related health problems is based on clinical signs and an awareness of the weather conditions, and forages and grains likely to produce phytoestrogens and/or favor fungal growth and zearalenone production (see **Table 1**). However, of the enzootic reproductive diseases discussed in this article, xenoestrogen-induced effects in ruminants are likely to be the least anticipated and the most difficult to diagnose. Diagnostic testing for xenoestrogens involves identification of plants that are known to produce phytoestrogens, observation of moldy corn, wheat, oats, or barley; detection of significant concentrations of phytoestrogens (analyses not performed by all laboratories) and/or zearalenone and vomitoxin (DON) in suspect feedstuffs and bedding (ie, pastures, hays, processed feeds, and straw or other bedding); and, in areas where large numbers of sheep are raised, analyses for zearalenone metabolites in urine are often performed. Phytoestrogens, although concentrations are greatly reduced, can still be toxic in leguminous hays (see **Fig. 2**) and zearalenone can be present in some grasses, as well as both the grain and stems/straw of *Fusarium*-infected plants.

Formononetin concentrations greater than 0.5% in clovers have been associated with xenoestrogenic problems in sheep; however, other clinical reports have suggested that smaller concentrations of formononetin can cause endocrine disruption in ruminants.[8] It is not uncommon for alfalfa to contain coumestrol concentrations ranging between 1 and 20 ppm, during the early vegetative stages, and 25 and 65 ppm in later stages of growth. Adverse effects on cattle reproductive performance have been observed when coumestrol concentrations are in the range of 25 to 45 ppm or, depending on the reference cited and the analytical laboratory, 18 to more than 180 ppm.[8,29] Some studies report that cattle are relatively insensitive to zearalenone, whereas others have reported 25% lower pregnancy rates in heifers fed 12.5 ppm of zearalenone.[33,34] This disparity in these ranges attests to the likely importance that other enzootic predisposing factors and stressors, as well as the criteria used to evaluate impaired reproductive performance, play in determining the effect of xenoestrogen exposure on ruminant reproductive inefficiency.

The keys to successfully preventing and managing excessive exposure to xenoestrogens in ruminants include: (1) recognition of the potential for enzootic exposures, as well as predisposing factors and stressors; (2) the avoidance, if at all possible, of inexpensive feedstuffs containing grain screenings (fines) or moldy corn, wheat, oats, or barley; (3) when indicated by prevailing weather conditions and/or clinical circumstances, determination of the concentrations of common phytoestrogens and/or zearalenone and vomitoxin in suspect feedstuffs and bedding (ie, pastures, hays, processed feeds, and straw or other plant material used for bedding); (4) avoidance of grazing immature ruminants intended for breeding or pregnant sheep on leguminous pastures or feeding hays containing legumes, until analyses or other circumstances suggest that the pasture is safe; (5) early detection of the clinical signs and the removal of animals from the sources of xenoestrogens by pasture rotation or changes in grain or forage sources; (6) pasture/forage management, such as overseeding with nonleguminous forages, cutting legumes, particularly before the flowering stage, and drying for use in hay, enriching the phosphorus content of the soil, and limited application of nitrogen-based fertilizers; (8) semen evaluations, pregnancy examinations, and record keeping to detect diminished reproductive performance; (9) if possible, maintenance of dietary vomitoxin concentrations less than 1 ppm for dairy cattle and less than 2 ppm for breeding beef cattle to simultaneously limit vomitoxin and zearalenone concentrations; and (10) in the absence of vomitoxin, maintenance of dietary zearalenone concentrations less than 2 ppm for dairy cattle and less than 5 ppm for breeding beef cattle.

SUMMARY

This article was written from the perspective of a clinical and diagnostic toxicologist and theriogenologist. Reproduction is a critical biologic process and is essential for the production of important agricultural commodities. The article takes a novel, integrated approach to discuss the possible roles of reproductive toxicants, not only as the potential, primary causes of observed reproductive abnormalities but also in the context of other variables, including management, which can affect reproductive performance in ruminants. The rationale for this approach is to aid individuals involved in the livestock industry in understanding how less than optimal reproductive efficiency can develop within a given production system. Although impaired reproductive function can have a single, obvious toxic cause (ie, the smoking gun), the causes of diminished reproductive performance in ruminants are often multifactorial, involving various predisposing factors and/or stressors, including toxicants. Because these factors and stressors are common in normal livestock production, they can be classified as enzootic. It is critical that livestock producers, as well as their veterinarians, understand the potential contributions to diminished reproductive efficiency associated with physiologic and genetic predispositions and nutritional, environmental, infectious, and, in particular, toxic stressors. The adverse effects of these enzootic predispositions and stressors, which negatively affect animal production systems, can generally be prevented or greatly reduced with sound management practices. Reproductive toxicants, such as nitrate, mycotoxins, and xenoestrogens, can play primary or contributory roles in diminished reproductive efficiency in ruminant species. The recognition and prevention of the adverse effects of these enzootic toxic stressors are essential for optimal ruminant reproductive performance and production system profitability.

REFERENCES

1. Evans TJ. Reproductive toxicity and endocrine disruption. In: Gupta RC, editor. Veterinary toxicology: basic and clinical principles. New York: Academic Press/Elsevier; 2007. p. 206–44.
2. Senger PL. Pathways to pregnancy and parturition. 2nd revised edition. Moscow (ID): Current Conceptions; 2005.
3. Hafez B, Hafez ESE, editors. Reproduction in farm animals. 7th edition. Philadelphia: Lippincott Williams & Wilkins; 2000.
4. Youngquist RS, editor. Current therapy in large animal theriogenology. Philadelphia: WB Saunders; 1997.
5. Youngquist RS, Threlfall W, editors. Current therapy in large animal theriogenology. 2nd edition. Philadelphia: WB Saunders; 2001.
6. Casteel SW, Evans TJ. Nitrate. In: Plumlee KH, editor. Clinical veterinary toxicology. St Louis (MO): Mosby; 2004. p. 127–30.
7. Talcott P, Evans TJ. Nitrate toxicosis. In: Haskell SR, editor. Blackwell's five-minute veterinary consult: ruminant. Philadelphia: Wiley-Blackwell; 2008. p. 621–3.
8. Burrows GE, Tyrl RJ. Toxic plants of North America. Ames (IA): Iowa State University Press; 2001.
9. Evans TJ, Rottinghaus GE, Casteel SW. Fescue. In: Plumlee KH, editor. Clinical veterinary toxicology. St Louis (MO): Mosby; 2004. p. 243–50.
10. Evans TJ, Rottinghaus GE, Casteel SW. Ergot. In: Plumlee KH, editor. Clinical veterinary toxicology. St Louis (MO): Mosby; 2004. p. 239–43.
11. Cheeke PR. Natural toxicants in feeds. 2nd edition. Danville (IL): Interstate Publishers; 1998.
12. Jones KL, King SS, Iqbal MJ. Endophyte-infected tall fescue diet alters gene expression in heifer luteal tissue as revealed by interspecies microarray analysis. Mol Reprod Dev 2004;67(2):154–61.

13. Schuenemann GM, Edwards JL, Hopkins FM, et al. Fertility aspects in yearling beef bulls grazing endophyte-infected tall fescue pastures. Reprod Fertil Dev 2005;17(4):479–86.
14. Subcommittee on Beef Cattle Nutrition. Committee on Animal Nutrition, Board on Agriculture, National Research Council. Nutrient Requirements of Beef Cattle. 7th revised edition. Washington, DC: National Academy Press; 2000.
15. Subcommittee on Dairy Cattle Nutrition. Committee on Animal Nutrition, Board on Agriculture and Natural Resources, National Research Council. Nutrient Requirements of Dairy Cattle. 7th revised edition. Washington, DC: National Academy Press; 2001.
16. Committee on Nutrient Requirements of Small Ruminants. Board on Agriculture and Natural Resources, Division on Earth and Life Studies, National Research Council of the National Academies. Nutrient Requirements of Small Ruminants: Sheep, Goats, Cervids, and New World Camelids. Washington, DC: National Academies Press; 2007.
17. Spoiled feeds, molds, mycotoxins and animal health. Manitoba agriculture, food and rural initiatives. Available at: http://www.gov.mb.ca/agriculture/livestock/beef/baa05s27.html. Accessed February 22, 1011.
18. Aflatoxins and dairy cattle. AgNews TAMU. Available at: http://agnewsarchive.tamu.edu/drought/drghtpak98/drght30.htmlwebsite. Accessed February 22, 1011.
19. Henry MH. Mycotoxins in feeds: CVM's perspective. FDA. 2006. Available at: http://www.fda.gov/AnimalVeterinary/Products/AnimalFoodFeeds/Contaminants/ucm050974.htm. Accessed February 22, 1011.
20. Anderson ML, Blanchard PC, Barr BC, et al. A survey of causes of bovine abortion occurring in the San Joaquin Valley, California. J Vet Diagn Invest 1990;2(4):283–7.
21. Zralý Z, Bendová J, Svecová D, et al. Effects of oral intake of nitrates on reproductive functions of bulls. Vet Med (Praha) 1997;42(12):345–54.
22. Manassaram DM, Backer LC, Moll DM. A review of nitrates in drinking water: maternal exposure and adverse reproductive and developmental outcomes. Environ Health Perspect 2006;114(3):320–7.
23. Evans TJ. Endocrine disruptors. In: Gupta RC, editor. Reproductive and developmental toxicology. London: Academic Press/Elsevier; 2011. p. 873–91.
24. Looper ML, Rorie RW, Person CN, et al. Influence of toxic endophyte-infected fescue on sperm characteristics and endocrine factors of yearling Brahman-influenced bulls. J Anim Sci 2009;87(3):1184–91.
25. Burke JM, Spiers DE, Kojima FN, et al. Interaction of endophyte-infected fescue and heat stress on ovarian function in the beef heifer. Biol Reprod 2001;65(1):260–8.
26. Browning R Jr. Effects of endophyte-infected tall fescue on indicators of thermal status and growth in Hereford and Senepol steers. J Anim Sci 2004;82(2):634–43.
27. Al-Haidary A, Spiers DE, Rottinghaus GE, et al. Thermoregulatory ability of beef heifers following intake of endophyte-infected tall fescue during controlled heat challenge. J Anim Sci 2001;79(7):1780–8.
28. Jones KL, King SS, Griswold KE, et al. Domperidone can ameliorate deleterious reproductive effects and reduced weight gain associated with fescue toxicosis in heifers. J Anim Sci 2003;81(10):2568–74.
29. Mostrom M, Evans TJ. Phytoestrogens. In: Gupta RC, editor. Reproductive and developmental toxicology. London: Academic Press/Elsevier; 2011. p. 707–722.

30. Minervini F, Dell'Aquila ME. Zearalenone and reproductive function in farm animals. Int J Mol Sci 2008;9(12):2570–84.
31. Hassan M, Fatemeh R, Kobra B. Zearalenone is bioactivated in the river Buffalo (*Bubalus bubalis*): hepatic biotransformation. Trop Anim Health Prod 2010;42(6): 1229–34.
32. Weaver GA, Kurtz HJ, Behrens JC, et al. Effect of zearalenone on the fertility of virgin dairy heifers. Am J Vet Res 1986;47(6):1395–7.
33. Meerdink GL. Zearalenone. In: Plumlee KH, editor. Clinical veterinary toxicology. St Louis (MO): Mosby; 2004. p. 243–50.
34. Jouany J-P, Diaz DE. Effects of mycotoxins in ruminants. In: Diaz DE, editor. The mycotoxin blue book. Nottingham (UK): Nottingham University Press; 2005. p. 295–321.

Commercial and Industrial Chemical Hazards for Ruminants

Robert H. Poppenga, DVM, PhD

KEYWORDS

• Commercial • Industrial • Ruminant • Poisoning

For the purposes of this article, commercial and industrial chemical hazards are defined as any chemical hazard associated with nondrug commercial products, such as fertilizers, pesticides, feed additives, construction materials, or disinfectants used in or near ruminant livestock environments. Industrial chemical hazards also include those associated with the close proximity of a livestock operation to an industrial activity, such as manufacturing, mining, or recycling. Emphasis is placed on those chemical hazards that are not covered elsewhere in this issue.

The sources of toxicant exposure and the specific toxicants of concern can change over time. For example, used motor oil is not a common source for livestock exposure to lead because it was removed from gasoline in the mid-1970s. Also, although lead-containing paint on old farm buildings still poses a risk of intoxication for livestock, the gradual elimination of lead-based paint, along with the repainting or replacement of old farm buildings, has decreased the potential for livestock exposure to lead from this source. The use of certain wood preservatives, such as chromated copper arsenate (CCA), creosote, and pentachlorophenol, has also been curtailed in recent years due to concern about potential adverse human health and environmental effects, although exposure of ruminants can still occur if precautions are not taken to properly dispose of older treated materials.

Possible exposure pathways include inhalation, ingestion from various media (water and feed), and dermal contact. Some hazardous materials are actively ingested by livestock. For example, some minerals, such as lead and arsenic, are reportedly attractive due to a salt-like taste; this might be especially problematic in salt-deprived animals. The ingestion of potentially hazardous materials can result from pica induced either by nutritional deficiencies or boredom.[1]

The author has nothing to disclose.
California Animal Health and Food Safety Laboratory, School of Veterinary Medicine, University of California at Davis, West Health Sciences Drive, Davis, CA 95616, USA
E-mail address: rhpoppenga@ucdavis.edu

Vet Clin Food Anim 27 (2011) 373–387
doi:10.1016/j.cvfa.2011.02.011
vetfood.theclinics.com

Veterinarians might be asked to investigate producer claims of decreased livestock productivity, illness, and death after alleged exposure to commercial and industrial toxicants. In the majority of cases, losses can be attributed to other disease conditions or management deficiencies, although it is sometimes difficult to convince producers that they themselves might be primarily responsible for the situation. Investigation of such cases requires an open mind, thoroughness, and early consultation with outside sources of expertise. Patience in such cases is also a virtue, because their resolution can take years and often involves litigation.

This discussion focuses on several commercial or industrial toxicants of concern. It is not possible to cover all potential hazards because many products or chemicals are used around livestock. Documented cases of intoxication can occur, however, from unexpected sources. For example, in one case, 10 of approximately 340 lactating dairy cows suddenly developed depression, diarrhea, and incoordination.[2] A total of 18 cows was noted to have a reddish brown stain on their dorsal hair coats with welts noted below the stains. The welts were believed to have resulted from full-thickness burns of the skin; no other significant lesions were noted in one animal that died and was examined by necropsy. Routine toxicologic testing revealed high liver and kidney concentrations of chromium. Subsequent investigation revealed that a leaking container of 99.7% chromic acid had been stored above the area through which the cows walked to enter the milking parlor. This case illustrates the need for thorough examination of the premises in disease outbreaks of unknown etiology.

PETROLEUM EXPLORATION AND PRODUCTION

In certain regions of the country, oil exploration and production occur in close proximity to animal agriculture. Oil and petroleum–related compounds can be introduced into the environment of livestock in several ways, including via oil drilling and refining activities, oil or oil product spills, and many petroleum product uses. Crude oil is a complex mixture of hundreds of different chemical compounds or petroleum hydrocarbons and there is considerable variation in the specific chemical composition of oils from different sources.[3,4] In addition, livestock are potentially exposed to a variety of chemicals in drilling muds and additives used in oil exploration.[3,4]

Livestock intoxications from crude oil–related activity are well documented. Ruminants ingest crude oil or petroleum products when thirsty and water is unavailable, when food or water is contaminated, or when adequate feed and salt are not provided.[3,4] The toxicity of crude oil and clinical signs associated with its ingestion can vary depending on its chemical composition. The toxicity of crude oil, however, seems to correlate with its content of volatile components, such as kerosene, naphtha, and gasoline. Thus, sweet crude oil, which is relatively high in volatiles, is more toxic than sour crude oil, which is higher in less volatile components, such as gas oil, lubricating distillates, residue, and sulfur.[5] The process of weathering decreases the volatile and water soluble components in crude oil, which can further alter its toxicity and clinical effects. Acute clinical signs are attributed to the more volatile components of crude oil.

The major components of crude oil have different mechanisms of toxic action. The volatile components of crude oil have anesthetic properties, are more irritating, and are more likely to be aspirated into the lungs.[3] Volatile components may also sensitize the heart to catecholamines. Crude oil destroys rumen microflora and enzymatic activity, which perhaps contributes to the onset of bloat.

The effect of ingesting crude oil ranges from no clinical signs to sudden death. Reported signs include a petroleum smell on the breath, hypoesthesia or hyperesthesia, depression, mydriasis, ptyalism, epiphora, muscle and head tremors, ataxia, tonic-clonic seizures, hypothermia or hyperthermia, and gastrointestinal (GI) signs, such as emesis, bloat, rumen atony, abomasal displacement, and loose to hard feces with a petroleum smell or visible oil present. Aspiration pneumonia is a commonly reported sequel and hyperpnea, dyspnea, and moist rales can occur.

Necropsy findings include detection of crude oil in the GI tract contents and lung lesions consistent with aspiration pneumonia. The portions of the lungs lowermost at the time of aspiration are most severely affected (ie, caudoventral apical, cardiac and cranioventral diaphragmatic and intermediate lobes).

Diagnosis of intoxication is based on a history of possible access to a source, evidence of consumption, and analysis of GI contents and tissues. Mixing rumen or stomach contents with warm water allows oil or petroleum products, such as kerosene, to rise the surface, making identification easier.[5] Because of the unique chemical nature of each crude oil source, chromatograms or fingerprints from GI content and tissue analyses can be matched with those from different potential sources of exposure to assist in confirming the origin of exposure.[3]

Drilling fluids are used to facilitate the drilling of oil wells and serve several purposes, including clearing the bore hole of debris, lubrication, and maintenance of the drill hole wall.[4] Drilling fluids are liquids that contain suspended solids. The liquids used include fresh or salt water, a water-oil emulsion, or oil. The suspended solids are mixtures of clays and barite (barium sulfate). Various chemicals are added to drilling fluids to change their physical and chemical properties depending on specific needs. Additives are numerous and range from pulverized hard nut shells to organophosphate (OP) radicals. In addition to containing various chemical components, drilling fluids can be highly acidic or alkaline.[3,4]

Livestock exposure to drilling fluids can result in acid or alkaline burns. The toxicity of drilling fluids and the clinical sequelae after their ingestion can vary due to their chemical complexity. Intoxications have been attributed to caustic soda, arsenic, zinc chromate, and organic acids.[3] The potential for residues varies depending on the specific chemical composition of the fluids; there is likely an increased chance of harmful residues if certain metals are ingested.

Although proximity of livestock to oil or other petroleum hydrocarbon production facilities is a well-recognized hazard, exposure to petroleum products stored on farms can also present hazards. In one case, a herd of 1600 Angus beef cattle were placed in a new paddock that contained diesel fuel tanks surrounded by a low concrete barrier filled with rainwater.[6] Animals reaching for the water broke a fuel line, allowing diesel fuel to contaminate the water source. Eighteen animals were found dead with a strong diesel odor, froth exuding from the nose and mouth, and severe, diffuse pulmonary hemorrhage noted on postmortem examination. Affected animals had histologic lesions consistent with inhalation or aspiration pneumonia. The diesel fuel separated into an upper layer within the water source, which was apparently readily consumed by some individuals. In another case, kerosene intoxication of grazing dairy heifers occurred as a result of contamination of a stream serving as a water source for the animals.[7] The contamination was believed to have originated from an upstream airfield. These cases provide evidence that ruminants (eg, cattle, sheep, and goats) voluntarily ingest petroleum hydrocarbons, such as diesel fuel or kerosene.

Because crude oil and petroleum products contain compounds suspected of being human carcinogens, meat or milk from exposed animals should not be used for human consumption. Also, the possibility exists that rumen microflora metabolize chemicals found in crude oil or petroleum products to form carcinogenic metabolites. A concentration of total petroleum hydrocarbons as crude oil in drinking water for cattle that does not result in a meat concentration exceeding a human health-based safe consumption level has been determined to be 1120 mg/L (1120 ppm).[8] This is above a concentration of total petroleum hydrocarbons in water for cattle that does not cause an adverse health effect (355 mg/L, or 355 ppm). Thus, meat concentrations of concern most likely are associated with clinically affected cattle. Any petroleum hydrocarbon concentration detected in milk likely results in the milk considered adulterated.

MINING AND SMELTING

Lead

Lead is a nonessential, highly toxic heavy metal that is ubiquitous in the environment. It is widely used in batteries, solder, pigments, piping, ammunition, paints, ceramics, and caulking.[9] Lead is one of the easiest metals to mine and smelting requires only moderate temperatures. Most anthropogenic emissions of lead occur as a result of mining, smelting, and refining of lead and other metal ores; vehicle emissions; and industrial emissions resulting from the production, use, recycling, and disposal of lead-containing products.

Currently, the most common sources of exposure of livestock to lead are from ingestion of lead plates found in storage batteries and lead-based paint or grazing of pastures contaminated by lead mine tailings. The ingestion of lead-contaminated motor oil is much less likely to occur now than in the past because lead has been removed from gasoline. Accidental releases of lead from industrial and other point sources can result in significant water contamination, and local soil contamination can occur around storage battery reclamation plants, near mines, and around older buildings where leaded paint has been used and is flaking or has been sanded or scraped. One source of exposure of cattle to lead occurred when rice bran became contaminated with zinc ore during its shipment; one sample of finished feed incorporating the contaminated rice bran contained almost 2200 ppm lead (expressed on a dry weight basis).[10] More than 1800 farms and 50,000 dairy cows were exposed.

Clinical signs associated with the diagnosis of lead intoxication are well described and are not discussed in this article. Once a diagnosis of lead intoxication is made, however, the source of exposure should be determined and, if people are likely to be exposed, it should be suggested that they are examined and tested by their physicians.

Because of the toxicity of very low levels of lead to people, especially children, there is justifiable concern about residues of lead in animal products intended for human consumption. Some states quarantine animals exposed to lead until tissue concentrations fall below levels of concern as determined by testing of whole blood samples. Lead accumulates in tissues, such as liver, kidney, and bone, but muscle and milk accumulate little. Thus, in reality, there is little reason to be concerned about significant lead exposure to humans from lead-intoxicated animals as long as their blood lead levels are normal. In addition, although blood lead concentrations rise in periparturient animals previously exposed to lead due to mobilization of lead from bone storage, there is no detectable rise in milk lead concentrations.[11]

Fluoride

Fluorine in a free form is uncommon in nature; it is most commonly found combined with another element, such as aluminum, calcium, or potassium, among others, to form a salt or fluoride. Fluorides are widely distributed in the environment. Although the essentiality of fluorine is unclear, it seems necessary for normal tooth development, and fluorides are added to most human drinking water to prevent dental caries.[12] Fluorides are emitted from industrial plants processing fluoride-containing raw materials, such as bauxite or phosphate rock; are found in rock phosphate used for livestock mineral supplementation or as fertilizer; and can be found in high concentrations in water obtained from deep wells and geothermal springs in certain geographic regions of the United States.[13,14] Fluoride exposure is most often from a localized source and most intoxications have been associated with ingestion of contaminated forages due to airborne emissions from industrial facilities. Current limits on industrial emissions of fluorides and removal of fluorine during the processing of rock phosphate intended for livestock mineral supplementation minimize exposure from these sources. Although fluorosis is not common, cases or alleged cases involving various animal species occur occasionally.[15,16]

Fluoride toxicosis can be either acute or chronic.[13,17] Acute toxicosis is uncommon and is generally associated with ingestion of sodium fluoroacetate or sodium fluorosilicate (rodenticides), sodium fluoride, or feeds with very high fluoride concentrations.[13] Chronic fluorosis is more common and is a slowly progressive, debilitating disease, primarily of herbivores, that involves teeth and bones. The toxicity of fluoride is dependent on several factors, including amount, duration, and timing of ingestion; form ingested; species, age, and nutritional and health status of the animal exposed; and normal biologic variation within a group of animals.[17]

In chronic fluorosis, fluoride damages ameloblasts and odontoblasts necessary for normal tooth development. Matrix laid down by the damaged cells does not mineralize normally. In bone, fluoride disrupts osteoblastic activity resulting in defective matrix formation and subsequent mineralization.

Acute fluorosis, resulting from the accidental ingestion of very high concentrations of fluoride-containing compounds, is generally manifested as excitement, clonic convulsions, urine and fecal incontinence, stiffness, weakness, salivation, emesis, depression, cardiovascular collapse, and death.[13,17] Chronic fluorosis is insidious and can be confused with other chronic debilitating diseases, such as osteoarthritis and degenerative joint disease. In chronic fluorosis, months to years may pass between the beginning of exposure to excessive fluoride and clinical manifestations of toxicosis.

Animals ingesting sufficient fluoride at the time of permanent tooth development exhibit tooth mottling, brown staining or discoloration (chalky white or creamy yellow to brownish black), hypoplasia, pitting and loss of enamel with exposure of dentine, and increased and uneven wear.[13,17] Excessive tooth involvement secondarily results in difficult mastication, decreased feed intake, slow growth or poor performance, and signs associated with dental pain, such as lapping of water. Once teeth have calcified and erupted, fluoride ingestion has little to no effect on them. Bone lesions of chronic fluorosis are manifested grossly as hyperostotic, chalky-white lesions. Lesions can occur at any age. Therefore, depending on the age at which exposure occurs, an animal may have both dental and bone lesions or only bone lesions. Bone lesions are generally bilateral and symmetric and appear first on the medial surfaces of the proximal one-third of the metatarsal bones. As the condition progresses, the mandible, metacarpals, and ribs become involved. Bone involvement results in characteristic, intermittent lameness.

Long-term dietary fluoride tolerances have been established for various livestock species based primarily on controlled feeding trials. Dairy or beef heifers are the most sensitive category of livestock and have the lowest tolerance whereas poultry are the least sensitive.[17] There is some controversy with regard to established tolerances. Some investigators believe that current tolerances are too high to protect animal health.[18]

Most soft tissues do not accumulate fluoride, even during high intakes. Kidney, however, usually exhibits elevated fluoride concentrations during high intakes due to excretion of fluoride in urine. Milk fluoride concentrations are affected only minimally by dietary intake. Thus, there is unlikely to be significant human health concern about ingestion of meat or milk from affected animals.

Barium

Barium intoxication has been documented in range cattle driven through an old lead, silver, and zinc mine.[19] Clinical signs included protruding tongues, hypersalivation, mild muscle tremors, hypermotility of the rumen, watery mucoid diarrhea, tachycardia, and tachypnea. High concentrations of barium were found in serum, liver, and kidney samples from affected animals; all other metal concentrations were within acceptable ranges. The source of barium was determined to be a clay-like material found in the abomasums of dead animals and which was also found in a tailings pond to which the animals had access. The material contained high concentrations of barium. There are several barium salts (eg, acetate, carbonate, chloride, nitrate, and sulfide), all of which are considered highly toxic. Only barium sulfate is relatively nontoxic. Barium causes direct stimulation of smooth, striated, and cardiac muscle and blockage of potassium channels leads to severe hypokalemia. There are no characteristic gross or microscopic lesions noted on postmortem examination and a diagnosis of intoxication relies on tissue and environmental (eg, feed, water, or other potential sources) testing.

AGRICULTURE

Pesticides

There are a variety of pesticides in the farm environment to which livestock can be exposed, including herbicides, insecticides, fungicides, and fertilizers. Most herbicides, fungicides, and fertilizers have low toxicity and are not discussed further. Many OP and carbamate insecticides, often collectively referred to as cholinesterase-inhibiting insecticides due to their common mode of action, however, pose a significant hazard because of their extreme toxicity. Most problems occur when farm chemicals are not stored properly or are accidentally incorporated into livestock feed.

Chlorinated Insecticides

Chlorinated insecticides include dichlorodiphenyltrichloroethane (DDT), dieldrin, aldrin, endrin, chlordane, toxaphene, endrin, heptachlor, methoxychlor, and lindane. Most are no longer used in developed countries because of their environmental persistence, devastating effects on certain wildlife species, and development of insect resistance. They are still used, however, in many underdeveloped countries and are ubiquitous environmental contaminants. There have been few documented cases of livestock intoxication in recent years due to their unavailability, although there are occasional unpublished cases where livestock have been exposed to old containers of insecticide and intoxicate themselves.

Perhaps of more concern than acute intoxication is the possibility of contamination of meat, milk, and eggs with residue levels above current tolerances. Because of the long half-lives of these insecticides, decontamination after exposure can take a prolonged amount of time and cause considerable economic impact.[20]

Organophosphate and Carbamate Insecticides

OP and carbamate insecticides are still widely used in the farm environment. They can be applied by the dermal route or orally administered to livestock or applied to soils and crops for pest control. Those that are applied to animals directly are much less toxic than those applied to crops. For example, chlorpyrifos, used by dermal application to cattle, has a rat oral median lethal dose (LD_{50}) of 96 to 270 mg/kg whereas fonofos, an insecticide incorporated into soil, has a rat oral LD_{50} of 8 to 17.6 mg/kg.[21] Some OP and carbamate insecticide uses or formulations have been banned due to potential for intoxicating animals. For example, granular diazinon and carbofuran use has been curtailed due to concern about wildlife intoxications. Acute intoxication of livestock still occurs, most often through accidental incorporation of the chemicals into feed or misuse on animals.

As the name cholinesterase implies, these insecticides inhibit cholinesterase enzymes. Specifically, when acetylcholinesterase enzyme is inhibited, the neurotransmitter acetylcholine accumulates within synapses, resulting in continued stimulation of muscarinic and nicotinic postsynaptic receptors. The clinical signs and diagnosis of intoxication have been extensively discussed elsewhere.[22,23]

Unlike the chlorinated insecticides, OPs and carbamates are rapidly metabolized and generally do not cause persistent residues in meat, milk, or eggs. Those intended for use on livestock have recommended withdrawal times on product labels. When products are used in an extralabel manner or accidental exposures occur, there are no established withdrawal times. Dermal application of OPs to livestock can persist for extended periods on hair or in skin and subcutaneous fat depots.[24]

It is likely that with the development of safer insecticides, such as pyrethroids or insect growth regulators, availability of genetically engineered, insect-resistant crops, and introduction of integrated pest management techniques, the more toxic OP and carbamate insecticides are used less frequently in the future and, therefore, pose less of a hazard to livestock and wildlife.

Grain Fumigants

Currently, only three fumigants are labeled for use in stored grain: phosphine, chloropicrin, and methyl bromide. Each of these products has special limitations and restrictions governing its use.

Chloropicrin

Chloropicrin is still registered for grain fumigation as well as empty bin fumigation to combat insect infestations. It is especially useful for the control of insects in the subfloor aeration area of empty bins. Chloropicrin has also been used as a soil fumigant and as a riot control agent and is classified as a lacrimator.[25] Undiluted chloropicrin is severely and immediately irritating to the upper respiratory tract, eyes, and skin on direct contact. In humans, exposure to airborne concentrations of chloropicrin exceeding 0.15 ppm (1 mg/m^3) can cause tearing and eye irritation, which is reversible on termination of exposure.[26] Prolonged inhalation exposures at airborne concentrations above 1 ppm may cause symptoms of respiratory system damage, including irritation of the airways, shortness of breath and/or tightness in chest, and difficulty in breathing. Inhalation exposure to very high levels, even if brief, can lead to pulmonary edema, unconsciousness, and even death. No documented cases of chloropicrin intoxication of livestock were identified.

Methyl bromide (bromomethane)

Methyl bromide is an effective grain fumigant for the control of stored grain insects at all stages of development. It evolves into a gas at temperatures above 39°F and has virtually no odor or irritating qualities to indicate its presence. Because methyl bromide is a gas at ambient temperatures, the most significant route of exposure is via inhalation.[27] Methyl bromide can be highly irritating on contact to the mucous membranes of the eyes and airways and to skin. Approximately 1000 human poisoning incidents caused by methyl bromide exposure have been documented, with effects ranging from skin and eye irritation to death. Most fatalities and injuries occurred when methyl bromide was used as a fumigant. The lowest inhalation level found to cause toxicity in humans is 0.14 mg/L in air. The use of methyl bromide has been or is being phased out in many regions, but in the United States there remain some critical use exceptions. No documented cases of methyl bromide intoxication of livestock were identified.

Aluminum phosphide

Phosphine-producing materials (primarily aluminum phosphide) have become the predominant fumigants used for the treatment of bulk-stored grain throughout the world. Zinc phosphide is used primarily as a rodenticide and is likely of less concern to livestock. Fumigant phosphides are available in solid formulations of aluminum phosphide or magnesium phosphide. When exposed to heat and moisture, the formulations release phosphine, a highly toxic gas. The time required for release of phosphine varies with temperature, grain moisture, and formulation. Phosphine gas is heavier than air and has a distinct odor that has been described as similar to rotten fish or acetylene. Intoxication can occur via ingestion of solid formulations or via inhalation of phosphine gas. Documented instances of livestock intoxication from phosphides have involved the contamination of feed with aluminum phosphide.[28,29]

Intoxication is believed, in part, due to inhibition of oxidative phosphorylation.[30] Peroxidation of cell membranes and other cellular oxidative damage might also occur and contribute to disease pathogenesis. An acute oral LD_{50} of zinc phosphide for ruminants is reportedly 60 mg/kg body weight; presumably, toxic dosages of the other phosphides are similar.[30]

Clinical signs in ruminants can include rumen tympany and bloat followed by ataxia, weakness, recumbence, hypoxia, and struggling. Central nervous system stimulation, characterized by hyperesthesia and seizures, might also be noted. Acidosis, circulatory shock, and liver damage are possible as well. Intoxication by phosphine does not cause any characteristic postmortem lesions. A diagnosis relies on a history of exposure and the detection of phosphine in GI contents or tissues, such as liver and kidney. Due to the rapid hydrolysis of aluminum or zinc phosphide, along with rapid dissipation of phosphine gas once formed, samples should be placed in airtight containers and kept frozen when shipped to a diagnostic laboratory for testing.

There is no specific antidote or therapeutic regimen to treat intoxication. Appropriate decontamination procedures, such as administration of activated charcoal and a cathartic, might be useful if instituted early after exposure. Otherwise, symptomatic and supportive care is provided as needed.

Fertilizers

Fertilizers are soil amendments used to promote plant growth. The three primary macronutrients in fertilizers are nitrogen, phosphorus, and potassium. Secondary macronutrients in fertilizers are calcium, sulfur, and magnesium. Fertilizers can also contain several micronutrients, including boron, chlorine, manganese, iron, zinc, copper, molybdenum, and selenium. Fertilizers are available in various forms, including granular and liquid forms. Fertilizers can be broadly categorized as inorganic or organic. Inorganic fertilizers are composed of synthetic chemicals and minerals, whereas organic fertilizers are composed of plant or animal organic matter. Examples of synthetic agricultural fertilizers are granular triple superphosphate, potassium chloride, urea, and anhydrous ammonia.

Toxicosis from phosphorus is rare in food-producing animals.[31] Phosphates are readily excreted via the urine and animals tolerate a wide range of phosphorus intakes, particularly if diets are appropriately balanced with calcium. Phosphorus intoxication is associated with metabolic disorders of calcium absorption and function (ie, hypocalcemia).[31] The maximum tolerable level of dietary phosphorus for cattle is 0.7% (expressed on a dry matter basis). Likewise, potassium toxicosis in healthy animals is rare due to the ability of the body to readily excrete the mineral. Potassium toxicosis is associated with potentially fatal arrhythmias. A conservative safe maximum tolerable level for ruminants is 20,000 mg/kg.[32]

Urea intoxication of ruminants is well described in the veterinary literature and is not discussed in this article. Another common nitrogen source, anhydrous ammonia, is a clear, colorless gas at standard temperature and pressure conditions and has a characteristic odor. The odor is the strongest safety feature of the product. At a concentration of only 50 ppm, it is readily identified. Normally, the odor at that concentration drives a person away from the area. Anhydrous ammonia combines with moisture in mucous membranes of the mouth, respiratory tract, and cornea to form ammonium hydroxide, a strong alkaline caustic. At concentrations greater than 5000 ppm, people become incapacitated such that escape is impossible and suffocation results.

Intoxication of cattle unable to escape exposure has been documented. In one case, 72 dairy cows and replacement heifers died acutely after they were exposed to anhydrous ammonia leaking from a nurse tank.[33] Most animals died within several minutes of exposure. Animals surviving the acute exposure developed red and peeling skin on the nose and udder, severe damage to the respiratory tract resulting in dyspnea and copious nasal discharge, and corneal opacity. Several animals died up to 4 weeks after exposure due to bacterial pulmonary infections, which were believed secondary to extensive epithelial damage to the respiratory tract.

CONSTRUCTION MATERIALS

Wood Preservatives

Chromated copper arsenate

CCA is a chemical wood preservative containing chromium, copper, and arsenic. CCA is used in pressure treated wood to protect wood from rotting due to insects and microbial agents. The United States Environmental Protection Agency has classified CCA as a restricted use product, for use only by certified pesticide applicators. CCA has been used to pressure treat lumber since the 1940s. Since the 1970s, the majority of the wood used in outdoor residential settings has been CCA-treated wood. Pressure-treated wood containing CCA is no longer produced for use in most residential settings. CCA-treated wood can still be used by animal production facilities, however, and is not considered hazardous when used in structures to house animals. The greatest risk to ruminants occurs after exposure to ashes from burning treated wood, which serves to concentrate arsenic in the ashes.[34] Cattle, especially if salt deprived, readily ingest the ashes due to a salty taste.

Arsenic intoxication is typically acute with major affects on the GI and cardiovascular systems.[35] Arsenic has a direct damaging effect on capillaries, which leads to transudation of plasma, hemorrhage, and circulatory shock. Signs include severe watery and hemorrhagic diarrhea, severe colic, dehydration, weakness, depression, and a weak pulse. Postmortem lesions include necrosis of epithelial and subepithelial tissues along the GI tract and diffuse inflammation of the liver, kidneys, and other visceral organs. Fatty degeneration and necrosis can be noted in the liver and tubular damage is noted in the kidneys. Diagnosis of arsenic intoxication requires analysis of whole blood or urine sample ante mortem or liver and kidney samples postmortem. Analysis of potential sources of exposure is recommended as well.

Treatment of affected animals is largely symptomatic and supportive with particular attention paid to fluid replacement and cardiovascular support. Although dimercaprol is used to chelate arsenic, its efficacy in large animals when used alone is questionable. The water-soluble analog of dimercaprol, succimer, is less toxic and more effective, but its use in ruminants is cost prohibitive. D-Penicillamine is also an arsenic chelator that has been used successfully in people.

Pentachlorophenol

The use of pentachlorophenol as a wood preservative was cancelled in 1986. Because of its toxicity, agricultural and residential use is prohibited. Pentachlorophenol can be absorbed through the skin and lungs and is irritating to skin and mucous membranes. Animals fed in troughs made from lumber treated with pentachlorophenol salivate and have irritated oral mucosa.[36] Inhalation of pentachlorophenol from enclosed animal holding areas has caused illness and death. Acutely toxic doses are reported to range from 27 to 350 mg/kg.[36]

Once absorbed, pentachlorophenol uncouples oxidative phosphorylation. Clinical signs of intoxication include nervousness, tachycardia, tachypnea, weakness, muscle tremors, fever, and convulsions, followed by death. Chronic exposure results in fatty liver, nephrosis, and weight loss. A diagnosis of intoxication relies on a history of exposure, occurrence of compatible clinical signs, and, in some cases, identification of pentachlorophenol in source materials or biologic samples.

There is no specific treatment for pentachlorophenol intoxication. Termination of exposure, dermal decontamination, administration of activated charcoal, and symptomatic and supportive care are recommended. Possible violative meat and milk residues can occur with exposure.

Creosote

The distillation of coal tar results in the production of cresols (phenolic compounds), crude creosote (cresols, heavy oils, and anthracene), and pitch. Cresols can be used as disinfectants whereas creosote has been used as a wood preservative. Exposure of ruminants to creosote is most often due to ingestion of a product or treated material in contrast to exposure via food or water contamination. Phenol is the most toxic chemical in coal tar products with an approximate acute oral LD_{50} for most species of 0.5 g/kg. The LD of creosote in calves is reported to be 4 g/kg.[37]

There is no specific treatment for phenol intoxication. Appropriate decontamination and symptomatic and supportive care are recommended.

IRRIGATION

In many areas of the western United States, irrigation wastewater can accumulate in confined shallow aquifers. If not drained away, the accumulated wastewater rises to levels that adversely affect crop production. Systems for the drainage and disposal of the wastewater have been constructed and in many areas the water is either discharged directly into surface aquatic systems or to evaporation ponds. Irrigation drainage water can contain several chemicals that are either applied to crops or leached from native soils. The most troublesome leachate in many irrigated areas is selenium. The concentration of selenium in evaporation ponds in the San Joaquin Valley in southern California and its subsequent bioaccumulation in aquatic food chains resulted in substantial aquatic bird mortality in the early 1980s.[38] To prevent further wildlife mortality, the ponds were filled and the area converted into grassland habitat.[39] Although there has been no documented livestock morbidity or mortality from ingestion of selenium from irrigation sources, the possibility exists that animals could be chronically exposed to elevated selenium in water or pasture plants, resulting in chronic selenosis.

POLYCHLORINATED BIPHENYLS, POLYBROMINATED BIPHENYLS, DIOXINS, AND FURANS

Polychlorinated biphenyls (PCBs), polybrominated biphenyls (PBBs), dioxins, and furans belong to a group of related chemical compounds widely distributed in the environment. They are not single compounds but each group includes several chemically similar compounds, or congeners. For example, there are 209 different congeners of PCBs. Not all of the congeners within each group are toxic; only 30 of the 209 PCBs are considered toxic.

PCBs and PBBs were used in many commercial applications due to their inertness; they resist acids and alkalis, they have low dielectric constants and are thermally stable. PCBs were used as heat exchange and hydraulic fluids, lubricants, dielectric fluids in transformers and capacitors, and plasticizers in applications where flame resistance was important. PCBs and PBBs are no longer manufactured in the United States although they continue to be manufactured and used in other countries. Unfortunately, due to their environmental persistence and wide atmospheric distribution, PCBs are now ubiquitous and found throughout the world. PCBs serve as an example of a class of compound that can still be of concern in the United States due to their widespread distribution even though they are no longer manufactured in this country.

Widespread exposure of food animals to PBBs occurred in the mid-1970s as a result of contamination of feed with a fire retardant when it was confused with a similarly packaged feed supplement, magnesium oxide.[40] Dairy cattle, pigs, sheep, and chickens were exposed. More recently, Belgian livestock were exposed to PCBs and dioxins as a result of contaminated fat being incorporated into livestock feed. In the United States, poultry and catfish were found contaminated with dioxins; the ultimate source was determined to be ball clay used as an anticaking agent for soybean meal.[40]

In contrast to PCBs and PBBs, dioxins and furans have no commercial use. The most infamous of these compounds is 2,3,7,8-tetrachlorodibenzodioxin (TCDD). TCDD is one of the most toxic compounds yet encountered.[41] Dioxins and furans have been released into the environment primarily as contaminants of chemical and combustion processes. With the exception of the dioxin-contaminated clay from a site in Mississippi, they are not known to occur naturally.

The mechanisms of toxic action of these compounds have not been clearly established, but clinical affects are multiple. Toxic congeners bind a cytosolic receptor, called the Ah receptor, which in turn affects gene regulation.[41] The Ah receptor is found in a variety of species and is expressed in multiple tissues. Ah receptor binding and subsequent induction of aryl hydrocarbon hydroxylase activity and other cytochrome P450-dependent enzymes affect the metabolism of steroids and other hormones. Toxic effects can be manifested in several organ systems, including the immune, reproductive, and nervous systems. These compounds are also teratogenic and have tumor-promoting effects.

These chemicals are either not considered very toxic (PCBs and PBBs) or are quite toxic but present at extremely low concentrations (TCDD). Thus, acute intoxications are unusual. Animal and human health effects after chronic exposure, however, are well documented. Dairy cattle exposed to PBBs in Michigan exhibited many nonspecific clinical signs, such as unthriftiness, decreased milk production, abscesses, abnormal hoof growth, and decreased appetite.[40] A wasting syndrome is well described in several animal species.[40,41] In Missouri, horses unintentionally exposed to TCDD-contaminated oil exhibited a progressive deterioration in health including anorexia, listlessness, loss of body weight and emaciation, dermatitis, weakness, an unsteady gait, and chronic cough.[42] There is a case report of dioxin intoxication of horses after chronic exposure to pentachlorophenol-contaminated wood shavings.[43]

Residues are a major concern with these chemicals. They are extremely lipophilic and resistant to metabolic transformation. Once ingested, they have long half-lives; the estimated half-life of PBBs in human serum is 10.8 years.[40] Because of their lipophilicity, they are found in muscle and milk fat and egg yolks. Tolerances have been established for PCBs in foods and feed ranging from 0.2 ppm for finished feed for food-producing animals and human infant and junior foods to 10 ppm for paper food-packaging material.[40] No safe level, tolerance, or action level has been established for dioxins or furans in animal feed, feed components or food, although an interim level of concern for TCDD of 1 part per trillion was established for catfish, eggs, and poultry exposed to dioxin-contaminated ball clay. The extremely low tolerance set for TCDD compared with that for PCBs reflects its much greater toxicity.

ETHYLENE GLYCOL

There is one case report of ethylene glycol (EG) intoxication of a calf.[44] Oxalate crystalluria is often found in ruminant urine or kidney tissue due to exposure to soluble oxalate-containing plants, such as *Sarcobatus vermiculatus* (greasewood), *Halogeton glomeratus* (halogeton), *Rumex* spp (dock), *Amaranthus* spp (pigweed), and *Oxalis* spp, among others.[45] Because both EG and soluble oxalate-containing plants might be present in a ruminant environment, they should be considered in cases of acute renal failure. Clinical signs in cattle include dyspnea, incoordination, paraparesis, recumbence, and hypocalcemia. A toxic dose for adult cattle and nonruminating calves is reported to be 5 to 10 mL/kg body weight and 2 mL/kg body weight, respectively.[44]

Tests are readily available for the identification of EG in antemortem or postmortem samples to help differentiate between the two, although the rapid metabolism of EG might result in failure to detect the toxicant in biologic samples. Laboratory indicators of EG poisoning include hypocalcemia, acidosis, elevated EG blood levels, positive urine oxalate crystals, and renal oxalosis detected by histopathology.

If a diagnosis of EG exposure or intoxication is made soon after ingestion, ethanol or fomepizole is antidotal, although the use of fomepizole is most likely cost prohibitive in food production animals. Additional treatment involves correction of acid-base imbalances and attempting to maintain urine flow; other therapeutic interventions are symptomatic and supportive.

REFERENCES

1. Radostits OM, Gay CC, Hinchcliff KW, et al. Disturbances of appetite, food intake and nutritional status. In: Veterinary medicine: a textbook of the diseases of cattle, horses, sheep, pigs and goats. 10th edition. Edinburgh (UK): Saunders Elsevier; 2007. p. 112–4.
2. Talcott PA, Haldorson GJ, Sathre P. Chromium poisoning in a group of dairy cows. In: 48th Annual Conference Proceedings of the American Association of Veterinary Laboratory Diagnosticians. Hershey (PA); 2005. p. 45.
3. Edwards WC, Coppock RW, Zinn LL. Toxicoses related to the petroleum industry. Vet Hum Toxicol 1979;21:328–37.
4. Edwards WC. Toxicology of oil field wastes: hazards to livestock associated with the petroleum industry. Vet Clin North Am Food Anim Pract 1989;5: 363–74.
5. Osweiler GD, Carson TL, Buck WB, et al. Crude oils, fuel oils and kerosene. In: Clinical and diagnostic veterinary toxicology. Dubuque (IA): Kendall-Hunt; 1985. p. 177–8.
6. Gailbreath KL, Talcott PA, Baszler TV. Fibrinosuppurative pneumonitis associated with diesel ingestion in a herd of beef cattle. In: 52nd Annual Conference Proceedings of the American Association of Veterinary Laboratory Diagnosticians. San Diego (CA); 2009. p. 60.
7. Barber DM, Cousin DA, Seawright D. An episode of kerosene poisoning in dairy heifers. Vet Rec 1987;120:462.
8. Ryer-Powder J, Scofield R, Lapierre A, et al. Determination of safe levels of total petroleum hydrocarbons as crude oil in cattle's drinking water and in meat from cattle. In: Proceedings of the Petroleum Hydrocarbons and Organic Chemicals in Ground Water: Prevention, Detection and Remediation Conference. Westerville (OH): Ground Water Publishing; 1996. p. 99–109.
9. Keogh JP, Boyer LV. Lead. In: Sullivan JB, Kreiger GR, editors. Clinical environmental health and toxic exposures. Baltimore (MD): Lppincott, Williams and Wilkins; 2001. p. 879–88.
10. Allen WM. Environmental accidents: the assessment of the significance of an environmental accident due to the feeding of lead-contaminated feedstuffs to several hundred cattle farms. Bovine PR 1999;33:76–9.
11. Galey FD, Slenning BD, Anderson ML, et al. Lead concentrations in blood and milk from periparturient diary heifers seven months after an episode of acute lead toxicosis. J Vet Diagn Invest 1990;2:222.
12. National Academy of Sciences. Fluorine. In: Mineral tolerance of domestic animals. Washington, DC: National Academy of Sciences; 2005. p. 154–81.
13. Osweiler GD, Carson TL, Buck WB, et al. Fluoride. In: Clinical and diagnostic veterinary toxicology. Dubuque (IA): Kendall-Hunt; 1985. p. 183–8.
14. Shupe JL, Olson AE, Peterson HB, et al. Fluoride toxicosis in wild ungulates. J Am Vet Med Assoc 1984;185:1295–300.
15. Botha CJ, Naude TW, Minnaar PP, et al. Two outbreaks of fluorosis in cattle and sheep. J S Afr Vet Assoc 1993;64:165–8.
16. Jubb TF, Annand TE, Main DC, et al. Phosphorus supplements and fluorosis in cattle—a northern Australian experience. Aust Vet J 1993;70:379–83.
17. Shupe JL. Clinicopathologic features of fluoride toxicosis in cattle. J Anim Sci 1980;51:746–58.
18. Crissman JW, Maylin GA, Krook L. New York State and U.S. federal fluoride pollution standards do not protect cattle health. Cornell Vet 1980;70:183.

19. Richards T, Erickson DL, Talcott PA, et al. Two cases of barium poisoning in cattle. In: 49th Annual Conference Proceedings of the American Association of Veterinary Laboratory Diagnosticians. Minneapolis (MN); 2006. p. 155.
20. Raisbeck MF, Kendall JD, Rottinghaus GE. Organochlorine insecticide problems in livestock. Vet Clin North Am Food Anim Pract 1989;5:391.
21. Crop protection handbook. Willoughby (OH): Meister Publishing; 2005. p. 85, 204.
22. Meerdinck GL. Anticholinesterase insecticides. In: Plumlee KH, editor. Clinical veterinary toxicology. St Louis (MO): Mosby; 2004. p.178–80.
23. Meerdink GL. Organophosphorous and carbamate insecticide poisoning in large animals. Vet Clin North Am Food Anim Pract 1989;5:375.
24. Henny CJ, Blus LJ, Kolbe EJ, et al. Organophosphate insecticide (famphur) topically applied to cattle kills magpies and hawks. J Wildl Manag 1985;49:648.
25. Suchard JR. Chemical weapons. In: Flomenbaum NE, Howland MA, Goldfrank LR, et al, editors. Goldfrank's toxicologic emergencies. 8th edition. New York: McGraw-Hill; 2006. p. 1775–91.
26. EXTOXNET. Available at: http://extoxnet.orst.edu/pips/chloropi.htm. Accessed December 15, 2010.
27. EXTOXNET. Available at: http://extoxnet.orst.edu/pips/methylbr.htm. Accessed December 15, 2010.
28. Easterwood L, Chaffin MK, Marsh PS, et al. Phosphine intoxication following oral exposure of horses to aluminum phosphide-treated feed. J Am Vet Med Assoc 2010;236:446.
29. Morgan S, Niles GA, Edwards WC. Case report: phosphine gas detected in the rumen content of dead calves. Bovine Practitioner 2000;34:127.
30. Albretson JC. Zinc phosphide. In: Plumlee KH, editor. Clinical veterinary toxicology. St Louis (MO): Mosby; 2004. p. 456–8.
31. National Academy of Sciences. Phosphorus. In: Mineral tolerance of domestic animals. Washington, (DC): National Academy of Sciences; 2005. p. 290.
32. National Academy of Sciences. Potassium. In: Mineral tolerance of domestic animals. Washington, (DC): National Academy of Sciences; 2005. p. 306.
33. Carson TL, Till DJ, Quinn WJ, et al. Anhydrous ammonia fertilizer poisoning in cattle: peracute death loss and sequelae. In: 39th Annual Conference Proceedings of the American Association of Veterinary Laboratory Diagnosticians. Little Rock (AR); 1996. p. 66.
34. Hullinger G, Sangster L, Colvin B, et al. Bovine arsenic toxicosis from ingestion of ashed copper-chrome-arsenate treated lumber. Vet Hum Toxicol 1998;40:147–8.
35. Merck Veterinary Manual. Arsenic. In: Kahn CM, editor. Merck veterinary manual. 9th edition. Whitehouse Station (NJ): Merck & Co; 2005. p. 2346–8.
36. Merck Veterinary Manual. Pentachlorophenol poisoning. In: Merck veterinary manual. 9th edition. Whitehouse Station (NJ): Merck & Co; 2005. p. 2429.
37. Merck Veterinary Manual. Coal-tar poisoning. In: Merck veterinary manual. 9th edition. Whitehouse Station (NJ): Merck & Co; 2005. p. 2352–3.
38. Ohlendorf HM. Bioaccumulation and effects of selenium in wildlife. In: Selenium in agriculture and the environment. Madison (WI): Soil Science Society Special Publication No. 23; 1989. p. 133–77.
39. Clemings R. Of drainage and baby ducks. In: Mirage: the false promise of desert agriculture. San Francisco (CA): Sierra Club Books; 1996. p. 51.
40. Headrick ML, Hollinger K, Lovell RA, et al. PBBs, PCBs, and dioxins in food animals, their public health implications. Vet Clin North Am Food Anim Pract 1999;15:109–32.

41. Koss G, Wolfle D. Dioxin and dioxin-like polychlorinated hydrocarbons and biphenyls. In: Marquardt H, Schafer SG, McClellan R, et al, editors. Toxicology. San Diego (CA): Academic Press; 1999. p. 699–728.
42. Case AA, Coffman JR. Waste oil: toxic for horses. Vet Clin North Am 1973;3:273.
43. Kerkvliet NI, Wagner SL, Schmotzer WB, et al. Dioxin intoxication from chronic exposure to pentachlorophenol-contaminated wood shavings. J Am Vet Med Assoc 1992;201:296.
44. Crowell WA, Whitlock RH, Stout RC, et al. Ethylene glycol toxicosis in cattle. Cornell Vet 1979;69:272.
45. Knight AP, Walter RG. Plants causing kidney failure. In: A guide to plant poisoning of animals in North America. Jackson (WY): Teton New Media; 2001. p. 263–77.

Safety of Antibiotic Drugs in Food Animals: Comparison of Findings from Preapproval Studies and Postapproval Experience in the United States with Safety Information in Published Literature

Tomislav Modric, DVM, PhD[a,*], Sanja Modric, DVM, PhD[b], Michael J. Murphy, DVM, JD, PhD[a], Susan J. Bright, DVM[a], Stacey Shults, DVM[a]

KEYWORDS

- Antibiotic drugs • Safety • Adverse events • Toxic
- Food animals

Antibiotic drugs are among the most widely prescribed drugs in both human and veterinary medicine. Based on many years of use and experience, they are generally considered safe and of tremendous benefit to both human and animal health. Their safety record is based at least in part on the fact that antimicrobial drugs target microbes, rather than the host species. Because the microbial targets are generally different from the host species, toxicity for the host species at therapeutic doses is

---

The authors have nothing to disclose.
[a] Office of Surveillance and Compliance, FDA Center for Veterinary Medicine (CVM), 7519 Standish Place, Rockville, MD 20855, USA
[b] Office of New Animal Drug Evaluation, FDA CVM, 7500 Standish Place, Rockville, MD 20855, USA
* Corresponding author.
E-mail address: tomislav.modric@fda.hhs.gov

Vet Clin Food Anim 27 (2011) 389–405
doi:10.1016/j.cvfa.2011.02.005
0749-0720/11/$ – see front matter. Published by Elsevier Inc.

not expected. However, antimicrobials may exert various adverse toxicologic effects in target animals (animal species/class for which the animal drug is intended and approved for use), some of which have been described in the literature.

The Center for Veterinary Medicine (CVM) within the Food and Drug Administration (FDA) ensures that animal drugs approved for use in food animals are effective and safe for the animals, the environment, and for humans consuming edible products derived from animals treated with these drugs. Determining adverse effects is part of both the preapproval process and postapproval monitoring responsibilities of CVM.

Many of the toxic effects observed either in the preapproval evaluation or postapproval monitoring are shared among various members of an antibiotic class. For example, fluoroquinolones are known for their ability to cause retinal degeneration and arthropathies in young animals, cephalosporins for gastrointestinal (GI) disturbances, and phenicols for bone marrow toxicities. These effects depend on the animal species and class, the antibiotic drug, and the dose and dosing regimen of the antibiotic used to treat or control an infection (however, it should be noted that toxicities are less likely to occur if the drug is used as per the FDA-approved drug label). The ideal antibiotic has maximal therapeutic effect and minimal adverse effects in the treated animal. In selecting the optimal antimicrobial therapy for a given infection and target species, it is important to determine the risk-to-benefit ratio, which assumes a fundamental understanding of possible adverse reactions associated with that therapy. In this article, the authors aim to enhance the knowledge and understanding of possible adverse reactions associated with the use of selected antibiotic therapies in food animals by correlating the preapproval and postapproval safety data with those reported in the peer-reviewed literature and veterinary pharmacology textbooks. The need to discuss the abundant CVM repository of Adverse Drug Experience (ADE) data is augmented by the fact that the published literature provides very limited information in this area.

DRUG SAFETY EVALUATION DURING THE DRUG APPROVAL PROCESS

As part of the preapproval process for food animals, a drug sponsor must provide evidence that a drug is safe for the target animal and the environment, has the intended effect, can be manufactured adequately to preserve the product's identity, strength, quality, and purity, and that the edible products derived from treated animals are safe for human consumption (21 CFR 514). Sponsors systematically address each of these components by completing 7 elements (commonly referred to as technical sections). The 7 technical sections are: Chemistry, Manufacturing, and Controls (CMC), Effectiveness, Target Animal Safety (TAS), Human Food Safety (HFS), Environmental Safety, All Other Information, and Labeling. This article focuses on the TAS element of the new animal drug evaluation process for food animals.

The specific TAS information needed for approval of a particular drug depends on the type of drug, species and class of animal, route of administration, indication, dose and frequency of administration, available scientific knowledge about the drug, and other potential factors. The principles of TAS evaluation are outlined in the FDA-CVM Guidance for Industry (GFI) #185 (VICH GL43): *Target Animal Safety for Veterinary Pharmaceutical Products*. This document was developed and implemented as part of the VICH (International Cooperation on Harmonization of Technical Requirements for Registration of Veterinary Medicinal Products) program, aimed at harmonizing technical requirements for veterinary product registration among its member countries, which are the European Union, the United States, and Japan.

The components of the TAS technical section are described here. For some drugs each of these components will be necessary whereas for others, for which a lot of information is already available and drug action and safety are well understood, less information will be needed. In addition, alternative approaches for obtaining TAS data, which are not listed here, are also acceptable.

Pharmacologic/Toxicologic Characterization

The pharmacologic/toxicologic characterization includes any information submitted by the sponsor that may help design the pivotal TAS study. In addition, it can help to better predict and understand any potential adverse effects that may occur in the target animal. Data in the pharmacologic/toxicologic characterization package may include published literature and preliminary studies, including various target and nontarget laboratory animal studies, as well as pharmacokinetic, pharmacodynamic, and toxicology studies.

Pivotal Margin of Safety Study

Margin of safety studies have historically been used to support the safety of an investigational new animal drug. These studies are generally characterized by a small sample size, relative homogeneity of study animals, limited study duration, and the use of healthy young animals. Although the use of multiple doses is commonly needed to extrapolate safety findings of new animal drugs to their use under various clinical conditions, the actual multiples of the 1× dose in a margin of safety study are not strictly defined. Most typically, however, the margin of safety is demonstrated in a 0×-, 1×-, 3×-, and 5×-dose study with the drug administered for 3 times the intended duration. The product safety is then established by demonstrating an acceptable level of safety (above 1× dose) and identifying (if present) the toxic syndrome. Variables that are typically assessed in a margin of safety study include: physical examinations and observations, various clinical pathology tests (hematology, blood chemistry, and urinalysis), necropsy, and histopathology. Other information, such as toxicokinetic data, may also be collected if deemed necessary.

Other Laboratory Safety Studies

Additional safety studies may be needed to answer specific safety questions in the intended target species or class of animal. Examples of such specialized studies include reproductive safety studies, specific animal class safety studies (eg, neonatal, geriatric), injection/administration-site safety studies, and mammary gland safety studies.

Safety Information from Field Effectiveness Studies

Additional safety information needed is gathered from field (clinical) effectiveness studies. Unlike the margin of safety studies, the field studies are conducted under clinical conditions representative of the intended use of a new animal drug (eg, client-owned diseased animals of various breeds, classes, and ages). These studies allow detection of some adverse findings that occur at low frequencies and may have been missed in small-scale margin of safety studies. More importantly, these studies provide data on drug safety in diseased animals.

Safety Data from Foreign Approvals

If an investigational drug is already approved in other countries, CVM will also evaluate foreign adverse reports, if available, to learn about these adverse findings under clinical conditions of use (see Draft Guidance for Industry #188: *Data Elements for Submission of Veterinary Adverse Event reports to the Center for Veterinary Medicine*).

In general, the preapproval safety evaluation is based on the principles of risk assessment, which are used to integrate the available body of evidence to weigh the severity of an adverse effect (harm), the potential of reversibility, and the probability that it will occur. Once all the data required for approval of a new animal drug have been generated, the sponsor submits a New Animal Drug Application. If all requirements have been met and CVM determines that the drug is safe and effective for its intended use, the drug is approved, a notice of approval is published in the Federal Register, and the new animal drug can be legally marketed, promoted, and used. More information on the veterinary drug approval process is available on CVM's Web site (http://www.fda.gov/AnimalVeterinary/ResourcesforYou/AnimalHealthLiteracy/ucm219207.htm). At the time of the approval, CVM publishes a Freedom of Information (FOI) Summary (http://www.fda.gov/AnimalVeterinary/Products/ApprovedAnimalDrugProducts/FOIADrugSummaries/default.htm), which contains a summary of the preapproval studies submitted by the sponsor that formed the basis for the Center's approval.

POSTAPPROVAL MONITORING AND ADVERSE DRUG EXPERIENCE REPORTING

Pharmacovigilance is defined by the World Health Organization (WHO) as "the science and activities relating to the detection, assessment, understanding, and prevention of adverse effects or any other drug-related problems" (WHO *Safety Monitoring of Medical Products: Guidelines for Setting Up and Running a Pharmacovigilance Center*. Uppsala Monitoring Center, Sweden, 2006). CVM's Division of Veterinary Product Safety is responsible for postapproval monitoring of ADEs for drugs intended for use in animals, medicated feeds, and veterinary devices. Although CVM employs a rigorous preapproval process for animal drugs, well-conducted, randomized, controlled clinical trials cannot uncover every safety problem, nor are they expected to do so. In most cases clinical trials are not large enough, diverse enough, or long enough in duration to provide all of the information on a product's performance and safety. It is only after a drug has been out on the market for a year or several years, and a large number of animals have been treated, that potentially serious adverse events, not observed during preapproval studies, may manifest. Consequently, ADEs are monitored after the drug is approved.

Adverse drug experience is defined in the Code of Federal Regulations (21 CFR 514.3) as "any adverse event associated with the use of a new animal drug, whether or not considered to be drug related, and whether or not the new animal drug was used in accordance with the approved labeling." An ADE includes, but is not limited to: an adverse event occurring in animals in the course of the use of an animal drug product by a veterinarian or by a livestock producer or other animal owner or caretaker; failure of a new animal drug to produce its expected pharmacologic or clinical effect, or an adverse event occurring in humans from exposure during use of the drug. A *serious adverse drug experience* is also defined in 21 CFR 514.3, as "an adverse event that is fatal, or life-threatening, or requires professional intervention, or causes an abortion, stillbirth, infertility, or congenital anomaly, prolonged or permanent disability, or disfigurement." An *unexpected adverse drug experience* is any adverse drug experience that is not listed on the current drug labeling.

Adverse drug event reporting is mandatory for sponsors marketing animal drugs, and voluntary for veterinarians and animal owners. Regulations in 21 CFR 514.80 describe the reporting requirements for regulated industry. Sponsors report adverse events and product defects to CVM on FDA Form 1932. Veterinarians and animal owners usually report adverse events to drug sponsors (manufacturers), but may also report directly to FDA on Form 1932a, or via "hotline" calls to CVM. In addition, electronic submission of adverse event information has recently become possible, including via FDA's Safety Reporting Portal.

Data mining, which is the use of computer algorithms to analyze data in large, complex databases, is used to help signal potential problems quickly, and generate hypotheses regarding possible drug safety problems. Once a signal is identified, individual review of cases is always necessary to further investigate a potential safety issue. CVM can use this information to evaluate trends and relative frequencies of reported ADEs.

ADE reports received by CVM from individuals and drug manufacturers are forwarded to the Division of Veterinary Product Safety for evaluation. ADE reports are reviewed by CVM safety reviewers, who are experienced clinical veterinarians. ADEs are prioritized in a way that those received for recently approved drugs, as well as those that are subject to an ongoing investigation, are reviewed before those received for drugs that have been marketed for a long time. All relevant information from each report is manually entered into a searchable ADE database, considering age, breed, gender, preexisting conditions, and concomitant drugs. At present, the reviewers evaluate each clinical sign reported using a scoring system that is a modified version of the Kramer algorithm.[1,2] With this system, every reported clinical sign is evaluated for each of the following criteria in the algorithm: previous experience with the drug, alternative etiologic candidates, timing of events, evidence of overdose, dechallenge (effects of drug withdrawal), and rechallenge (effects of drug readministration). A summary causality assessment score for each clinical sign is determined and entered into the database as part of the evaluation process. The summary score corresponds to the strength of the association between the drug and the clinical sign, and ranges between −9 and +7. Clinical signs with summary scores of zero or greater are considered possibly, probably, or definitely drug-related.

In this manner, CVM scientists use the ADE database to make decisions about product safety, which may lead to label revisions or other regulatory actions. Postapproval Experience sections are periodically added to drug labeling as data regarding adverse events are gathered. Interventions to help enhance safe drug use include "Dear Doctor" letters (letters to veterinarians notifying them of potential steps to mitigate risks associated with drug use), risk mitigation programs, or additional labeling components such as Client Information Sheets. Cumulative veterinary ADE reports are posted on CVM's Web site (http://www.fda.gov/AnimalVeterinary/SafetyHealth/ProductSafetyInformation/ucm055394.htm) and updated at regular intervals.

Underreporting occurs with most adverse event reporting systems. The frequency of reporting for a given new animal drug product varies over time, with time from first marketing, and with periods of media activity surrounding a product. Given the variability in reporting and the many factors that affect reporting, it is generally well accepted that reporting rates cannot be used to reliably estimate incidence rates of adverse events, and that comparison of reporting rates between products or between countries may not be reliable. The apparent usefulness of ADE data for understanding drug safety also illustrates the importance of reporting all suspected adverse drug events for the veterinary community.

INTEGRATION OF PREAPPROVAL AND POSTAPPROVAL SAFETY FINDINGS WITH PUBLISHED LITERATURE

Methods

The authors have limited their focus to antibiotics originally approved after 1990, because the processes and level of review of new animal drug approval have changed over time and older FOI summaries are not readily available on the CVM's Web site (the intent was to focus the analyses on the data that are readily available). Also, this report is limited to systemically administered antibiotics approved in the United States for therapeutic uses in food animals. Furthermore, the authors have limited this report for the preapproval safety evaluation of pioneer drugs only because typically no new TAS information is gathered in the approval of generic drugs. However, postapproval data from generic drugs are included in the ADE and literature review portions of the report. The focus is also limited to drugs containing single antibiotic ingredients as opposed to combination drugs, because it would be difficult to differentiate adverse effects among the single ingredients within a combination. Included are cattle, swine, chickens, sheep, and goats in a 3-way comparison (literature vs preapproval vs postapproval findings), to take into account all economically important food animals. Finally, in the search of the postapproval ADEs, the authors have limited their focus to those ADEs with positive causality. Positive causality is not proof of causal effect, but provides a reasonable suspicion that a drug has caused an adverse event, because most confounding factors have been evaluated on a case-by-case basis. When ADEs have been found to be associated with a drug, they are listed in the order of reporting frequency. However, no quantitative assessment of ADEs is provided because it would require inclusion of individual product sales data, which is proprietary information (individual products sales data are not available to the public). Because this report is limited to the publicly available information on the CVM Web site, all the assessments are qualitative.

Safety in target animals was assessed using 3 different methods:

1. Evaluation of published literature using the PubMed and Web of Science search engines and general pharmacology/veterinary pharmacology textbooks; the search terms were "safety," "adverse," and "toxic" (a separate search was conducted for each), as well as the appropriate species and established drug name
2. Use of FOI summaries from the FDA-CVM Web site
3. Postapproval cumulative Veterinary ADE reports sorted by reporting frequency for individual antibiotics, as available on the FDA-CVM Web site (generally truncated to approximately 10 most frequently reported signs) (http://www.fda.gov/AnimalVeterinary/SafetyHealth/ProductSafetyInformation/ucm055394.htm).

Results and Discussion

Very few literature reports specifically address the safety of antibiotic drugs in food animals. The majority of "hits" in literature searches using the terms "safety," "adverse," or "toxic" are related to HFS findings, development of antimicrobial resistance, or the effects of antibiotics on the intestinal flora. In this report all such findings were excluded, unless they were specifically linked to safety of antibiotics in the target species. It should also be noted that the published literature reports specific to safety of the target species are not only scarce but provide very limited information, as compared with the CVM's preapproval and postapproval drug evaluation. In most published literature, the main objective of the study is usually an evaluation and/or description of a product's effectiveness, while any adverse reactions and safety concerns in the target species are only mentioned briefly as secondary findings.

Before listing and discussing specific drug results, it should be emphasized that the results of the TAS evaluation completed during the preapproval process are based on a limited number of studies and very few animals per study. Moreover, the preapproval findings in this report are grouped together irrespective of the dose in which they were observed because the focus is on the comparative assessment of various sources of safety information on antibiotics in food animals, rather than quantitative analyses. This approach differs from the findings reported in the FOI summaries, which are listed by dose (treatment) group.

It should also be noted that the postapproval ADEs are based on voluntary reporting from veterinarians and animal owners, and thus are generally underreported, which makes any quantitative assessment unreliable. In addition, various extraneous factors are by design carefully excluded from preapproval studies, but not from the postapproval use, thus confounding the ADE data and making interpretation of ADEs difficult. Various comorbidities and concurrent drug usage are both likely to affect the outcome of drug treatment and make the evaluation of ADEs more complex. For example, the concomitant use of nonsteroidal anti-inflammatory drugs (NSAIDs) with antibiotics could make it difficult to determine whether an ADE is caused by the primary (antibiotic) or ancillary (NSAID) drug use. In addition, adverse reports are often associated with drug use outside the approved label, for example, different dose, regimen, species, animal class, route of administration, and so forth. The adverse findings associated with extralabel uses are routinely reported on the ADE site and are important for estimation of overall drug safety under clinical conditions of use. Finally, as already noted, there is no absolute certainty that the reported drug caused the ADEs.

Because of all the stated differences in methods and processes for evaluation of drug safety between preapproval and postapproval monitoring, it becomes clear that the adverse reactions might not be the same when comparing the two sources. For example, occurrence of death during the preapproval process is a relatively rare finding and is always taken seriously, requiring further evaluations and steps to assure drug safety in the target animal. On the other hand, death is a frequently reported adverse event in the postapproval monitoring. This finding could be attributable to the fact that the animals included in postapproval monitoring are sick and managed under clinical conditions of use, so they may be concomitantly exposed to multiple other diseases as well as to multiple drugs, which may all greatly affect an animal's reaction to the drug. However, this does not mean that drugs included in this report are considered unsafe or less safe than others for which no reports of death (or other serious adverse events) were listed. All of the drugs included in this report are deemed safe and effective by the FDA, and no drug (or class) comparisons should be drawn from this report. The objective of this study was to compare the various sources of TAS findings (published literature vs preapproval safety studies vs postapproval monitoring) to evaluate their importance and value for an overall safety determination of antibiotics in food animals.

Finally, it should be emphasized that a finding of "no adverse effects" in the preapproval process does not mean that one drug is safer or less toxic than others in the same class (or in one species vs another) for which there are reports listed. As a result, no across-drugs or across-class comparisons should be attempted with these data. Drugs included in this report have been approved over a 20-year span, and the differences observed are at least partly due to the noncontemporaneous nature of data collection. It has been well documented that the number of postapproval ADEs has steadily increased over the years; in addition, more recent drug approvals receive greater attention, may be used more frequently, and are given a higher priority. Therefore, the ADE database available for these drugs is much more complete, further complicating interpretation of the results.

The adverse events associated with the approval and clinical use of antibiotics in cattle, swine, poultry, sheep, and goats are listed in **Tables 1–6**. Antibiotics are grouped together in the following classes: cephalosporins, macrolides, phenicols, lincosamides, fluoroquinolones, and pleuromutilins.

Table 1
Adverse events associated with the use of the cephalosporin, ceftiofur, in cattle, swine, poultry, sheep, and goats

	AE Reported by Source		
Species (Dosage Form)	**FOI Summary (Preapproval)**	**CVM's ADE Database (Postapproval)[a]**	**Published Literature**
Cattle (injection)	None	Death, ineffectiveness, IS swelling, collapse, anaphylaxis/toid, IS abscess, death (Tx failure), dyspnea, Pr-lung(s), lesion(s), recumbency etc	Cutaneous reaction[6]
Swine (injection)	Anemia, transient pain (limping), discoloration at IS	Death, anaphylaxis/toid, diarrhea, death (Tx failure), dyspnea, peritoneal effusion, ineffectiveness, Pr-lung(s), edema, vomiting	No AEs found
Chickens (injection)	Depression, ataxia and prostration, death, reduced weight gain	No ADEs reported	No AEs found
Sheep (injection)	None	Anaphylaxis/toid, ataxia, fever, hypersalivation, polyuria, trembling	No AEs found
Goats (injection)	None	Death, anaphylaxis/toid, ataxia, collapse, hyperactivity, nervousness, nystagmus, vocalization	No AEs found

Abbreviations: ADE, adverse drug experience; AE, adverse event; anaphylaxis/toid, anaphylactic or anaphylactoid reaction; CVM, Center for Veterinary Medicine; FOI, freedom of information; IS, injection site; Pr-, pathology report; Tx, therapy.
[a] If "etc" is listed in the tables, it indicates that only the most frequent (approximately the first 10) signs are included. If there is no "etc" the list is all-inclusive.

Cephalosporins

Cephalosporins are a class of β-lactam antibiotics derived from 7-aminocephalosporanic acid. Similar to penicillins, cephalosporins bind to penicillin-binding proteins located beneath the cell wall and interfere with transpeptidase and other cell-wall enzymes. Each of the 3 cephalosporin generations exhibits an increasingly broad spectrum of activity and resistance to β-lactamase activity. One first-generation cephalosporin, cephapirin, and one third-generation cephalosporin, ceftiofur, are approved in the United States for food animal use. As a class, cephalosporins are among the most widely prescribed antibiotics in both human and veterinary medicine, and are generally considered very safe. Adverse reactions are typically limited to local reactions associated with dosing; specifically, gastrointestinal signs when orally administered or skin-related reactions when an injectable dosage form is used. Hypersensitivities are reported in humans but are rare in veterinary species.[3–5]

Ceftiofur is the only antibiotic from the cephalosporin class approved since 1988 in cattle, swine, poultry, sheep, and goats. Ceftiofur-associated ADEs were identified during preapproval studies in swine and chickens but not in cattle, sheep, or goats. Postapproval ADEs were reported for cattle, swine, sheep, and goats, but not in poultry (see **Table 1**).

Table 2
Adverse events associated with the use of the macrolide, tulathromycin, in cattle and swine

Species (Dosage Form)	AE Reported by Source: FOI Summary (Preapproval)	CVM's ADE Database (Postapproval)[a]	Published Literature
Cattle (injection)	IS swelling, head-shaking, pawing at the ground and jumping immediately postdose, decreased feed intake, transient urine color change, IS congestion, edema, hemorrhage, subacute inflammation, vascular thrombosis	Ineffectiveness, death (Tx failure), death, lung lesions, IS swelling, recumbency, anaphylaxis/toid, collapse, abortion, IS alopecia, etc	No AEs found
Swine (injection)	Transient elevation in serum aspartate aminotransferase and IS-related discomfort, IS discoloration and injury (Zenker's degeneration)	Death, IS abnormalities, death (Tx failure), discomfort, ineffectiveness, IS pain, anaphylaxis/toid, distress, dyspnea, IS abscess, etc	No AEs found

Injection-site reactions were the predominant sign reported in cattle both preapproval and postapproval. Adverse skin reaction was also reported in literature as a case study of a 4-year old Limousin cow[6] with an injection-site reaction including hair loss and pruritus. Intradermal allergy testing supported the allergenicity of the animal to ceftiofur. Despite several reports of injection-site reactions associated with ceftiofur, no difference in meat quality was found between ceftiofur-injected and placebo-injected cattle.[7] Neurologic signs were seen in cattle (postapproval) and chickens (preapproval), as well as in sheep and goats (both postapproval). When compared with known class toxicity the neurologic signs of lethargy, ataxia, and nystagmus were unique and new findings, which emphasize the need to carefully evaluate the safety of new animal drugs through both preapproval studies and postapproval monitoring. Diarrhea, which is commonly associated with cephalosporin use, was the predominant postapproval adverse event in swine, and has been frequently reported in cattle as well. In swine, no overlap was observed between the signs reported before and those reported after drug approval (see **Table 1**).

Except for injection-site discoloration and pain, no typical signs related to cephalosporin use (such as diarrhea) were reported postapproval in any species except for swine. Anaphylaxis/anaphylactoid reactions and edema were the only signs that were consistently observed in all species (except chickens). In addition, completely different signs were observed for swine in the preapproval and postapproval periods. These observations clearly illustrate the importance of monitoring drug reactions for each species that the drug is approved in, and that the ADEs reported during the postapproval period may reveal species-specific safety concerns that were not observed during the preapproval TAS studies.

Macrolides

Macrolides are a group of closely related antibiotics with a typical large lactone ring and chemical substitutions on the various carbon atoms in the structure. Macrolides are primarily bacteriostatic; their mechanism of action involves inhibition of bacterial protein synthesis by binding to the 50S subunit of the ribosome. All macrolides diffuse

Table 3
Adverse events associated with the use of the macrolide, tilmicosin, in cattle, swine, and sheep

Species (Dosage Form)	AE Reported by Source: FOI Summary (Preapproval)	CVM's ADE Database (Postapproval)[a]	Published Literature
Swine (feed)	One animal died (no abnormalities found, but possibly treatment-related), no other findings	Ineffectiveness, death, anorexia, death (euthanized), death (Tx failure), unpalatable—won't eat, alopecia, ataxia, coughing, enteritis, etc	Positive chronotropic effects, negative inotropic effects in overdosed swine, IS reactions at therapeutic doses[9]
Cattle (injection)	IS swelling (histology: noninflammatory subcutaneous edema sometimes accompanied by necrosis), histology: small foci of myocardial necrosis in the papillary muscle, death (when administered intravenously or at 15×)	Death, IS swelling, collapse, ineffectiveness, recumbency, dyspnea, anaphylaxis/toid, lameness, death (Tx failure), depression/lethargy, etc	Positive chronotropic effects, negative inotropic effects[9]
Sheep (injection)	Limited data (from pharmacokinetic bioequivalence study) indicate no AEs	Death, dyspnea, recumbency, anaphylaxis/toid, weakness, collapse, ataxia, hematuria, depression/lethargy, respiratory distress, etc	Death of one lamb with a septal defect,[13] No adverse cardiopulmonary effects when dosed at 10 mg/kg,[14] No AEs at 15 mg/kg once or twice 4 days apart in lambs <15 kg with decreased selenium status[15]

well into body fluids, except cerebrospinal fluid, and reach much higher concentrations in tissue than in plasma. Macrolides approved in the United States for use in food animal species include erythromycin, tylosin, tilmicosin, and tulathromycin, with the latter two being approved since 1990.

The most common safety concerns associated with macrolide therapies in veterinary medicine include GI disturbances (due to their motilin-receptor agonist activity), cardiac toxicity (including the QT-interval prolongation), and inhibition of hepatic metabolism (leading to numerous drug interactions).[3,8]

Among macrolides approved in the United States for food animals, tulathromycin is approved for use in cattle and swine, and tilmicosin for use in cattle, swine, and sheep. Injection-site reactions with tulathromycin use have been observed during preapproval and postapproval evaluation (see **Table 2**) in cattle and swine. Ineffectiveness, death (no cause listed), and death due to treatment failure have been reported postapproval for tulathromycin (see **Table 2**) and tilmicosin (see **Table 3**) in cattle and swine. However, these signs are likely related to the disease process for which the

Table 4
Adverse events associated with the use of the phenicol, florfenicol, in cattle and swine

	AE Reported by Source		
Species (Dosage Form)	**FOI Summary (Preapproval)**	**CVM's ADE Database (Postapproval)[a]**	**Published Literature**
Cattle (injection)	Decreased feed/water consumption and IS swelling, transient local reaction in the subcutaneous tissue and underlying muscle tissue at IS	Death, anaphylaxis/toid, recumbency, anorexia, diarrhea, collapse, death (euthanized), hyperpnea, hypersalivation, ineffectiveness, IS swelling, etc	Changes in antimicrobial susceptibility, increased ratio of neutrophils without pseudopodia at high concentrations, but normal neutrophil function[20]
Swine (feed or drinking water)	Decreased food/water consumption, decreased number of reticulocytes, increased serum Ca, urea N, and creatinine, decreased serum P, decreased bone marrow cellularity	Diarrhea, abdominal distention, ineffectiveness, skin inflammation	No AEs found

animals were being treated, and without having more information on the disease state and the animal condition prior to drug administration, no further implications can be drawn. Postapproval reports of death, dyspnea, recumbency, anaphylaxis/anaphylactoid reactions, weakness, collapse, ataxia, bloody urine, depression/lethargy, respiratory distress, hyperactivity, hyperpnea, injection-site swelling, and neurologic disorders have been documented in sheep treated with tilmicosin. The tilmicosin label contains the warning not to administer the drug to animals other than cattle or sheep (and swine in feed).

Macrolide toxicity observed in the preapproval study and reported postapproval could only partially be corroborated with the published literature. Of interest is that tilmicosin has not been associated with adverse cardiac effects in food animals except in overdosed swine,[9] although cardiac toxicity has been documented in several species, including humans,[10] horses,[9] dogs,[11] and swine.[12] A lamb with ventral septal defects died after receiving an injection of tilmicosin subcutaneously.[13] However, this death was confounded by the reported cardiac defect. A one-time subcutaneous injection of 10 mg/kg (approved dose) did not result in any cardiopulmonary effects of tilmicosin in sheep.[14] A case-report study illustrated that lambs with respiratory disease were not adversely affected by the use of tilmicosin at 15 mg/kg either once or twice given 4 days apart.[15] In discussion of the cardiac toxicity of tilmicosin in swine, it should be noted that one pig died in the preapproval safety evaluation of tilmicosin after receiving a 10× dose of tilmicosin in feed (see **Table 3**, and FOI summary [FOI Summary for NADA 141-064, PULMOTIL 90, dated December 17, 1996]), with no clinical signs of abnormalities found at necropsy. Because the mechanism of action for tilmicosin toxicity in dogs is a disruption of the electrical conduction in the heart, which is not associated with specific lesions (FOI Summary for NADA 140-929, MICOTIL, dated March 24, 1992), it was concluded that the death observed in the pig in the pivotal safety study could have potentially been treatment-related. Likewise, death is one of the most

Table 5
Adverse events associated with the use of fluoroquinolones in cattle and swine

Fluoroquinolone Antibiotic	Species (Dosage Form)	AE Reported by Source		
		FOI Summary (Preapproval)	CVM's ADE Database (Postapproval)[a]	Published Literature
Danofloxacin	Cattle (injection)	Lameness, ataxia, nystagmus, depression, recumbency, IS swelling, death	Death, anaphylaxis/toid, collapse, ineffectiveness, recumbency, hypersalivation, ataxia, dyspnea, mouth froth, staggering, etc	No AEs found
Enrofloxacin	Cattle (injection)	Depression, incoordination, muscle fasciculation, inappetence, transient reaction in the subcutaneous tissue and underlying muscle	Death, ineffectiveness, IS Swelling, anaphylaxis/toid, dyspnea, IS abscess, abortion, death (Tx failure), neck edema, epistaxis, etc	Changes in antimicrobial susceptibility[24,25]
Enrofloxacin	Swine (injection)	Depression, lameness, stiffness, osteochondrosis, transient diarrhea, transient IS swelling, discoloration and light scar formation	No AE's reported	Antibiotic-associated diarrhea, changes in antimicrobial susceptibility[26]

Table 6
Adverse events associated with the use of the pleuromutilin, tiamulin, in swine

Species (Dosage Form)	AE Reported by Source FOI Summary (Preapproval)	CVM's ADE Database (Postapproval)[a]	Published Literature
Swine (feed or drinking water)	None	Ineffectiveness, death, skin congestion, depression/ lethargy, ataxia, diarrhea, nervousness, pain, Pr-colon lesions, etc	No AEs found, except for interactions with monensin[28] and nitrovin[29]

frequently observed postapproval signs after tilmicosin treatment in all 3 species, and may also be treatment-related. However, as already stated, because of the presence of the disease for which the animals were treated under clinical conditions of use, the likelihood of this finding being treatment-related cannot be determined. Two studies evaluated safety of tulathromycin in goats, for which tulathromycin is currently not approved. A study in which goats were administered tulathromycin subcutaneously in a dose approved for swine and cattle (1×), as well as 0×, 3×, and 5×, the drug was found to be generally safe, except for coagulation parameters, which exhibited reduced prothrombin time and activated partial thromboplastin time in all treated groups.[16] The changes in coagulation parameters are potentially consistent with the observed vascular thrombosis observed in the preapproval studies in cattle (see **Table 2** and the FOI summary [FOI Summary for NADA 141-244, DRAXXIN, dated May 24, 2005]). Increased serum creatine kinase levels, injection-site lesions, and genotoxicity were reported in goats given a 10× tulathromycin subcutaneously.[17]

In conclusion, GI tract findings have been observed in both the preapproval and postapproval monitoring processes for macrolides, which is also consistent with the known class toxicities. All other class adverse signs have either not been reported (diarrhea, cholestatic hepatitis) or their cause has been found to be inconclusive (cardiac toxicity).

Phenicols

Phenicols inhibit bacterial protein synthesis by impairing peptidyltransferase activity at the 50S ribosomal subunit. Examples of drugs from this class include chloramphenicol and its derivatives. Chloramphenicol may potentially cause serious bone marrow toxicities and has been prohibited from use in many species. Moreover, there is a possibility that tissue residues of chloramphenicol in food animals might induce aplastic anemia in humans[3]; this risk has resulted in a prohibition of its use in food animals in the United States and several other countries.

Florfenicol is the only antibiotic from the phenicol class approved for use in cattle and swine in the United States. Aside from bone marrow suppression (which is typical of chloramphenicol, but not florfenicol), other class-related safety concerns associated with phenicol therapy include diarrhea and other GI disturbances, decreased feed consumption, anorexia, and an increased risk of toxicity in young animals due to an immature glucuronidation system.[3,4,8]

In the preapproval studies for florfenicol, decreased food and water consumption were reported in both cattle and swine (see **Table 4**). In addition, injection-site reactions were observed in cattle, both before and after the drug was approved. Ineffectiveness, diarrhea, and anaphylaxis/anaphylactoid reactions were among the signs reported postapproval in cattle and swine, all of which are not uncommon for florfenicol antibiotics. Some ADE reports of ineffectiveness may be associated with changes in antimicrobial susceptibility.[18]

Thiamphenicol and florfenicol were developed as safer alternatives to chloramphenicol by removing a nitro group, which is believed to prevent the development of aplastic anemia.[3] However, decreased bone marrow cellularity was observed in the preapproval safety evaluation of florfenicol in swine (see **Table 4** and FOI Summary for NADA 141-264, Nuflor [florfenicol] Type A Medicated Article, dated November 3, 2006). Neutropenia and bone marrow hypoplasia were also reported in a Thompson gazelle overdosed with 10× of the intended dose of florfenicol.[19] This adverse effect is supported by findings of in vitro studies, in which the morphology of bovine polymorphonuclear leukocytes was altered after treatment with high dose of florfenicol, although without any difference detected in function.[20]

In conclusion, florfenicol use in cattle and swine has been associated with multiple adverse effects commonly reported for the class, such as diarrhea, decreased food consumption, and anorexia, as well as possible suppression of bone marrow function. Injection-site reactions and pain are not typically associated with clinical use of phenicols but were reported in the preapproval and postapproval findings in food animals.

Fluoroquinolones

Fluoroquinolones are a family of synthetic broad-spectrum antibiotics that are rapidly bactericidal for a wide variety of clinically important bacteria in veterinary medicine. One of their advantages is that they can be administered by a variety of routes, making them ideal antibiotics for use in animals. Quinolones inhibit bacterial DNA replication and transcription by targeting the enzyme DNA gyrase. Danofloxacin (cattle) and enrofloxacin (cattle and swine) are the only quinolones approved for use in food animals.

Fluoroquinolones have a relatively good safety record in veterinary species. Major types of toxicities include GI disturbances, allergic reactions, phototoxicity, central nervous system (CNS) effects (including convulsions), retinal lesions, blindness, and arthropathies in young animals.[3,21]

Cattle treated with danofloxacin showed multiple signs of CNS toxicity in both the preapproval and postapproval periods, which is consistent with the class effect (see **Table 5**). Similar CNS effects were also observed for enrofloxacin in both cattle (both preapproval and postapproval) and swine (preapproval only). It is interesting that no ADEs were reported for the postapproval use of enrofloxacin in swine, although numerous ADE reports exist for a variety of other species (in which enrofloxacin is either approved or unapproved).

Fluoroquinolones are well recognized in literature and in practice for their arthropathogenic potential in young animals.[22] In humans and animals, the use of quinolones is not recommended for individuals whose bone growth is incomplete or for pregnant/nursing women.[23] There seems to be a species-specific susceptibility to this adverse effect, and food animals tend to be less prone to it than dogs and rats.[21] However, possible signs of arthropathies were observed in preapproval and postapproval monitoring of danofloxacin and enrofloxacin in cattle, as well as in preapproval studies of enrofloxacin in swine (see **Table 5**).

No reports of toxicity associated with danofloxacin use have been found in the literature, while enrofloxacin has been reported to change antimicrobial susceptibility in cattle[24,25] and has been related to antibiotic-associated diarrhea in swine.[26] Enrofloxacin inhibits cytochromes P4501A1 and P4501A2 in rat liver,[27] potentially affecting pharmacokinetics of concomitant drugs metabolized by these enzymes, and would be worth investigating further. The inhibition of the P450 enzymes could be a source of some ADEs, but this is difficult to determine because of confounding effects.

Pleuromutilins

Pleuromutilins are antibacterial drugs that inhibit protein synthesis in bacteria by binding to the peptidyl transferase component of the 50S subunit of ribosomes. Tiamulin is the only antibiotic from the pleuromutilin class approved since 1990, and is approved for use only in swine. Tiamulin is generally considered as safe,[3] and the only adverse effects reported in the literature include redness of skin,[4] possible reduction in feed intake, salivation, vomiting, and depression.

No adverse safety findings were observed during the preapproval safety studies of tiamulin in swine, but multiple ADEs have been reported in association with tiamulin use postapproval (see **Table 6**). Of those, depression and skin disorders are consistent with the expected class effects. These findings could not be corroborated with the published literature because no reports could be found. However, some published research suggests that interaction between tiamulin and either monensin[28] or nitrovin[29] may result in adverse events, possibly due to tiamulin-induced inhibition of CYP3A enzymes, which are responsible for metabolizing monensin.[30] Whether this effect has implications on ADEs should be subject to further investigations.

SUMMARY

Numerous and noticeable differences exist in observed adverse safety findings between the preapproval and postapproval periods and published literature for antibiotic agents used in food animals, although significant overlap was also observed (as expected). Some of the differences result from application of different methods employed in each of the evaluations and are thus complementary rather than contradictory to each other. Whereas the preapproval TAS studies are well controlled and performed in a small number of animals, postapproval safety data are generally reported from a large number of animals at conditions of use, but lack adequate controls and are often confounded with concomitant drug use and diseases. For example, injection-site reactions reported in postapproval ADE reports are generally more severe than reactions reported in preapproval studies, possibly because controlled drug studies are performed by more skilled personnel than in clinical practice and/or that the pivotal studies abide by the maximum injection-site volume per injection site, whereas this may not be the case in clinical practice.

The reported findings emphasize the need to continue applying both methods of safety evaluation in target species (with detailed preapproval characterization and vigilant postapproval monitoring) to obtain the most complete picture possible for an ultimate goal of approving and maintaining safe and effective drugs on the market. One of the limitations of this review is that it could not take into account individual patient variation, which has presumably contributed to several adverse events discussed in this article. This aspect is one that may be considered, as it already is in human medicine, for the future of animal safety evaluation and monitoring. A noted constant for all of the drugs included in this search is a scarcity of published literature on drug safety in target animals, which suggests that it is not a "hot topic" in veterinary drug research (unlike, for example, antimicrobial resistance). The findings of this article suggest that more research is needed to further elucidate the extent and nature of antibiotic toxicity in target animals in order to optimize a positive outcome of antibiotic treatment in veterinary species.

REFERENCES

1. Hutchinson TA, Leventhal JM, Kramer MS, et al. An algorithm for the operational assessment of adverse drug reactions. II. Demonstration of reproducibility and validity. JAMA 1979;242(7):633–8.

2. Kramer MS, Leventhal JM, Hutchinson TA, et al. An algorithm for the operational assessment of adverse drug reactions. I. Background, description, and instructions for use. JAMA 1979;242(7):623–32.
3. Merck Veterinary Manual. In: Kahn CM, Line S, editors. 10th edition. Whitehouse Station (NJ): John Wiley & Sons; 2010.
4. Plumb DC. Veterinary drug handbook. Ames (IA): Iowa State Press; 2002.
5. Vaden SL, Riviere JE. Penicillins and related b-lactam antibiotics. In: Adams HR, editor. Veterinary pharmacology and therapeutics. 8th edition. Ames (IA): Iowa State University Press; 2001. p. 818–27.
6. Tyler JW, Ruffin DC, Yu A. Probable ceftiofur-induced cutaneous drug reaction in a cow. Can Vet J 1998;39(5):296–8.
7. Sullivan MM, Vanoverbeke DL, Kinman LA, et al. Comparison of the Biobullet versus traditional pharmaceutical injection techniques on injection-site tissue damage and tenderness in beef subprimals. J Anim Sci 2009;87(2):716–22.
8. Papich MC, Riviere JE. Chloramphenicol and derivatives, macrolides, lincosamides, and miscellaneous antimicrobials. In: Adams HR, editor. Veterinary pharmacology and therapeutics. 8th edition. Ames (IA): Iowa State University Press; 2001. p. 868–97.
9. Jordan WH, Byrd RA, Cochrane RL, et al. A review of the toxicology of the antibiotic MICOTIL 300. Vet Hum Toxicol 1993;35(2):151–8.
10. McGuigan MA. Human exposures to tilmicosin (MICOTIL). Vet Hum Toxicol 1994; 36(4):306–8.
11. Main BW, Means JR, Rinkema LE, et al. Cardiovascular effects of the macrolide antibiotic tilmicosin, administered alone and in combination with propranolol or dobutamine, in conscious unrestrained dogs. J Vet Pharmacol Ther 1996;19(3):225–32.
12. Shen J, Li C, Jiang H, et al. Pharmacokinetics of tilmicosin after oral administration in swine. Am J Vet Res 2005;66(6):1071–4.
13. Christodoulopoulos G. Adverse outcome of using tilmicosin in a lamb with multiple ventricular septal defects. Can Vet J 2009;50(1):61–3.
14. Modric S, Webb AI, Derendorf H. Pharmacokinetics and pharmacodynamics of tilmicosin in sheep and cattle. J Vet Pharmacol Ther 1998;21(6):444–52.
15. Christodoulopoulos G, Warnick LD, Papaioannou N, et al. Tilmicosin administration to young lambs with respiratory infection: safety and efficacy considerations. J Vet Pharmacol Ther 2002;25(5):393–7.
16. Clothier KA, Jordan DM, Loynachan AT, et al. Safety evaluation of tulathromycin use in the caprine species: tulathromycin toxicity assessment in goats. J Vet Pharmacol Ther 2010;33(5):499–502.
17. Washburn KE, Bissett W, Fajt V, et al. The safety of tulathromycin administration in goats. J Vet Pharmacol Ther 2007;30(3):267–70.
18. Sawant AA, Hegde NV, Straley BA, et al. Antimicrobial-resistant enteric bacteria from dairy cattle. Appl Environ Microbiol 2007;73(1):156–63.
19. Tuttle AD, Papich MG, Wolfe BA. Bone marrow hypoplasia secondary to florfenicol toxicity in a Thomson's gazelle (*Gazella thomsonii*). J Vet Pharmacol Ther 2006;29(4):317–9.
20. Paape MJ, Miller RH, Ziv G. Effects of florfenicol, chloramphenicol, and thiamphenicol on phagocytosis, chemiluminescence, and morphology of bovine polymorphonuclear neutrophil leukocytes. J Dairy Sci 1990;73(7):1734–44.
21. Papich MC, Riviere JE. Fluoroquinolone antimicrobial drugs. In: Adams HR, editor. Veterinary pharmacology and therapeutics. 8th edition. Ames (IA): Iowa State University Press; 2001. p. 898–917.

22. Stahlmann R. Safety profile of the quinolones. J Antimicrob Chemother 1990; 26(Suppl):D31–44.
23. Wolfson JS. Quinolone antimicrobial agents: adverse effects and bacterial resistance. Eur J Clin Microbiol Infect Dis 1989;8(12):1080–92.
24. Catry B, Croubels S, Schwarz S, et al. Influence of systemic fluoroquinolone administration on the presence of *Pasteurella multocida* in the upper respiratory tract of clinically healthy calves. Acta Vet Scand 2008;50:36.
25. Katsuda K, Kohmoto M, Mikami O, et al. Antimicrobial resistance and genetic characterization of fluoroquinolone-resistant *Mannheimia haemolytica* isolates from cattle with bovine pneumonia. Vet Microbiol 2009;139(1–2):74–9.
26. Tsukahara T, Ushida K. Succinate accumulation in pig large intestine during antibiotic-associated diarrhea and the constitution of succinate-producing flora. J Gen Appl Microbiol 2002;48(3):143–54.
27. Vancutsem PM, Babish JG. In vitro and in vivo study of the effects of enrofloxacin on hepatic cytochrome P-450. Potential for drug interactions. Vet Hum Toxicol 1996;38(4):254–9.
28. Witkamp RF, Nijmeijer SM, Csiko G, et al. Tiamulin selectively inhibits oxidative hepatic steroid and drug metabolism in vitro in the pig. J Vet Pharmacol Ther 1994;17(4):317–22.
29. Noa M, Bulnes C, Valcarcel L, et al. Tiamulin-nitrovin interaction in pigs: a case report and experimental reproduction. Vet Hum Toxicol 2000;42(5):286–8.
30. Szucs G, Tamasi V, Laczay P, et al. Biochemical background of toxic interaction between tiamulin and monensin. Chem Biol Interact 2004;147(2):151–61.

Identifying Plant Poisoning in Livestock: Diagnostic Approaches and Laboratory Tests

Bryan L. Stegelmeier, DVM, PhD

KEYWORDS

• Plant • Livestock • Poisoning • Diagnosis • Laboratory

Local veterinarians are familiar with regional livestock management practices, livestock diseases, and many endemic plants, thus they should play a key role in diagnosing plant poisoning. However, as most training programs in veterinary medicine and surgery have minimal instruction in plant identification and toxicity, many veterinarians feel inadequate when called on to inspect feeds, pastures, or ranges. This may lead some to avoid such problems, forcing those with less training in infectious and metabolic diseases to interpret data. This article provides direction and information to allow veterinarians to find information, recruit needed expertise and help, and provide the means to analyze samples and identify problems caused by toxic plants.

SIGNALMENT AND HISTORY

As with any diagnostic investigation, the first and essential step is to collect information concerning the animals (signalment), clinical signs, lesions, and disease progression (**Box 1**). This information should be included with all samples when they are submitted for analysis. Once this information is gathered, differential diagnoses can be developed. As many infectious, degenerative, and immunologic diseases produce clinical signs, biochemical changes, and lesions identical to those caused by toxins and poisonous plants, all the appropriate experts should be included to ensure that the list is complete. Both veterinarians and producers should also develop working relationships with local, state, and regional experts to facilitate this cooperative effort.

The author acknowledges the thoughtful suggestions and input from J.O. Hall and N. F. Suttle.
The author has nothing to disclose.
USDA-Agricultural Research Service, Poisonous Plant Research Laboratory, 1150 East 1400 North, Logan, UT 84341, USA
E-mail address: Bryan.Stegelmeier@ARS.USDA.GOV

Vet Clin Food Anim 27 (2011) 407–417
doi:10.1016/j.cvfa.2011.02.014 vetfood.theclinics.com
0749-0720/11/$ – see front matter. Published by Elsevier Inc.

Box 1
Components essential for a good diagnosis in suspected plant-poisoning episodes

History and Clinical Disease:

Pertinent facts: breed, sex, age, number, condition, vaccination status, mineral supplements, feeding or pasture changes, and other treatments

Clinical disease: number affected, signs, clinical course and progression, lesions, mortality

Clinical tests: Blood tests to evaluate inflammation, organ function, and evaluate immunologic responses to infectious agents (blood cell counts and serum element, metabolite and biochemical analyses, and serologic tests)

Field Studies:

Animals: Condition, unusual behaviors, clinical signs, lesions. Additional clinical tests may be indicated: blood tests or chemical tests for plant toxins or metabolites in the tissues, blood, urine, or feces

Pasture:

1. Determine forage availability, plant species composition, and evidence of grazing patterns
2. Collection of potential problem plants or unidentified plants (dried samples for identification, frozen samples for chemical analysis)
3. Note weather conditions and their effect on forage and forage availability

Prepared feeds: Hay, silage, or concentrated feed samples (frozen for analysis)

Water, salt, and mineral supplements, including location and use (samples frozen for analysis)

Physical location, weather at time of incident, and other obstacles or pressures

Check for other potential hazards, such as old batteries, pesticide-laced feed, and so forth

Postmortem Examination:

Animal condition and lesions

Rumen and gastrointestinal tissues and contents

Tissues for histologic studies fixed in 10% neutral buffered formalin (brain, lung, heart, liver, spleen, gastrointestinal tract, kidney, skeletal muscle, and any gross lesions)

Tissues for chemical or microscopic studies stored in plastic bags and frozen (rumen and gastrointestinal contents, feces [from live animal], complete eye, liver, kidney, serum, whole blood, body fat, bone, urine, milk if lactating)

Extension agents and local pasture or range scientists generally have good working knowledge of plant communities and plant identification. Toxicologists, diagnosticians, and pathologists can contribute by identifying lesions or the lack of lesions that contribute to the diagnostic process. Additionally, there are several Web pages and inexpensive textbooks that approach poisonous plant problems by both plant and systemic methods that are invaluable resources for veterinarians (**Box 2**). A complete differential diagnosis allows selection of appropriate tests to confirm the cause of the clinical syndrome.

The differential diagnoses will lead to field investigations, definitive plant identification, physical or clinical examinations, biochemical or serologic evaluations of the blood, possible postmortem evaluations, and, at times, chemical or microscopic

Box 2
Resource list

USDA/ARS Poisonous Plant Research Laboratory, 1150 East 1400 North, Logan UT 84341, 435-752-2941. http://www.pprl.ars.usda.gov/

State Agricultural Extension Service. http://www.csrees.usda.gov/Extension/

State Animal Disease Diagnostic Laboratory. Contact your local or state veterinarian. http://www.aavld.org/mc/page.do?sitePageId=33930&orgId=aavld (laboratories accredited by American Association of Veterinary Diagnostic Laboratories)

Local Herbarium. Contact your local county agent or your Land Grant College or University. http://herba.msu.ru/mirrors/www.helsinki.fi/kmus/botmus.html (lists of public herbaria throughout the world)

Microscopic analysis of feces and ingesta. Texas Veterinary Medical Diagnostic Laboratories, 888-646-5623. http://tvmdlweb.tamu.edu

Toxic Plants of North America (2001). George E. Burrows and Ronald J. Tyrl. Wiley-Blackwell, 1340 pages. ISBN-10: 0813822661. $229.99. http://www.wiley.com/WileyCDA/WileyTitle/productCd-0813822661.html

A Guide to Plant Poisoning of Animals in North America (2001). Anthony P. Knight and Richard Walter. Teton New Media. 1st edition, 367 pages. ISBN-10: 1893441118. $75.00. http://www.tetonnm.com/cgi-bin/shopper.cgi?preadd=action&key=00031893441113

evaluations of plants or animal tissues. As a matter of review, these brief explanations are included.

FIELD INVESTIGATIONS

Field studies are an essential part of the investigation in which experts should be recruited and used. For example, county extension agents often are trained and experienced in plant identification. If not, they can be helpful in finding outside experts in plant taxonomy and identification who might assist in plant identification. Close examination of pastures and ranges will determine what plants are present in the community, and what plants the animals are eating (**Fig. 1**).

Good field studies also include close monitoring and examination of affected animals. As livestock producers and herders have the most contact with the animals, they may observe subtle changes that should be noted. Experienced observers are also valuable, as many toxic plants produce subtle changes that become obvious if they have been seen previously. For example, locoweed poisoning often produces characteristic "dull"-appearing eyes, whereas larkspur poisoning may result in muscular weakness and trembling that is often first seen as a failure to defecate completely.

Important information can also be obtained from sick animals. Blood or serum biochemical and serologic studies can help rule out many infectious and metabolic diseases. Some plant toxins produce characteristic damage to specific organ systems. Biochemical analysis of blood or serum for metabolites or enzyme activities can be useful in identifying damaged tissues. For example, pyrrolizidine alkaloid damaged livers typically result in increased serum activities of specific enzymes. These enzymes differ from those that increase with white snakeroot–induced muscle damage. Other diseases, such as kidney disease, cause increased concentrations of

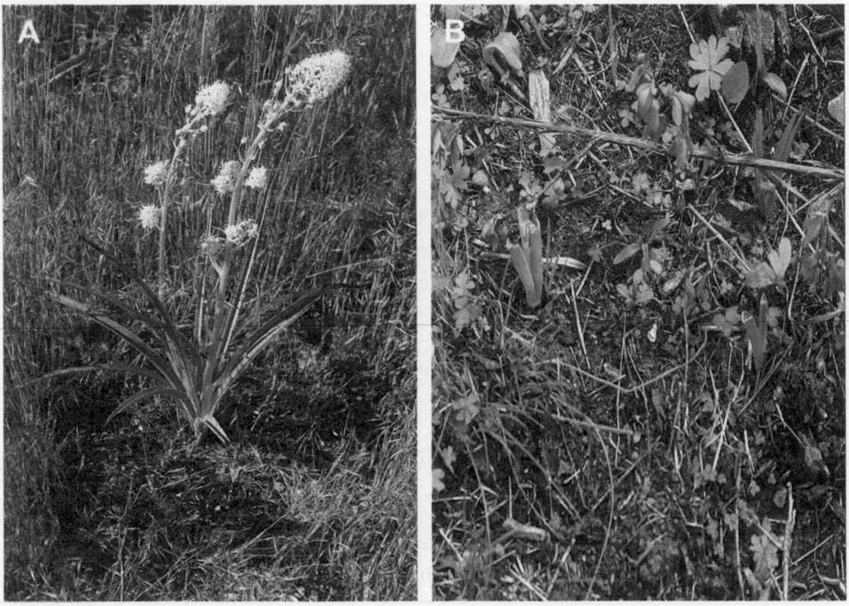

Fig. 1. Death camas (*Zigadenus* spp). (*A*) Intact plant, and (*B*) plant that has been grazed. Death camas is a perennial that has grasslike leaves that grow from a deeply buried bulb. Livestock are most commonly poisoned in the early spring when death camas can grow to 25 cm tall. Poisoning is less frequent when the plant senesces in the early summer.

specific metabolites, such as urea. Such biochemical changes are useful in identifying damaged tissues and ultimately support a specific diagnosis.

PLANT IDENTIFICATION AND PLANT AND FEED ANALYSIS

Unidentified plants or any potentially toxic plants should be collected for positive identification. Plant samples are best collected in paper bags. If plant samples are to be mailed to a local herbarium or the Poisonous Plant Research Laboratory, they should be pressed and dried. The entire plant should be collected if possible. Flowering plants are most easily identified. A convenient way to press plants is to place them for several days between 2 pages of a newspaper and press them under a couple of heavy books. Pressed plants are best mailed in a large envelope taped to a sheet of cardboard. Most state land grant or agricultural colleges have herbaria with experts in plant identification. The Poisonous Plant Research Laboratory, in collaboration with the Intermountain Herbarium at Utah State University, has taxonomic capabilities if other local options are unavailable.

Because the toxicity of a plant is often variable, plant samples may also be needed for a chemical evaluation. For example, the toxins in some larkspur plants of the same species can vary from nontoxic to so toxic than only grams are required to obtain a lethal dose (**Fig. 2**). It is best to carefully label (location, collection date, and species) and freeze freshly collected plant samples in plastic bags if the samples are to be analyzed chemically. Care should be taken to ensure the samples remain frozen during shipping. If freezing is not an option, then partially drying the plant by placing it in a paper bag, then drying the bagged plant in an oven at 150°F (65°C) for 12 hours, will preserve the sample until it can be analyzed. Do not microwave plant samples.

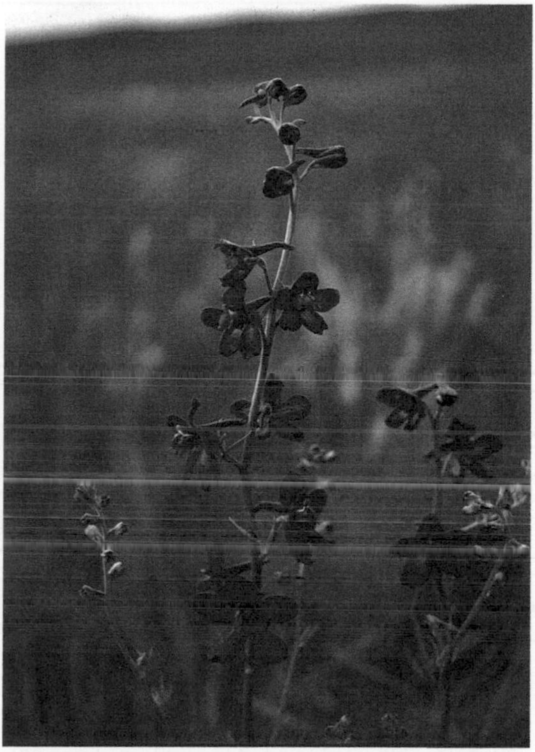

Fig. 2. Flowering portion of tall larkspur (*Delphinium occidentale*), a perennial toxic plant that, depending on the location, can have toxic methyllycaconitine concentrations ranging from 0 to 100 mg/kg. Toxicity appears to be location dependent, but variability suggests that plants must be sampled to determine their toxicity.

Refrigerated plants generally become moldy and rot; moldy samples are of little use for plant identification or chemical analysis. Because each laboratory has specific submission requirements, it is best to contact the laboratory before submission to ensure the sample is properly prepared and that an adequate sample size is being sent (see **Box 2** and **Table 1**).

Some field studies may include evaluation of prepared feeds or forages. Identifying toxic plants in hay is possible, but often problematic. Poisonous plant contaminants in harvested feeds are generally not distributed uniformly, so proper sampling is critical. For example, patchy invasion of weeds in new hay results in contamination of a few bales with the remaining portions of the crop contaminate free. Additionally, some symptoms of toxic plant ingestion are not manifested for days or even months after exposure. During the delay between ingestion and the display of symptoms, the contaminated feed may be consumed, making it unavailable for sampling. Consequently, it is often more productive to examine the area where the feed was harvested. Close examination of the hay field before cutting the first crop provides a better indication of contamination than trying to find patches of plants after harvest. If these more productive methods are not available, sampling of hay should include submission of at least 5 or 6 bales to maximize the chance of finding contaminating plants. Core samples of hay are often used for nitrate or chemical analysis, but they destroy plant morphology and therefore are of minimal use for plant identification. When more

Table 1
Partial list of tests, samples, sample size, and preservation for investigation of potential poisonous plant poisoning[a]

Test	Sample	Size	Shipping
Blood counts	Purple top blood tube	3–5 mL	Chilled shipped on ice
Serum biochemistries	Red top blood tube	5–10 mL	Chilled on ice or if frozen serum should be separated from the cells
Microscopic evaluation of tissues	Various tissues (see **Box 1**)	1 × 1 × 2 cm in pieces	Fixed in formalin
Postmortem or necropsy	Dead or moribund animal	Whole animal	Fresh
Chemical evaluation of serum, blood, urine, or milk	Serum, whole blood, urine, or milk	20 mL	Stored in plastic tubes and shipped on ice or frozen
Chemical evaluation of tissue	Various tissues (The complete eye is the best tissue to analyze for nitrate poisoning.)	2 × 2 × 4 cm in pieces	Stored in plastic bags and shipped frozen
Chemical evaluation of feces or gastrointestinal contents	Feces or ingesta	0.5–1.0 kg (about a sandwich-bag full)	Stored in plastic bags and shipped frozen
Plant identification	Whole plant	Whole plant including flowers, pods, eaves, stems and roots	Fresh if delivered that day, dried if hand delivered later, pressed and dried if sent through the mail
Plant chemical analysis	Whole plants	5 or 6 whole plants	Fresh if delivered that day, dried if mailed or frozen if they can be maintained frozen during shipping
Hay for weed contamination and weed identification	Stored baled hay	5 or 6 bales	Dry
Hay for nitrate analysis	Hay	Several representative samples. These can be core samples, 0.5–1.0 kg	Dry
Prepared feeds	Feeds	Representative feed samples such as cubed feed, 0.5–1.0 kg	Dry
Silage or green chopped feed	Feeds	Representative feed samples, 2–4 kg	Frozen

[a] Be sure to check with the laboratory, as they often require specific sampling, sample preparation, and shipping. Label all materials with indelible ink; provide date, owner, location, and contact information.

intensely prepared feed, such as pellets, are submitted for analysis, they should be randomly sampled, dried at low temperatures, and stored in paper bags so they do not mold.

POSTMORTEM EXAMINATION

Livestock producers often complain that the most expensive animals are the first to be poisoned and die. They should be reminded that if such early fatalities are used to prevent further losses, they indeed are the most valuable, as they may be used to minimize herd losses. A good postmortem examination, or necropsy, provides the most information needed to formulate a definitive diagnosis. At times, field necropsies are the only option in some investigations. The best and most diagnostic samples are obtained from animals that have recently died, or dying animals that are euthanized just before necropsy. Rotten carcasses provide little information, as some toxins degrade and the tissues become unsuitable for microscopic evaluation. When possible, submitting freshly dead or moribund animals to a diagnostic laboratory can increase diagnostic speed and accuracy and it ensures that correct samples are collected and properly preserved. Nearly all states have animal diagnostic laboratories that specialize in postmortem examinations and diagnosing animal diseases. These services are usually supported by state agriculture departments with minimal fees. The veterinary pathologists at these facilities have the experience and instrumentation to recognize, sample, and analyze postmortem tissue samples (see **Box 2**).

At necropsy (either a field necropsy or one performed in a diagnostic laboratory), animal tissue samples should be collected for microscopic studies (see **Box 1** and **Table 1**). These tissues should be small ($1 \times 1 \times 2$ cm) and preserved in fixative (10% neutral buffered formalin with volumes of about 10 times the volume of the tissues). Microscopic evaluation of animal tissues is helpful in identifying many plant-induced lesions; however, most of the plant-induced microscopic lesions are not specific for plant toxins. For example, halogeton forms oxalate crystals that damage kidney cells. There are other diseases and substances, like automotive antifreeze, that can produce similar crystals. However, in sheep that are eating halogeton (not drinking antifreeze), such crystal-induced kidney disease is highly diagnostic (**Fig. 3**). If there are no microscopic lesions or if information from microscopic studies does not specifically identify the cause, the results can always be used to exclude those toxins and diseases that would have produced lesions. For example, white snakeroot generally causes characteristic muscular degeneration and necrosis (**Fig. 4**). The absence of these lesions generally indicates that such causes can be excluded.

At necropsy, gastrointestinal contents should be collected for physical, microscopic, and chemical evaluations. Many plants have characteristic leaves or cellular structures that can be recognized in the rumen or upper intestines. For example, yew or oleander leaves can often be found in the rumen of animals that die of poisoning (**Fig. 5**). Other plants can be identified using microscopic analysis of rumen or gastrointestinal contents. Microscopic evaluation of ingesta for plant identification is a highly specialized field and samples must generally be sent to laboratories that support such analysis. The Texas Veterinary Medical Diagnostic Laboratory provides a service in which they identify plants in rumen or fecal material using microscopic techniques (see **Box 2**). Ingesta, tissues, urine, and blood can also be analyzed chemically for plant toxins. Samples for chemical analysis should be preserved by freezing all samples except whole blood, which should be refrigerated. Care should also be taken to ensure frozen samples do not thaw during transport to testing laboratories.

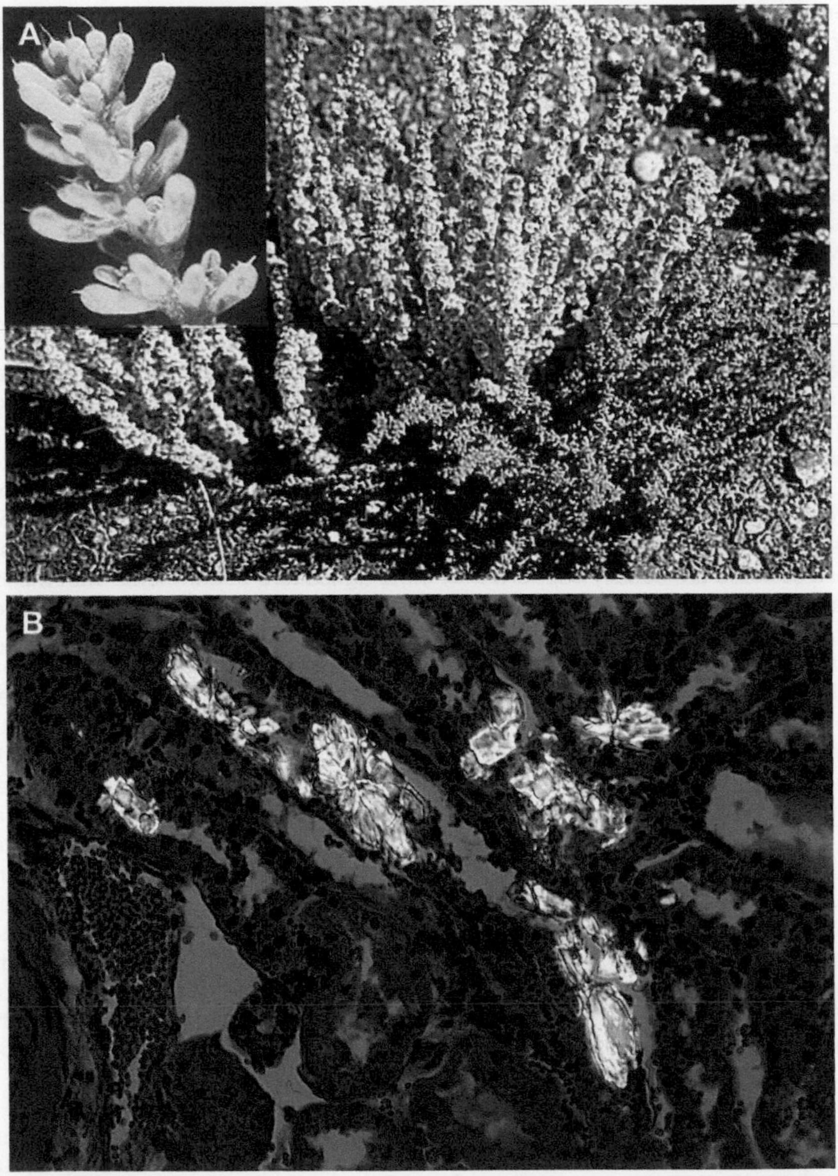

Fig. 3. (*A*) Halogeton (*Halogeton glomeratus*). (*B*) Photomicrograph of oxalate crystals in the renal tubules of a poisoned sheep. Halogeton poisoning occurs when unaccustomed livestock ingest large amounts of halogeton. Animals can adapt to halogeton and eat large quantities of plant without adverse effect if they are exposed to it gradually.

Presence of the plant or toxins in the gut provides definitive evidence of consumption, but does not prove that the plant caused death. As chemical analysis is expensive and specific for particular plant toxins, these assays must be directed and indicated by the clinical and necropsy findings. Screens of animal samples for unknown toxins are often unproductive, as specific instruments and conditions are required to analyze

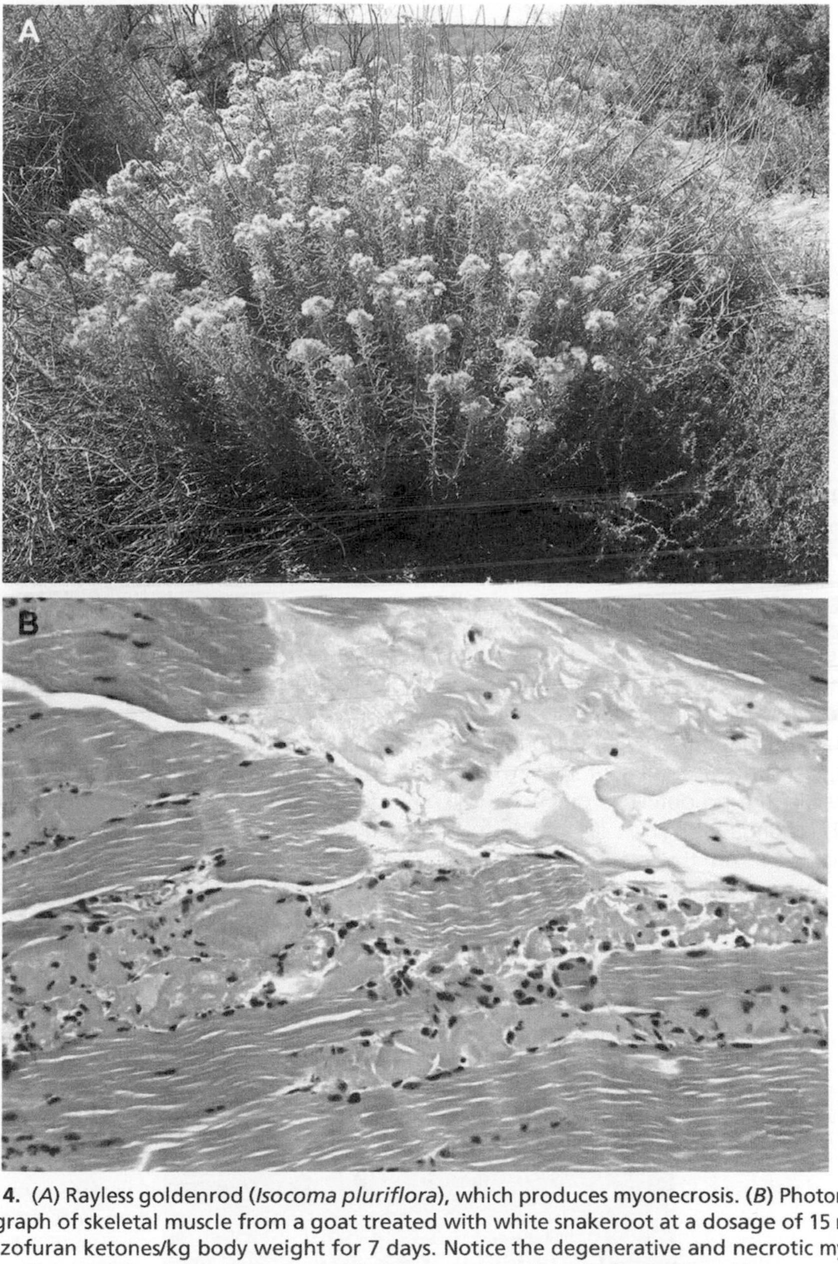

Fig. 4. (*A*) Rayless goldenrod (*Isocoma pluriflora*), which produces myonecrosis. (*B*) Photomicrograph of skeletal muscle from a goat treated with white snakeroot at a dosage of 15 mg benzofuran ketones/kg body weight for 7 days. Notice the degenerative and necrotic myocytes. These lesions produced remarkable increases in activities of creatinine kinase.

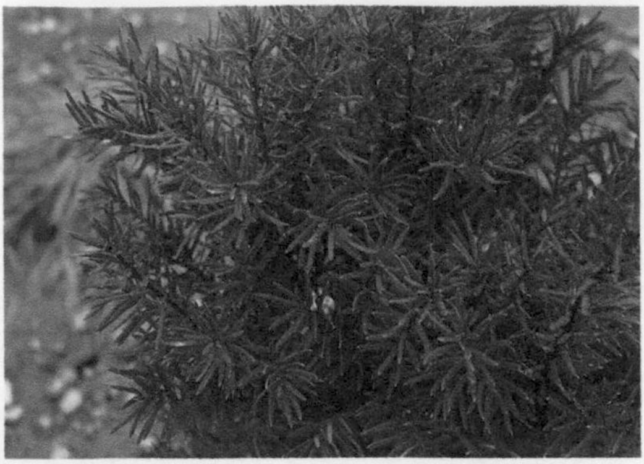

Fig. 5. Japanese yew (*Taxus cuspidata*), an ornamental plant that commonly poisons livestock when clippings are thrown into paddocks and pastures.

each class of toxin. Generally, chemical analyses for toxins are primarily used to document plant toxicity and confirm poisoning.

INTERPRETATION

Care should be taken in interpreting investigative results to ensure that the clinical disease, postmortem findings, and microscopic findings all support the chemical findings. When all information is accumulated and probable diagnoses are evaluated and compared, the information will often identify a most likely diagnosis. This can be difficult, as some portions of the investigative results may seem contradictory. It is possible that no definitive diagnosis will emerge. Despite the contradictions, a most likely diagnosis or short list needs to be made to formulate recommendations and treatment. From these consultations, a plan should be formulated to avoid additional poisoning. This step is often relatively easy and inexpensive. For example, livestock poisoning by consuming low larkspur, can be averted by delaying turning livestock into the pasture until after low larkspur has begun to senesce (**Fig. 6**). Other solutions

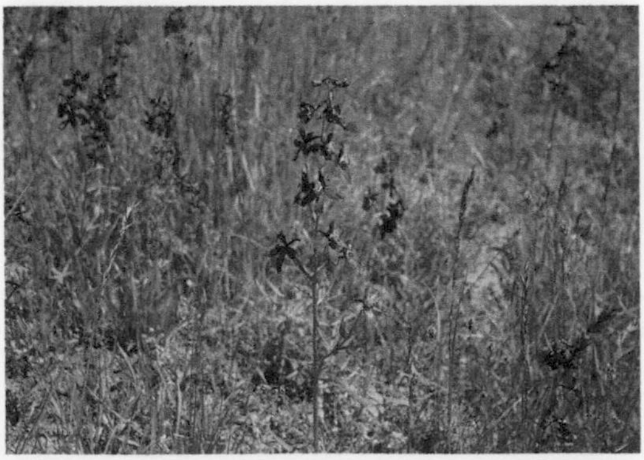

Fig. 6. Low larkspur (*Delphinium nuttallii*), an annual toxic plant that commonly poisons cattle in the spring. The plant grows to 12 to 20 cm tall in the spring. It quickly flowers, puts on seeds, and senesces in the early summer. Poisoning is avoided by delaying grazing until after the plant begins to senesce.

may involve changes in grazing or animal management, herbicidal control, or a variety of other options.

SUMMARY

In summary, correctly organizing, collecting, and preserving materials, and enlisting the proper experts and techniques in the correct manner are essential in arriving at accurate diagnoses and formulating practical solutions for livestock poisoning by toxic plants. A rapid and accurate diagnosis will not only aid in avoiding catastrophic losses, but is a valuable guide to avoiding future losses and ensuring safe and high-quality animal products.

Pyrrolizidine Alkaloid–Containing Toxic Plants (*Senecio, Crotalaria, Cynoglossum, Amsinckia, Heliotropium, and Echium* spp.)

Bryan L. Stegelmeier, DVM, PhD

KEYWORDS

• Pyrrolizidine • Alkaloid • Toxic plants • Senecio • Crotalaria
• Amsinckia

Many problematic pyrrolizidine alkaloid (PA)-containing plants are foreign invasive weeds that invade pastures, fields, and ranges, and contaminate feeds and food. Others are native plants that may increase or expand on field edges or in disturbed areas. Most are unpalatable, only becoming a problem for livestock when alternative forages are unavailable, or when they are included in hay and other harvested feeds. Human poisoning is most often a result of contaminated grain or flour, although several poisonings have resulted from the use of PA-containing herbal preparations. Major PA plants and their specific health-related characteristics are discussed individually.

INDIVIDUAL PYRROLIZIDINE PLANTS

Senecio *Species*

More than 3000 *Senecio* species are found throughout the world. Of these, reports document that approximately 30 have produced livestock and human poisoning such as "stomach staggers," "walking disease," "Pictou disease," "Winton disease," "Molteno," "dunziekte," and "sirasyke."[1,2] Although many other species contain PAs and have toxic potential, their growth patterns and lack of palatability makes

The author has nothing to disclose.
USDA-Agricultural Research Service, Poisonous Plant Research Laboratory, 1150 East, 1400 North, Logan, UT 84341, USA
E-mail address: Bryan.Stegelmeier@ARS.USDA.gov

Vet Clin Food Anim 27 (2011) 419–428
doi:10.1016/j.cvfa.2011.02.013
vetfood.theclinics.com
0749-0720/11/$ – see front matter. Published by Elsevier Inc.

poisoning infrequent. The "more toxic" species are expansive and invasive, allowing them to contaminate feeds and food and dominate plant communities. *Senecio* species that commonly poison livestock in North America include *S jacobaea, riddellii, douglasii* var. *longilobus*, and *vulgaris.* Other "less toxic" *Senecio* species have been suspected of poisoning, suggesting that their identity should be confirmed and their toxicity evaluated chemically (**Fig. 1**).

S jacobaea or tansy ragwort is an invasive noxious western European weed that was inadvertently introduced into Eastern Europe, South Africa, Australia, New Zealand, and North America. In the Pacific Northwest, tansy ragwort often invades pastures and fields. Although it is not very palatable and generally not eaten by livestock, poisoning occurs when plants or seeds contaminate feeds, when grazing animals cannot easily differentiate the early rosette from adjacent forage, or when no other forages are available. *S jacobaea* contains six toxic PAs. The chronic lethal dose in cattle is approximately 2.5 mg total PA per kilogram of body weight (bw) for 18 days, suggesting that a cow would need to eat approximately 1.7 kg of fresh plant per day for several weeks to obtain a lethal dose. Higher doses cause acute hepatocellular necrosis and liver failure, but these poisonings are rare because these doses are unpalatable.

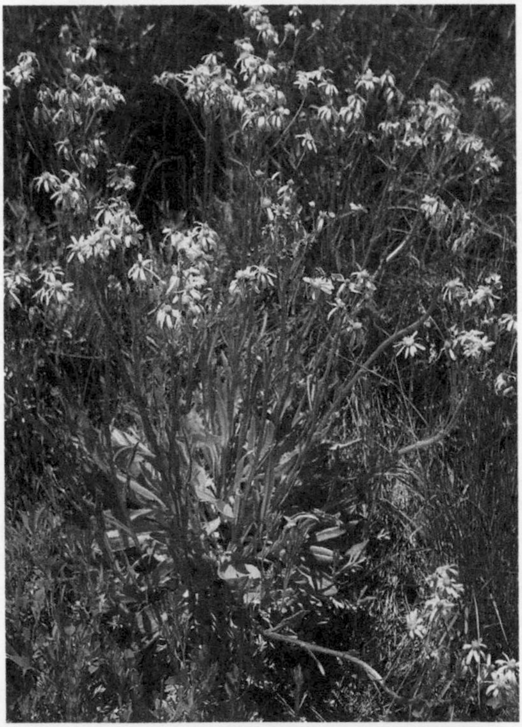

Fig. 1. *Senecio hydrophiloides* (stout meadow groundsel) in the flower. Notice the composite flower typical of most *Senecio* plants. This species is a less common pyrrolizidine alkaloid–containing plant that usually is a minor member of plant communities in the western states. However, it is toxic and under some conditions may proliferate or animals may be forced to eat it and poisoning is possible. Similar minor *Senecio* species can be found in most plant communities.

S riddellii or Riddell groundsel is found in Nebraska, New Mexico, Texas, Colorado, and Wyoming. *S riddellii* differs from other *Senecio* species in that it contains a single major alkaloid, riddelliine. Alkaloid concentrations vary, with PA concentrations in plants collected from the same site ranging from 0.2% to 18.0% (dry weight). *S riddellii* is toxic to cattle at PA doses of 15 mg/kg bw for 20 days or approximately 176 g of fresh *S riddellii* per day. Although riddelliine is less toxic than PAs from other *Senecio* species, the plant can contain more toxin, making the whole plant highly toxic. Riddelliine has also been shown to be carcinogenic to rodents.

S douglasii var. *longilobus*, or threadleaf or woolly groundsel (**Fig. 2**), is a perennial branched shrub that grows on abused or degraded arid rangelands of the southwestern states. It contains four alkaloids with concentrations varying from 0.63% to 2.02% of the plant dry weight, suggesting that approximately 750 g of green plant for 15 days would be lethal for cattle.

S vulgaris or common groundsel is an erect, annual or biennial plant that has been historically used for medicinal purposes. However, it can contaminate feeds and several reports exist of poisoning in horses. Plant PA concentrations vary from 0.63% to 2.02% of the plant dry weight, suggesting that approximately 250 g of green plant per day for 15 days will poison cattle.

Crotalaria Species

Most species of *Crotalaria* that contain PAs were introduced into North America as soil-enriching cover crops. Some escaped cultivation and often spread along fencerows and ditch banks where they may spread and contaminate pastures and fields. Most have long, kidney-shaped seeds that rattle in mature dry pods, resulting in the common name "rattle pod." The seeds can be harvested with grains to contaminate feeds and foods. *sagittalis* poisoning, originally called Missouri Bottom disease, produces liver disease, and causes horses to appear slow, emaciated, weak, and stuporous. Horses that are highly susceptible are most often poisoned when grazing *C sagittalis*–infested stubble fields. *Crotalaria* seeds contaminating grain have poisoned both livestock and poultry.

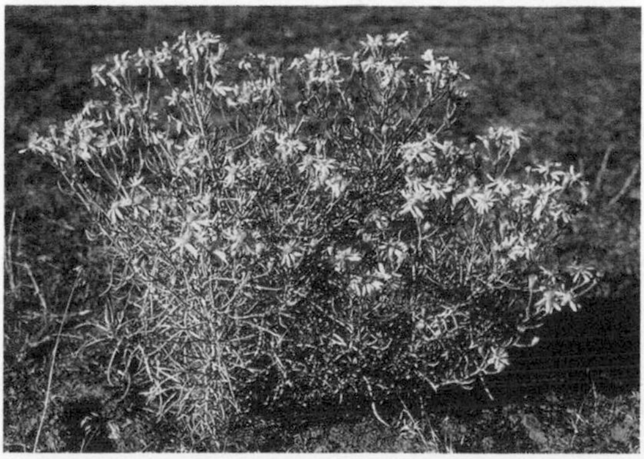

Fig. 2. *Senecio douglasii* var. *longilobus* (wooly groundsel) in the flower. Wooly groundsel is a woody bush that grows up to 1.5 m tall in the southwestern United States. Poisoning occurs when animals are forced to eat it or it is included in stored feeds.

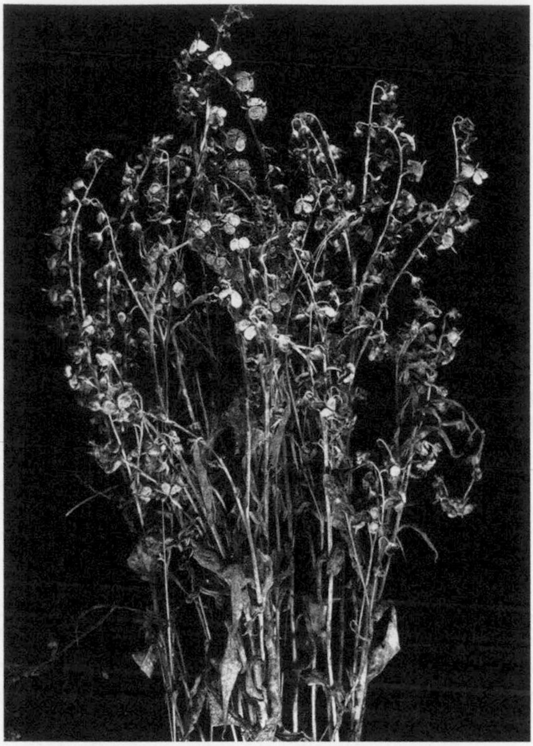

Fig. 3. *Cynoglossum officinale* (houndstongue) dry senescent plant. Houndstongue is a biennial noxious weed that has invaded fields, pastures, and many ranges. It grows approximately 0.5 m tall and produces small burrs that are easily transported on fur, tack, and clothing. As a noxious weed is has become a large concern because it has infested many national forests and public lands.

Cynoglossum Officinale

Cynoglossum officinale, or houndstongue, is a biennial European plant that invades pastures, rangelands, and fields (**Fig. 3**). It is generally unpalatable to livestock, and most poisoning occurs when animals are fed contaminated feed. Hound's tongue contains four PAs, with heliosupine the most abundant and toxic. PA concentrations range from 0.5% to 2.2%, suggesting that 680 g of green plant per day for 14 days would be lethal for cattle.

Heliotropium *and* Echium

Species of both are intermittently reported to poison Australian livestock. *Echium plantagineum,* commonly called Patterson's curse or Salvation Jane, is a noxious weed that can replace alternative forages and poison livestock. Sheep are relatively resistant, but horses and other livestock are susceptible. *Heliotropium europaeum* is a Mediterranean annual that can invade fields and contaminate feeds and food. In Australia it has been reported to poison pigs, cattle, and sheep. However, although it grows in the southern United States, it is rarely reported to cause poisoning. Recent studies documenting PA contamination to honey and wildlife intoxications have renewed interest in both *Echium* and *Heliotropium* toxicity.

Other PA-Containing Boraginaceae Plants

Amsinckia intermedia, commonly called tarweed or fiddleneck, is an annual weed that grows in waste areas and fields. *Amsinckia* is not highly toxic, but it has been reported to cause walking disease in horses and hard liver disease in cattle and swine.

Symphytum officinale, or comfrey, has been used as both forage and a medicinal herb. It contains several PAs and has been shown to cause disease in both experimental animals and humans. Low doses of comfrey have been shown to produce hepatic neoplasms in rodents. This finding has led to increased restriction of its sale, and most herbal companies no longer market comfrey-containing products. However, it continues to be used in herbal preparations on an individual basis.

Several other plants, including members of the *Borago* and *Trichodesma* genera, also contain small amounts of PAs (**Table 1**). Although some are used as medicinal plants and herbs, little information exists on the toxic effects of low-dose PA exposure associated with these plants.

TOXICOKINETICS AND MECHANISM OF ACTION

Plant PAs are composed of free base and *N*-oxides and, because both are toxic, should be analyzed and included when determining plant toxicity. PAs are not directly toxic. To become toxic they must be bioactivated by mixing function oxidases to toxic dehydropyrrolizidine alkaloids (*pyrroles*). Most activation occurs in the liver, which most often results in hepatic damage. Nontoxic metabolites are also produced and quickly excreted. The toxic species damage the adjacent tissues because they are potent electrophiles, and they bind to and cross-link DNA, proteins, amino acids, and glutathione. Depending on the extent and location of the damage, the results are both cytotoxic and antimitotic.[1] Some pyrrole–tissue adducts may persist for months or years and may even be recycled, producing additional damage.

TOXICITY AND RISK FACTORS

Despite similar structures, acute PA toxicity is highly variable and pyrrole-specific. For example, the reactive metabolites of seneciphylline and retrorsine are primarily hepatotoxic. Less-reactive PAs, such as trichodesmine and monocrotaline, produce more stable pyrrole intermediates, resulting in fewer hepatic changes with extensive extrahepatic lesions. Susceptibility to poisoning is influenced by species, age, sex, and other temporary factors, such as biochemical, physiologic, and nutritional status.

Different animal species have vastly different susceptibilities to PAs. For example, the toxic doses of some plants are estimated to be 20 times higher for sheep than those that kill cattle. Consequently, experts have suggested that sheep and goats be used to graze pastures that are dangerous to horses and cattle. The relative species susceptibilities to PA poisoning are: pigs = 1; chickens = 5; cattle and horses = 14; rats = 50; mice = 150; and sheep and goats = 200.[3] Some have suggested that these differences are because of rumen embolism, but it seems like it is a combination of metabolism and species-specific hepatic metabolism.

Age, gender, and nutritional status are also important factors. Young animals are generally more susceptible, and neonatal and nursing animals and humans may develop fatal hepatic disease while their lactating mothers were unaffected. Male rats are more susceptible to poisoning than females. Animals with marginal nutrition or stress with excessive hepatic copper are also more susceptible to PA poisoning. These differences have also been linked to metabolic rates, and toxicity is thought

Table 1
Pyrrolizidine alkaloid–containing Compositae, Leguminosae, and Boraginaceae plants that have been associated with poisoning

Compositae	
Senecio abyssinicus	Rats
S alpinus	Cattle
S bipinnatisectus	Calves
S brasiliensis	Cattle
S burchelli	Cattle
S cisplatinus	Livestock
S desfontainei	Poultry
S douglasii var. *longilobus*	Cattle, rodents
S erraticus	Cattle, horses, sheep
S glabellus	Livestock, rats
S heterotrichius	Cattle
S integerrimus	Livestock
S jacobaea	Livestock, rodents, poultry
S latifolius	Cattle
S lobatus	Cattle
S lautus	Cattle
S leptolobus	Cattle
S madagascariensis	Horses
S montevidensis	Cattle
S oxyphyllus	Cattle
S pampeanus	Cattle
S plattensis	Horses
S quadridentatus	Cattle
S raphanifolius	Yaks
S retrorsus	Wildlife
S riddellii	Livestock
S sanguisorbae	Sheep
S selloi	Cattle
S spartioides	Livestock
S spathulatus	Cattle
S subalpinus	Cattle
S tweediei	Cattle
S vernalis	Goats
S vulgaris	Horses, rodents
Leguminosae	
Crotalaria anagyroides	Cattle
C assamica	Mice
C equorum	Horses
C goreensis	Chickens
C incana	Man
C juncea	Cattle, horses, pigs

(continued on next page)

Table 1 (*continued*)	
C laburnoides	Man
C mucronata	Sheep, cattle
C nana	Man, rats
C retusa	Poultry, pigs
C sagittalis	Horses
C saltiana	Goats, mice, calves
C spectabilis	Livestock, rodents, poultry
C verrucosa	Man
Boraginaceae	
Amsinckia intermedia	Livestock, rodents
Cynoglossum officinale	Cattle, horses
Echium plantagineum	Livestock, rodents
Heliotropium amplexicaule	Cattle
H dasycarpum	Sheep
H europaeum	Livestock, poultry, rodents
H lasiocarpum	Man
H ovalifolium	Sheep, goats
H scottae	Mice
H supinum	Rats
Symphytum officinale	Man, rodents
S peregrinum	Poultry
Trichodesma ehrenbergii	Poultry

Data from Mattocks AR. Chemistry and toxicology of pyrrolizidine alkaloids. Orlando (FL): Academic Press; 1986. p. 1–13, 130–57, 158–90; and Stegelmeier BL, Edgar JA, Colegate SM, et al. Pyrrolizidine alkaloid plants, metabolism and toxicity. J Nat Toxins 1999;8(1):95–116.

to be linked to both the ability of the liver to synthesize and metabolize pyrroles and the hepatic ability to repair pyrrole-induced damage.

Plant and plant/animal interactions also contribute to toxicity. Palatability, the amount and rate that animals eat, varies with season, location, weather, and the availability of other forages. Usually plants are most toxic in the early bud stage when beginning to flower. However, huge variations exist in PA concentrations from year to year and from site to site, making it difficult to predict when a particular group of plants will contain toxic PA concentrations.[1]

Clinical, Biochemical, and Histologic Lesions

Cellular indications of PA intoxication are first seen as dose-dependent hepatocyte swelling. With continuing damage, cellular degeneration continues, with ultimate loss of cellular homeostasis and necrosis or cell death. Histologically, this is seen as acute hepatocellular necrosis or more chronic hepatic fibrosis and biliary proliferation. High PA doses ingested quickly cause acute intoxication, with panlobular hepatocellular necrosis accompanied by hemorrhage and minimal inflammation (**Fig. 4**). These animals show signs of acute liver failure, including anorexia, depression, icterus, visceral edema, and ascites. Serum biochemical changes include massive elevations in aspartate amino transferase (AST), sorbitol dehydrogenase (SDH), alkaline phosphatase (ALK), and gamma glutamyl transpeptidase (GGT) activities, with increased

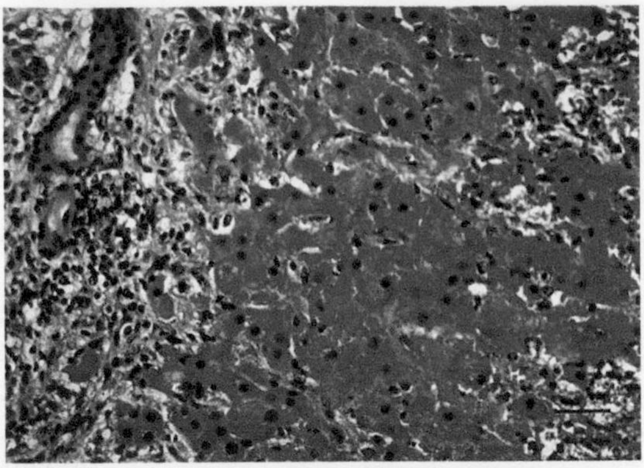

Fig. 4. Photomicrograph of the liver of a horse poisoned with 15 mg of *Cynoglossum officinale* pyrrolizidine alkaloids for 14 days. Notice the massive hepatocellular necrosis and hemorrhage (Hematoxylin-eosin, original magnification ×30 μm).

amounts of bilirubin and bile acids. These conditions must be differentiated from other toxic, viral, and immunologic diseases that cause extensive hepatic necrosis. Fortunately, these animals have high concentrations of tissue-bound pyrroles that can be extracted and detected chemically.

Chronic poisoning is caused by lower PA doses of longer duration. Initially these may not be apparent clinically, because animals develop transient elevations in serum enzymes (AST, SDH, ALK, and GGT). They may have mild elevations in serum bilirubin and bile acids. Hepatic biopsies often have focal hepatocyte necrosis (piecemeal necrosis), minimal peribiliary fibrosis, and mild bile duct proliferation. With time, damaged hepatocytes often develop into large megalocytes (**Fig. 5**). Animals may show no clinical signs, and serum biochemistries may be normal for several months or even years after PA ingestion. However, hepatocellular damage may continue, resulting in continued hepatocyte necrosis with subsequent inflammation, fibrosis, and ultimately cirrhosis. With loss of hepatic function, poisoned animals often do poorly. When these hepatic cripples are subjected to physiologic stresses, such as

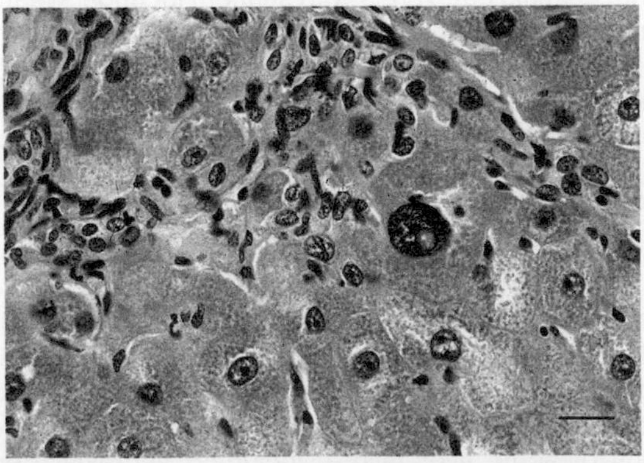

Fig. 5. Photomicrograph of liver from a horse dosed with 5 mg of *Cynoglossum officinale* pyrrolizidine alkaloids per kilogram of body weight for 14 days. Note the megalocytes (enlarged hepatocyte) with large nucleus and biliary proliferation (Hematoxylin-eosin, original magnification ×100 μm).

pregnancy or lactation, they develop clinical liver failure with photosensitivity, icterus, and increased susceptibility to hepatic lipidosis or ketosis. Because this can develop months after PA exposure, the PA-containing plant or feed contaminant is difficult to identify. Initial kinetic studies found that these animals had low concentrations of tissue-bound pyrroles that may not be detected.[4]

DIAGNOSTIC TESTING

Because clinical signs of poisoning can be delayed, exposure to PA-containing plants may be difficult to document. Many diagnoses are made using characteristic histologic changes alone (hepatic necrosis, fibrosis, biliary proliferation, and megalocytosis) (**Fig. 6**). Unfortunately, these are nonspecific changes and a definitive diagnosis is difficult. The ubiquitous nature of PA-containing plants suggests that PA intoxication is underdiagnosed. Although chemical methods using spectrophotometry and gas chromatography/mass spectrometry can identify tissue-bound pyrroles (PA-metabolites), these assays lack sensitivity and are not quantitative. Improved sensitive diagnostics, including enzyme-linked immunosorbent assay (ELISA)–based immunodiagnostics, are needed to definitively identify PA adducts and provide more information on pyrrole kinetics, possible pyrrole recycling, or the cumulative effects of poisoning.

TREATMENT AND PROGNOSIS

The progressive nature of chronic PA intoxication suggests that low chronic PA exposure has cumulative effects. Little is known about what doses or durations are damaging, or the effect of subclinical intoxication on growth or productivity. Although various treatments and diet supplements have been suggested, none have been effective in livestock. Poisoned animals that show clinical signs rarely recover.

PREVENTION AND CONTROL

Prevention is the best control measure. Because most poisonings are attributed to contamination of forages or feed, careful inspection of feed is recommended.

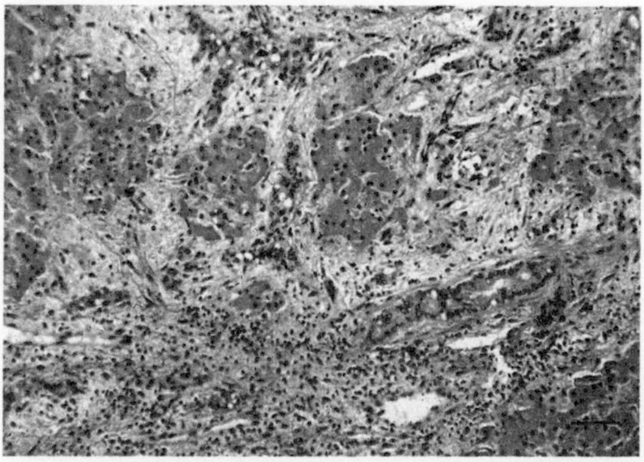

Fig. 6. Photomicrograph of liver from a cow dosed with 15 mg of *Senecio longilobus* pyrrolizidine alkaloids per kilogram of body weight for 14 days. Notice the extensive fibrosis with adjacent hepatocellular degeneration and necrosis. Extensive proliferation of biliary epithelium is also present (Hematoxylin-eosin, original magnification ×50 μm).

Contaminated feeds should be discarded or fed to less-susceptible species. Inspection of fields before harvest provides the best chance of detecting PA-containing plants. Although most PA-containing plants are not highly palatable, eliminating them from pastures and ranges is also recommended. Species-specific herbicide regimens have been developed for most plants and are widely available through county weed and extension services.

REFERENCES

1. Mattocks AR. Chemistry and toxicology of pyrrolizidine alkaloids. Orlando (FL): Academic Press; 1986. p. 1–13, 130–57, 158–90.
2. Johnson AE, Molyneux RJ, Ralphs MH. *Senecio*: a dangerous plant for man and beast. Rangelands 1989;11:261–4.
3. Hooper PT. Pyrrolizidine alkaloid poisoning- Pathology with particular reference to differences in animal and plant species. In: Keeler RF, editor. Effects of poisonous plants on livestock. New York: Academic Press; 1978. p. 161–76.
4. Stegelmeier BL, Edgar JA, Colegate SM, et al. Pyrrolizidine alkaloid plants, metabolism and toxicity. J Nat Toxins 1999;8(1):95–116.

Effects of Xenobiotics and Phytotoxins on Reproduction in Food Animals

Kip E. Panter, PhD*, Bryan L. Stegelmeier, DVM, PhD

KEYWORDS

• Phytotoxins • Plants • Xenobiotics • Reproduction • Animals

The influence of natural toxicants and anthropogenic compounds on reproduction in food animals is significant in its economic impact, and the subject requires more research and further experimental substantiation. Confounding factors such as stress, nutritional status, season of the year, animal species involved, genetic variability, disease conditions, management factors, and so forth exacerbate the difficulty of making an accurate diagnosis and thereby may impede progress to improve reproductive performance on an individual operation. The interaction between the reproductive system and xenobiotics (reproductive toxicology) is a relatively new area of study and a subject of increasing interest, especially in the area of environmental exposures and potential work place toxicants affecting human health and reproduction.[1] Much of the experimental literature about this subject comes from rodent models designed to replicate human exposure; however, the extrapolation to food-producing animals is limited at best. The list of compounds in this article with known effects on reproductive function is extensive and represents most classes of chemicals in the environment; however, this list is not intended to be exhaustive.

Investigation of reproductive dysfunction, especially infertility, abortions, and teratogenesis, should center on a thorough examination of animal condition and health, management practices, and infectious agents while potential toxicants are sought. This method requires a systematic approach including individual animal and herd/flock history, veterinary examination of individual animals, testing of blood, urine, feces, or tissues, gross and pathologic/histologic postmortem examination, and

The authors have nothing to declare.

Poisonous Plant Research Laboratory, USDA-Agricultural Research Service, 1150 East 1400 North, Logan, UT 84341, USA
* Corresponding author.
E-mail address: Kip.panter@ars.usda.gov

Vet Clin Food Anim 27 (2011) 429–446
doi:10.1016/j.cvfa.2011.02.010 vetfood.theclinics.com

toxicologic screening of samples of feed and or tissue. In livestock production systems, these investigations are often limited by economics, and the extent of the battery of tests must be determined in consultation between the animal producer, veterinarian, and diagnostician. Reproductive dysfunction includes all facets of reproduction, and when such dysfunction occurs failure to conceive, abortion, stillbirths, and anomalous fetuses may result.

Although the following discussion focuses on abnormal embryonic and fetal development (teratogenesis), many of the principles and methods outlined in this article may be used to investigate the other causes of reproductive dysfunction.

DEVELOPMENTAL TOXICOLOGY (TERATOGENESIS)

Although the exact molecular mechanism(s) is (are) unknown for many developmental anomalies, the production of an abnormal phenotype may be the result of a single (or multiple) defect(s) in the genotype, environmental insult, or animal-environmental interaction. This process results in tissues either failing to differentiate and develop or in incorrect tissue-tissue interactions. Subsequently, these failures impair normal development. Abnormal development occurs when a threshold of genetic and environmental insults is reached and the fetal compensatory mechanisms are overwhelmed; however, abnormal development is only part of the story of reproductive toxicology.

Six basic principles of teratology were originally described by Wilson[2] in 1959 and further defined in 1977. These principles have withstood the test of time and are applicable for not only developmental toxicology but for other types of reproductive dysfunction.

1. *Genetic susceptibility*. Embryonic/fetal susceptibility to teratogens depends on the interaction of genotype and putative teratogen.
2. *Time of exposure*. Developmental stage of the embryo/fetus at exposure or insult often determines the type of defect. The embryo is often more sensitive than the fetus because this is the stage of organogenesis. However, there are numerous examples whereby the teratogen adversely affects fetal development at various stages of pregnancy, such as lupine-induced "crooked calf disease."[3]
3. *Pathogenesis of defective development.* Teratogenic agents may act on cells or tissues by specific biochemical mechanisms to induce the abnormal development.
4. *Definition of abnormal development.* The final manifestation of abnormal development may include death with subsequent resorption or abortion, morphologic malformations, growth retardation, behavioral anomalies, or organ system dysfunction.
5. *Chemical nature of the teratogen.* The access and adverse influence to embryonic or fetal tissues or organs depend on the biologic, chemical, or physical nature of the teratogen.
6. *Dosage.* The amount of teratogen and size of dam influence the degree of insult from little or no effect to lethality. The effects and/or severity of the toxin or teratogen is dose dependent.

Many genetic, bacterial, and viral factors are responsible for certain malformations, and some of these may mimic defects induced by plant or chemical teratogens, thus confounding a diagnosis.

Causes of many human congenital malformations remain obscure, with estimates of 20% to 25% of developmental defects being attributable to genetic anomalies, 5% to identifiable toxicants, and the vast majority (40%–60%) to unknown causes associated with gene-toxicant interactions.[4,5] While Wilson's principles defining abnormal development have been validated consistently over time, the mechanisms responsible for xenobiotic-induced congenital defects remain elusive, and few studies have identified the pathways of the abnormalities. However, this area of research is rapidly progressing by using molecular tools superimposed on toxins with known effects.[6,7] **Table 1** outlines teratogenic plants and **Table 2** documents other xenobiotics with teratogenic effects.

ABORTION-INDUCING TOXICANTS

Certain natural toxins from plants, fungi, and man-made toxicants have been implicated or associated with abortion, embryonic death, or neonatal loss. In **Tables 3–6** the toxicants of significance to animals are listed, accompanied by the chemical name of the toxicant (if known), the clinical effects, and species affected. **Table 4** specifically lists pines, junipers, and other tree and shrub species that contain the abortifacient toxin isocupressic acid (ICA) or ICA derivatives associated with the so-called pine-needle abortion syndrome in cattle.[10,11] ICA was identified as the primary abortifacient in cattle from Ponderosa pine,[10] and since its discovery numerous tree and shrub species have been screened and found to contain ICA or related compounds (see **Table 4**). As toxin-induced abortions are relatively rare, more frequent causes should be excluded first. The differential diagnosis should also include bacterial or viral agents such as salmonellosis, brucellosis, leptospirosis, mycotic placentitis, bovine viral diarrhea (BVD), infectious bovine rhinotracheitis (IBR), and so forth, and nutritional factors such as deficiencies in β-carotene, selenium, copper, iron, iodine, and so forth.[12–15] Other factors may also be considered such as removal of corpus luteum by palpation or pharmacologically, insemination of the pregnant uterus, multiple fetuses, maternal anemia, uterine or umbilical torsion, rupture of amniotic vesicle, and so forth.

Unfortunately, identifying the exact diagnosis of abortion has a relatively low success rate (<40%). Of course, with improved clinical history, physical examination of affected animals and premises, blood tests, and postmortem evaluation, successful identification of the abortifacient is much better. There obviously is a need to advance methods and techniques to improve the exact diagnosis and to thoroughly identify causes of abortion. Readers are referred to Miller[12] for details of the diagnosis of abortion in livestock.

TOXICANTS AFFECTING FERTILITY

Toxicants causing infertility may result in a temporary reduction in reproductive function or may result in permanent dysfunction. Temporary infertility usually returns to normal when the source is removed and a period of time passes. Subtle changes in herd fertility are difficult to diagnose. Until production records are carefully evaluated and compared with past records, reductions in conception rates of 10% or less may go unrecognized. Even with good records, it is difficult to retrospectively implicate a toxicant when many other factors such as nutrition, stress, genetics, disease, and management may all contribute to such a reduction.

Toxins affecting reproduction may cause dysfunction through one or more mechanisms of action. Toxins may act directly by destroying oocytes or spermatocytes as do some alkylating agents; xenobiotics may act as hormone agonists or antagonists; or toxins may be metabolized to toxic intermediates or to putative compounds with

Table 1
Teratogenic plants

Plant	Toxicant	Effects	Specie and Stage (days) of Development
Veratrum californicum (skunk cabbage, false hellebore)	Steroidal alkaloids cyclopamine, jervine, cycloposine	Cyclopia, cleft palate, limb defects, tracheal stenosis, embryonic death	Cattle, goats, sheep: day 14 cyclopia; day 28–31 limb reductions; day 31–33 tracheal stenosis (sheep)
Veratrum eschscholtizi	Unknown, possibly as above	Cyclopia	Horses
Veratrum album	As above	Cyclopia	Llamas and alpacas
Oxytropis/Astragalus (locoweeds)	Swainsonine, swainsonine *N*-oxide	Bowed limbs, embryo/fetal death	Sheep, cattle, horses; most stages of pregnancy
Lupinus spp *L caudatus* *L sericeus* *L nootkatensis* *L sulphureus*	Anagyrine	Cleft palate, contracture-type skeletal defects	Cattle, 40–100 d
L formosus *L arbustus* *L argenteus*	Ammodendrine	Cleft palate, contracture-type skeletal defects	Cattle, 40–100 d; goats, 30–60 d
Nicotiana tabacum *N glauca*	Anabasine	Cleft palate, contracture-type skeletal defects	Pigs, 30–60 d; cattle, 40–100 d; sheep/goats, 30–60 (35–41 d cleft palate only)
Conium maculatum (poison-hemlock)	Coniine and γ-coniceine	Cleft palate, contracture-type skeletal defects	Pigs, 30–60 d; sheep/goats, 30–60 d; cattle, 40–100 d

Prunus serotina (wild black cherry)	Cyanogenic compounds suspected	Cleft palate, contracture-type skeletal defects	Pigs
Datura stramonium (jimsonweed)	Unknown; possibly alkaloids	Cleft palate, contracture-type skeletal defects	Pigs
Sorghum vulgare *S sudanese*	Cyanogen compounds suspected	Contracture-type skeletal defects	Horses
Lathyrus spp *L cicera* *L odoratus*	Lathyrogens	Skeletal defects	Cattle and sheep
Ipomoea carnea	Calystegines and or Swainsonine	Fetal growth reduced	Rats, goats, rabbits: organogenesis
Luffa acutangula	Proteins; luffin b and lufaculin	Fetal growth reduced; cleft palate	Rats; postimplantation
Mimosa tenuiflora	Unknown	Skeletal defects, brachygnathia, cranial deformities	Sheep, goats, cattle
Caulophyllum thalictroides (Blue cohosh)	Unknown	Cardiovascular and craniofacial cartilage defects	Japanese Medaka embryos
Aspidosperma pyrifolium	Unknown	Delayed fetal development	Rats, goats
Senna occidentalis	Anthraquinones	Delayed behavioral development	Goats

Data from Refs.[3,8,19–36]

Table 2
Teratogenic xenobiotics[a]

Toxicants	Source	Effect	Species
Parbendazole	Anthelmintic	Vertebral column and other skeletal defects	Sheep, goats, cattle, pigs
Methallibure	Pituitary inhibitor	Contracture-type defects	Pigs, 30–50 d gestation
Riboflavin deficiency	Vitamin	Cleft palate, limb reductions	Mammals, birds
Sulfonamides	Sulfur bacteriostatic agents	Beak and feet defects	Chickens
Tetrahydrophthalimide	Captan fungicides	Skull, limb, and visceral defects	Chickens
Tryptophane	Amino acid	Limb and visceral defects	Chickens
Trichlorfon	Organophosphoric insecticide	Cerebral hypoplasia	Pigs
Aminoacetonitrile	Synthetic osteolathyrogen	Skeletal defects	Cattle, sheep
Vitamin A deficiency	Vitamin	Ocular, facial, and central nervous system (CNS) defects	Pigs, cattle, rabbits
Copper deficiency	Trace element	Skeletal and brain defects	Sheep, pigs, horses
Manganese	Trace element	Limbs and vertebrae defects	Rabbits, calves
Molybdenum excess	Trace element	Demyelination resulting in CNS defects	Sheep
Selenium toxicity	Trace element	Fetal hoof defects	Cattle, horses
Aflatoxins	*Aspergillus* spp	Skeletal defects	Rats, goats
Cyanide (cyanogenic glycosides)	Plants	Skeletal contracture defects	Goats

[a] Many other teratogens with reference to rodent models are found in Shepard and Lemire[8] and Szabo.[9]

Data from Refs.[8,9,20,34,35,37–39]

structural similarities to endogenous compounds. These biologic imposters may compete at active sites or alter clearance of natural hormones.

Over the last 30 years, most of the reproductive toxicology research has focused on human reproductive vulnerability to disruption by drugs or workplace and environmental xenobiotics.[1] This research and the risk assessments in humans are generally determined using rodent models, primarily mice or rats. Although research using a rodent model clearly demonstrates potential problems, the direct extrapolation of results from these models to predict toxin-induced reproductive dysfunction or sex-dependent differences in xenobiotic toxicity in livestock species or humans can be inadequate or misleading.

More than 50 years ago sex-linked differences were identified in xenobiotic metabolism. This difference was first observed in rats, where the female was found to be more sensitive to the effects of barbiturates than the male.[5] Subsequent studies

Table 3
Abortifacient plants

Plant	Toxicant	Effect	Species
Pinus, Juniperus, and other woody spp needles and bark: see **Table 4** for specific information on multiple species	Isocupressic acid (ICA) and other ICA derivatives or labdane resin acids	Induced premature parturition	Cattle and bison; anecdotal information suggests llamas also susceptible
Gutierrezia sarothrae or *microcephala*	Unknown	Abortion when grown on sandy soil	Cattle, sheep, goats
Oxytropis and *Astragalus* (locoweeds)	Swainsonine (indolizidine alkaloid)	Abortion, embryonic death	All livestock
Swainsona spp (Australia)	Swainsonine	Similar to locoweeds	Cattle, sheep
Vicia villosa (hairy vetch)	Unknown	Abortion	Cattle
Leucaena leucocephala	Mimosine	Infertility, abortion	Pigs
Aspidosperma pyrifolium	Unknown	Abortion, resorptions	Small ruminants, rats
Tetrapterys spp	Unknown	Abortion	Goats
Artemisia monosperma	Ethanol extracts	Abortion, resorptions	Rats
Bambusa vulgaris	Aqueous extracts	Abortion, resorptions	Rabbits
Ateleia glazioviana	Green or dried leaves	Abortion, stillbirth	Sheep

Other suspected abortifacient plants: *Veratrum californicum* (false hellebore), *Cupressus macrocarpa* (Monterey cypress), *Indigofera spicata* (creeping indigo), *Raphanus raphanistrum* (wild radish), *Lantana camara*, *Iva augustifolia* (narrow-leaf sumpweed), hybrid Sudan (*Sorghum* spp).

Data from Refs.[10,20,23,27,32,37,40–46]

Table 4
Concentration of isocupressic acid or other related metabolic compounds from selected species and locations

Species	Common Name	Location	Isocupressic Acid Conc. (% Dry Weight)[a]
Abies concolor	White fir	Arizona	n.d.[b]
		California	n.d.
		Colorado	0.04
		Utah	n.d.
Abies grandis	Grand fir	Idaho	n.d.
		Oregon	n.d.
Abies lasiocarpa	Subalpine fir	Oregon	n.d.
		Colorado	n.d.
		Idaho	0.04
		Utah	n.d.
Abies magnifica	Red fir	California	0.05
Cupressus macrocarpa	Monterey cypress	California	n.d.–0.06
		New Zealand	0.89–1.24
Cupressus ovensii	—	New Zealand	0.81
Juniperus californica	California juniper	California	0.93 needles
		—	0.05 bark
Juniperus communis	Mountain common juniper	Colorado	2.05–2.88
		Utah	1.50–5.0
Juniperus monosperma	One-seed juniper	Arizona	0.14
		New Mexico	n.d.
Juniperus occidentalis	Western juniper	Oregon	0.10
		—	Imbricatoloic acid = 1.0
Juniperus osteosperma	Utah juniper	Utah	n.d.
		Nevada	0.07
		Arizona	n.d.
		Colorado	n.d.
		Utah	Agathic acid = 1.50
Juniperus scopulorum	Rocky Mountain juniper	Utah	0.84
		New Mexico	0.33
		Arizona	0.42
Juniperus virginiana	Eastern red cedar	Nebraska	needles, low
			bark, <0.10–high
Larix occidentalis	Western larch	Oregon	n.d.
Libocedrus decurrens	Incense cedar	Oregon	0.07
Picea engelmannii	Engelmann spruce	California	0.27
		Colorado	n.d
		Idaho	0.04
		Montana	0.31
		Oregon	n.d.
		Utah	n.d.
Picea pungens	Colorado blue spruce	Utah	0.17
		Colorado	n.d.
Pinus aristata	Bristle cone pine	Colorado	0.01–0.05
Pinus arizonica	Arizona pine	California	n.d.
		Arizona	n.d.

(*continued on next page*)

Table 4
(continued)

Species	Common Name	Location	Isocupressic Acid Conc. (% Dry Weight)[a]
Pinus contorta	Lodgepole pine	Oregon	0.28
		Idaho	0.11
		Colorado	0.29–0.47
		Utah	0.66
		Canada (BC)	0.45
Pinus densiflora	Japanese redpine	Korea	n.d.
Pinus echinata	Short-leaf pine	Arkansas	n.d.
Pinus edulis	Pinyon pine	Arizona	n.d.
		Colorado	0.12
		New Mexico	0.10
		Utah	0.45
Pinus elliottii	Slash pine	Arkansas	n.d.
Pinus flexilis	Limber pine	Colorado	n.d.-0.06
		Utah	n.d.
Pinus halepensis	Aleppo pine	California	n.d.
Pinus jeffreyi	Jeffrey pine	California	0.04–0.54
Pinus koraiensis	Korean pine	Utah	Positive
		Korea	0.02
Pinus monophylla	Single-leaf pinyon	Nevada	0.32
Pinus montezumae	Montezuma pine	California	n.d.
Pinus palustris	Long-leaf pine	Arkansas	n.d.
Pinus patula	Patula pine	South Africa	<0.10
Pinus ponderosa	Ponderosa pine	Oregon	0.74–1.30
		Arizona	0.49
		California	0.08–1.35
		Utah	0.51
		Colorado	0.49–0.58
		South Dakota	0.10–1.30
		Wyoming	0.58–1.11
		Germany	0.62
Pinus radiata	Radiata pine	New Zealand	n.d.–0.26
Pinus taeda	Loblolly pine	Arizona	n.d.
		Arkansas	n.d.
Pseudotsuga menziesii	Douglas fir	Utah	0.04
		Colorado	0.05
		California	n.d.
		Idaho	n.d.
		Arizona	n.d.
		Oregon	n.d
Thuja plicata	Western red cedar	Arizona	0.42
		New Mexico	0.33
		Utah	0.84
		Germany	n.d.
Tsuga mertensiana	Mountain hemlock	Oregon	n.d.

[a] Values are for measured concentrations of isocupressic acid, or where otherwise noted, may include the measurement of a similar related diterpene in samples where the indicated compound was identified and was also the major labdane acid present in the sample.

n.d., not detected (<0.01%).

Data from Gardner DR, Molyneux RJ, James LF, et al. Ponderosa pine needle-induced abortion in beef cattle: identification of isocupressic acid as the principal active compound. J Agric Food Chem 1994;42:756; and Yakubu MT, Bukoye BB, Oladiji AT, et al. Toxicological implication of aqueous extract of *Bambusa vulgaris* leaves in pregnant Dutch rabbits. Hum Exp Toxicol 2009;28:591.

Table 5
Mycotoxins associated with abortions

Fungi	Toxicant	Effect	Species
Claviceps spp (infected grains and grasses)	Ergot alkaloids	Vasoconstriction, abortion	Pigs, cattle, horse, sheep
Acremonium coenophialum (endophyte-infected fescue)	Perloline, peramine, formylloline	Stillbirths, abortion	Cattle, horses, sheep, pigs, rabbits
Balansia spp (infected grasses)	Ergot alkaloids	Similar to *Claviceps* spp	Cattle
Fusarium spp (trichothecenes)	Diacetoxyscirpenol (DAS)	Feed refusal, nausea, abortion	Cattle, pigs
Aspergillus spp and *Penicillium* spp	Ochratoxins (isocoumarins and phenylalanine derivatives)	Nephropathy, enteritis in swine; abortion in cattle	Pigs, cattle

Other mycotoxins suspected to cause abortion include: *Penicillium roqueforti* contaminated grains and corn silage reported in cattle; *Stachybotrys alterrans* contaminated hay or straw reported to cause anorexia, necrotic dermatitis, ulcerative lesions in horses, cattle, sheep and swine, and abortions in swine and cattle in terminal stages; and phomopsins from infected sweet lupines.
Data from Refs.[15,20,37,47,48]

demonstrated that in general, male rats have higher rates of xenobiotic metabolism than do females. This finding was further supported when experiments determined that female rats have 10% to 30% less total cytochrome P450 enzymes than male rats.[13] These sex-dependent differences are further demonstrated in the expression of cytochrome P450 isoforms that catalyze the hydroxylation of steroids.[16] While most literature on sex-dependent differences uses the rat model, there is some limited research suggesting similar sex-dependent differences in metabolism in mice, rabbits, dogs, monkeys, and humans.[1] In livestock there is very little if any research demonstrating similar differences.

Certain reproductive disorders in male children have been increasing in the last decade.[17] Reproductive tract abnormalities such as cryptorchidism, hypospadias, and testicular cancer are increasing in certain human populations. Declining sperm counts have also been reported in certain areas of the world. Similar reproductive disorders have been reported in wildlife species, and have been suggested to be caused by highly contaminated ecosystems. Although few of these types of reproductive disorders in livestock species have been associated with environmental toxicants, more and more anecdotal links are sure to come forth in this regard.

Where xenobiotic-induced reproductive dysfunction is suspected in livestock species, if at all possible the suspected toxicant should be evaluated in the target species. More research is needed to identify toxicants that have adverse impact on livestock reproduction. Toxicants known to affect male and female fertility are listed in **Tables 7** and **8**, and those affecting fowl are listed in **Table 9**.

Table 6
Other xenobiotics associated with abortion

Toxicant	Source	Effect	Species
Nitrates/nitrites	Plants, water, fertilizers	Poor growth, infertility, abortion, death	Ruminants most susceptible
High protein diets, excess urea	Immature high protein pastures, high urea added to diet	Abortion, embryonic death	Cattle
Carbon monoxide	Incomplete combustion, poor ventilation	Inhibited respiratory function, abortion, stillbirths	Pigs; all species potentially affected
Estrogens/phytoestrogens	Plants, silage, pharmaceuticals	Abortion, infertility, anestrus	Sheep sensitive; other species affected
Glucocorticoids	Pharmaceuticals	Abortion, retained placenta	All species
Halogenated dioxins and related compounds	Wood preservatives, lubricants, solvents	Hypovitaminosis, abortion	Cattle
Lead	Discarded materials, paint, greases, batteries	Ataxia, head pressing, encephalopathy, abortion suspected	All species
Phenothiazine	Anthelmintic	Primary photosensitization, abortion suspected	Cattle, sheep, horses, pigs
Prostaglandins	Pharmaceuticals	Abortions, retained placenta	All species
Oxytocin	Pharmaceuticals	Induced parturition	Horses
DDT, dieldrin, heptachlor	Pesticides	Residues detected in aborted fetuses	Cattle
Warfarin (coumarin)	Rodent bait	Abortion	Cattle

Data from Refs.[14,15,20,37]

Table 7
Toxicants causing infertility

Toxicant	Source	Effect	Species
Phytoestrogens Coumestrol Daidzein Biochanin A Formononetin	*Trifolium subterraneum* (subterranean clover), *Medicago sativa*, *Medicago truncata* (alfalfa)	Infertility, decreased conception, irregular estrous cycles	Sheep, cattle, horses
Zearalenone	*Fusarium* molds	Vulvovaginitis	Pigs most susceptible; other species affected
Zearalenol A and B	*Fusarium roseum*	Anestrus, uterine hypertrophy, anovulatory estrus	Pigs
Steroidal estrogens	Rayless goldenrod	Lactation in unbred ewes and wethers; dystocia, infertility	Sheep
Diethylstilbestrol (DES)	Pharmaceutical (discontinued)	Transplacental carcinogen, abnormal development in fetal reproductive tract	All species
Wheat germ	Wheat grains	Estrogenic effects	Unknown
o,p′-DDT	DDT metabolite	Estrogen effects (egg shell thinning)	Avian species
Ergot	*Ergot sclerotia* (seed grains)	Infertility, abortion, agalactia, decreased prolactin	Cows, sheep, goats, pigs, horses
Swainsonine	Locoweeds, *Swainsona* spp	Early embryonic loss, decreased estrus behavior, reduced ovulation rate, abortion	All species
Mimosine	*Leucaena leucocephala*	Infertility, abortion	Pigs
Selenium	Grasses and forbs on seleniferous soils	Inhibits estrous cycle in excess and may increase spontaneous abortion if deficient	Pigs, cattle
β-Carotene	Excess vitamin A	Reduced conception rates	Dairy cattle
Glucosinolates	*Brassica* spp	Infertility	All species
Ethanol extract	*Abrus precatorius* L.	Infertility/DNA damage to spermatozoa	Mice
Alcohol extract	Neem flower	Blocks ovulation	Rats

Treatment generally involves removal of source and recovery is usually spontaneous.
Data from Refs.[17,20,37,48–50]

Table 8
Toxicants affecting male reproduction

Toxicant	Source	Effect	Species
Swainsonine	Locoweed	Decreased libido, reduced sperm production, increased abnormal sperm	All species
Gossypol	Cotton seed meal	Blocks spermatogenesis, reduces sperm motility, male infertility, testicular degeneration	All species
Phytoestrogens	Clover and alfalfa (see **Table 6**)	Mammary development in wethers, reduced libido in rams	Sheep most susceptible; cattle affected
Boric acid	Commercial applications (roach control, therapeutic and industrial products)	Altered spermatogenesis, decreased sperm motility, increased abnormal sperm	Laboratory species
Anabolic steroids and androgenic hormones	Pharmaceuticals	Prolonged use results in masculinization, testicular degeneration	Horses; most species
Halogenated dioxins	Solvents, lubricants	Masculinization	Horses
Chlorinated naphthalene	Solvents, wood preservatives, lubricants	Testicular degeneration	All species
Acute cadmium toxicosis	Industrial contaminant, anthelmintic	Testicular degeneration	All species

Treatment: Observed changes in spermatogenesis are usually delayed 30 to 60 days, whereas changes in libido may be immediate; treatment usually involves removal of the source and recovery will occur spontaneously. With anabolic steroids, halogenated dioxins, chlorinated naphthalenes, and cadmium toxicosis, the effects may be permanent.

Data from Refs.[8,20,32,37]

Table 9
Toxicants affecting fowl reproduction

Toxicant	Source	Effect	Species
Gossypol	Cotton seed meal	Green yolks, pink albumin, decreased hatchability of eggs	Poultry
Aflatoxin, citrinin, patulin	*Aspergillus* spp	Thickened egg shells	Chickens (residues)
DAS (diacetoxyscirpenol) and others in *Fusarium*; DON (deoxynivalenol) and zearalenone	*Fusarium roseum*	Decreased hatchability, reduced egg production and egg shell weight	Chickens
Ammonia	Pit gases	Decreased egg production	Chickens
Lindane	Organochlorine pesticide	Smaller clutch size, reduced yolk protein	Ducks
DDT (DDE)	Organochlorine pesticide (illegal); residue still in environment	Reduced egg shell thickness, poor hatch, lighter eggs, delayed ovulation, reduced clutch size	All fowl
Lead	Lead-containing products	Reduced egg production	Chickens, quail
Thiocarbamates (thiram, ziram, ferbam, maneb, zineb)	Fungicides	Retarded testicular growth, abnormal seminiferous tubules, infertility	Chickens and other fowl
Selenium	Runoff from Se soils and additives to feeds	Decreased hatchability	All fowl
Glucosinolates	*Brassica* spp, crambe meal rapeseed, etc	Decreased egg production, off-flavored eggs, embryo thyroid enlargement	Chickens, turkeys
Linatine, linamarin	Raw soybean meal	Decreased growth	Chickens
Phytoestrogens	Red clover, subterranean clover (phytoestrogens during dry conditions)	Decreased reproduction rate	California quail
Mimosine	*Leucaena leucocephala*	Infertility at >10% *Leucaena* in diet	Chickens

Data from Refs.[18,20,51–56]

SUMMARY

With the technological advances made in molecular biology, biochemistry, chemical detection, and toxicology, reproductive toxicology has made significant progress in the identification of toxins and mechanisms of action. However, much of the reproductive toxicology research has been done in rodent models and may or may not be totally applicable to food-producing animals or humans. Novel molecular and biochemical probes will enable investigators to move to higher levels of sophistication in their search for mechanisms of action.[18] The charge to protect human health, animal health, and the environment from reproductive toxicants is a challenging one. An effective response will require the talents of multidisciplinary teams of scientists applying novel ideas and techniques. In this article the authors attempt to provide brief information in tabular form for rapid reference with regard to food-producing species. Although this list is undoubtedly incomplete, it demonstrates the extent and complexity of diagnosing the causes of reproductive dysfunction.

REFERENCES

1. Kedderis GL, Mugford CA. Sex-dependent metabolism of xenobiotics. Chemical Industry Institute of Toxicology 1998;18(7–8):1.
2. Wilson JG. Current status of teratology. In: Wilson JG, Fraser FC, editors. Handbook of teratology. New York: Plenum Press; 1977. p. 476.
3. Panter KE, James LF, Gardner DR. Lupine, poison-hemlock and *Nicotiana* spp: toxicity and teratogenicity in livestock. J Nat Toxins 1999;8:117.
4. Nelson K, Holmes LB. Malformations due to presumed spontaneous mutations in new born infants. N Engl J Med 1989;320:19.
5. Nelson DR, Koymans L, Kamataki T, et al. P450 superfamily: update on new sequences, gene mapping, accession numbers and nomenclature. Pharmacogenetics 1996;6:1–42.
6. Gaffield W. The *Veratrum* alkaloids: natural tools for studying embryonic development. In: Atta-ur-Rahman, editor, Studies in natural products chemistry, vol. 23. Amsterdam: Elsevier; 2000. p. 563–89.
7. Gaffield W, Keeler RF. Steroidal alkaloid teratogens: molecular probes for investigation of craniofacial malformations. J Toxicol Toxin Rev 1996;15:303.
8. Shepard TH, Lemire RJ. Catalog of teratogenic agents. 13th edition. Baltimore (MD): John Hopkins University Press; 2011.
9. Szabo KT. Congenital malformations in laboratory and farm animals. San Diego (CA): Academic Press; 1989. p. 8–93.
10. Gardner DR, Molyneux RJ, James LF, et al. Ponderosa pine needle-induced abortion in beef cattle: identification of isocupressic acid as the principal active compound. J Agric Food Chem 1994;42:756.
11. Welch KD, Davis TZ, Panter KE, et al. The effect of poisonous range plants on abortions in livestock. Rangelands 2009;31:28.
12. Miller RB. Bovine abortion. In: Morrow AA, editor. Current therapy in theriogenology: diagnosis, treatment and prevention of reproductive diseases in small and large animals. Philadelphia: WB Saunders; 1986. p. 291.
13. Holch HG, Munir AK, Mills LM, et al. Studies upon the sex-difference in rats in tolerance to certain barbiturates and to nicotine. J Pharmacol Exp Ther 1937;60:323.
14. Norton JH, Campbell RS. Non-infectious causes of bovine abortion. Vet Bull 1989;60:1137.

15. Osweiler GD, Carson TL, Buck WB, et al. Diagnostic toxicology. In: Clinical and diagnostic veterinary toxicology. 3rd edition. Dubuque (IA): Kendall/Hunt; 1985. p. 44–51.
16. Waxman DJ, Dannan GA, Gurngerich FP. Regulation of rat hepatic cytochrome P-450: age-dependent expression, hormonal imprinting, and xenobiotic inducibility of sex-specific isoenzymes. Biochemistry 1985;24:4409.
17. Mylchreest E, Foster PM. Antiandrogenic effects of Di(n-Butyl) phthalate on male reproductive development: a nonreceptor-mediated mechanism. Chemical Industry Institute of Toxicology 1998;1:181.
18. Edema FW, Garlick JD. Lead-induced egg production decrease in leghorn and Japanese quail hens. Poult Sci 1983;62:1757.
19. Barbosa-Ferreira M, Pfister JA, Gotardo AT, et al. Effects of *Senna occidentalis* seeds ingested during gestation on kid behavior. In: Riet-Correa F, Pfister J, Schild AL, et al, editors. Poisoning by plants, mycotoxins, and related toxins. Wallingford (CT): Oxfordshire: CAB International; 2011. p. 264–9.
20. Cheeke PR. Natural toxicants in feeds, forages and poisonous plants. Danville (IL): Interstate Publishers; 1998. p. 479.
21. Dugoua JJ, Perri D, Seely D, et al. Safety and efficacy of blue cohosh (*Caulophyllum thalictroides*) during pregnancy and lactation. Can J Clin Pharmacol 2008;15:66.
22. Fernandes LC, Cordeiro LA, Soto-Blanco B. Evaluation of the abortifacient effect of *Luffa acutangula* Roxb. in rats. In: Riet-Correa F, Pfister J, Schild AL, et al, editors. Poisoning by plants, mycotoxins, and related toxins. Wallingford (CT): Oxfordshire: CAB International; 2011. p. 270–3.
23. Figueiredo AP, Dantas FP, Medeiros RM, et al. Determination of teratogenic effects of *Aspidosperma pyrifolium* ethanolic extract in rats. In: Riet-Correa F, Pfister J, Schild AL, et al, editors. Poisoning by plants, mycotoxins, and related toxins. Wallingford (CT): Oxfordshire: CAB International; 2011. p. 280–4.
24. Gaffield W, Indardona JP, Kapur RP, et al. Mechanistic investigation of *Veratrum* alkaloid-induced mammalian teratogenesis. ACS Symposium Series #745. In: Tu AT, Gaffield W, editors. Natural and selected toxins: biological implications. Washington, DC: American Chemical Society; 2000. p. 173–87.
25. Hueza IM, Guerra JL, Haraguchi M, et al. Assessment of the perinatal effects of maternal ingestion of *Ipomoea carnea* in rats. Exp Toxicol Pathol 2007;58:439.
26. Keeler RF. Congenital malformations caused by poisonous plants. Comp Pathol Bull 1991;23:1.
27. Kingsbury JM. Poisonous plants of the United States and Canada. Englewood Cliffs (NJ): Prentice Hall; 1964. p. 460–1.
28. Lima MCJS, Soto-Blanco B. Experimental studies of poisoning by *Aspidosperma pyrifolium*. In: Riet-Correa F, Pfister J, Schild AL, et al, editors. Poisoning by plants, mycotoxins, and related toxins. Wallingford (CT): Oxfordshire: CAB International; 2011. p. 274–9.
29. Lippi LL, Santos FM, Moreira CQ, et al. Toxic effects of *Ipomoea carnea* on placental tissue of rats. In: Riet-Correa F, Pfister J, Schild AL, et al, editors. Poisoning by plants, mycotoxins, and related toxins. Wallingford (CT): Oxfordshire: CAB International; 2011. p. 251–5.
30. Medeiros RM, Figueiredo AP, Benicio TM, et al. Teratogenicity of *Mimosa tenuiflora* seeds to pregnant rats. Toxicon 2007;51:316.
31. Panter KE, Bunch TD, Keeler RF, et al. Multiple congenital contracture (MCC) and cleft palate induced in goats by ingestion of piperidine alkaloid-containing plants: reduction in fetal movement as the probable cause. J Toxicol Clin Toxicol 1990; 28:69.

32. Panter KE, James LF, Stegelmeier BL. Locoweeds: effects on reproduction in livestock. J Nat Toxins 1999;8:53.
33. Panter KE, Keeler RF. Induction of cleft palate in goats by *Nicotiana glauca* during a narrow gestational period and the relation to reduction in fetal movement. J Nat Toxins 1992;1:25.
34. Rousseaux CG, Blakley PM. Fetus. In: Haschek W, Rousseaux CB, editors. Handbook of toxicologic pathology. San Diego (CA): Academic Press; 1991. p. 937.
35. Rousseaux CG, Ribble CS. Developmental anomalies in farm animals II. Defining etiology. Can Vet J 1988;28:30.
36. Wu M, Hu Y, Ali Z, et al. Teratogenic effects of blue cohosh (*Caulophyllum thalictroides*) in Japanese medaka (*Oryzias latipes*) are probably mediated through GATA2/EDN1 signaling pathway. Chem Res Toxicol 2010;23:1405.
37. Putnam MR. Toxicologic problems in food animals affecting reproduction. Vet Clin North Am Food Anim Pract 1989;5:325.
38. Soto-Blanco B, Gorniak SL. Prenatal toxicity of cyanide in goats: a model for teratological studies in ruminants. Theriogenology 2004;62:1012.
39. de Carvalho PR, Pita MC, Loureiro JE, et al. Manganese deficiency in bovines: connection between manganese metalloenzymes dependent in gestation and congenital defects in newborn calves. Pakistan J Nut 2010;9:488.
40. Hijaza AM, Salhab AS. Effects of *Artemisia monosperma* ethanolic leaves extract on implantation, mid-term abortion and parturition of pregnant rats. J Ethnopharmacol 2010;128:446.
41. Panter KE, James LF. A review of pine needle and broom snakeweed abortion in cattle. Proceedings: Symposium on Plant-Herbivore Interactions. Washington, DC: USDA Forest Service General Technical Report INT-222;1987. p. 125.
42. Panter KE, James LF, Molyneux RJ. Ponderosa pine needle-induced parturition in cattle. J Anim Sci 1992;70:1604.
43. Peixoto PV, Caldas SA, Franca TN, et al. Chronic heart failure and abortion caused by *Tetrapterys* spp. in cattle in Brazil. In: Riet-Correa F, Pfister J, Schild AL, et al, editors. Poisoning by plants, mycotoxins, and related toxins. Wallingford (CT): Oxfordshire: CAB International; 2011.
44. Raffi MB, Barros RR, Graganca JFM, et al. The pathogenesis of reproductive failure induced in sheep by the ingestion of *Ateleia glazioviana*. Vet Hum Toxicol 2004;46:233.
45. Riet-Correa G, Riet-Correa F, Schild AI, et al. Abortion and neonatal mortality in sheep poisoned to *Tetrapterys multiglandulosa*. Vet Pathol 2009;46:960.
46. Yakubu MT, Bukoye BB, Oladiji AT, et al. Toxicological implication of aqueous extract of *Bambusa vulgaris* leaves in pregnant Dutch rabbits. Hum Exp Toxicol 2009;28:591.
47. Lynch GP. Biological effects of mycotoxins on ruminants. In: National Research Council, editor. Interaction of mycotoxins in animal production. Washington, DC: National Academy of Sciences; 1979. p. 96–117.
48. Porter JK, Thompson FN Jr. Effects of fescue toxicity on reproduction in livestock. J Anim Sci 1992;70:1594.
49. Gbotolorun SC, Osinubi AA, Noronha CC, et al. Antifertility potential of neem flower extract on adult female Sprague-Dawley rats. Afr Health Sci 2008;8:168.
50. Jahan S, Rasool S, Khan MA, et al. Antifertility effects of ethanolic seed extract of *Abrus precatorius* L. on sperm production and DNA integrity in adult male mice. J Med Plants Res 2009;3:809.

51. Abdelhamid AM, Dorra TM. Study on effects of feeding laying hens on separate mycotoxins (aflatoxins, patulin or citrinin)-contaminated diets on egg quality and tissue constituents. Arch Tierernahr 1990;40:305 Berlin.
52. Branton SL, Deaton JW, Hagler WM Jr, et al. Decreased egg production in commercial laying hens fed zearalenone- and deoxynivalenol-contaminated grain sorghum. Avian Dis 1989;33:804.
53. Chakravarty S, Mandal A, Lahiri P. Effect of lindane on clutch size and level of egg yolk protein in domestic duck. Toxicology 1986;39:93.
54. Chowdhury SD, Davis RH. Lathyrism in laying hens and increases in egg weight. Vet Rec 1988;123:272.
55. Deaton JW, Reece FN, Lott BD. Effect of atmospheric ammonia on laying hen performance. Poult Sci 1982;61:1815.
56. Serio R, Long RA, Taylor JE. The antifertility and antiadrenergic actions of thiocarbamate fungicides in laying hens. Toxicol Appl Pharmacol 1984;72:333.

Southeastern Plants Toxic to Ruminants

Steven S. Nicholson, DVM*

KEYWORDS

• Intoxication • Toxic plants • Ruminants • Nitrates • Cyanide
• Cattle • Sheep • Goats

In this article the southeast includes East Texas and Arkansas east to the Atlantic. It is a wide and diverse area, with many species of toxic plants and various potentially toxic agronomic crops that are used by ruminants. The author attempts to include in some detail the major plant hazards and briefly highlights those of lesser importance. Some toxic plants are not mentioned because they are rarely eaten by ruminants. To save space, routine recommendations such as removal of animals from the source of the toxicant, treatment with activated charcoal, there being no specific antidote, and so forth, are not mentioned for every toxicant. Space does not allow detailed botanic description of the plants. Plant images and general information about distribution can be found at the United States Department of Agriculture plants (http://www.plants.usda.gov) and state university herbarium Web sites.

APLASTIC ANEMIA

Bracken Fern

Bracken (*Pteridium aquilinum*) is an upright fern that grows up to 1.5 m tall, with triangular fronds. Bracken grows in colonies with a connecting network of roots and underground stems called rhizomes, which are the most toxic parts of the plants. Unlike most ferns, bracken grows in well-drained soils. Toxicants include a thiaminase compound and ptaquiloside, the bone marrow toxin and carcinogen. Sheep are susceptible to ptaquiloside and may develop intestinal and jaw tumors, progressive retinal damage, and aplastic anemia, but cases have not been reported in the region. There are no reports involving goats and whitetail deer of which the author is aware. Cattle develop bone marrow failure after consuming amounts greater than 30% of their body weight over a period of weeks or months. Poisoning is not common, but cattle confined to pastures in spring and early summer where bracken is prevalent and grass is scarce are at greatest risk. Bracken toxicosis mimics to some degree radiation sickness, anthrax, bacillary hemoglobinuria, and blackleg. Suckling calves

The author has nothing to disclose.
LSU School of Veterinary Medicine and the Department of Veterinary Science, Louisiana State University Agricultural Center, Louisiana State University (retired), Baton Rouge, LA, USA
* 9940 North Parkview Drive, Baton Rouge, LA 70815.
E-mail address: ssntox@cox.net

doi:10.1016/j.cvfa.2011.02.008

as young as 4 months may be affected. Signs include high fever, blood in the stool, epistaxis, petecchiae in vulvar mucosa, prolonged bleeding from tabanid bites, and hematuria. Severe neutropenia and platelet counts of less than 20,000 are present, but marked anemia is not present because of the long life span of red blood cells. Necropsy lesions include multiple large hemorrhages in the epicardium, plura, peritoneum, intestines, and urinary bladder. There is no recognized effective treatment for aplastic anemia. Extended antibiotic therapy to reduce bacterial infection in the face of neutropenia has been suggested. New cases may appear up to 3 weeks after the animals are removed from the source of bracken fern. The toxicant may remain in hay in the unlikely event that someone might cut and bale a sufficient amount to poison cattle. Neoplasia of the urinary bladder mucosa is possible, but is seen as a separate entity called "enzootic hematuria" in 3- to 4-year-old cattle in other countries. Enzootic hematuria, common in some countries, is the result of smaller amounts of bracken consumed over months or years, likely in conjunction with infection with bovine papilloma viruses.

CYANIDE

Bermudagrass, Johnsongrass, Sorghum Forage, Laurel Cherry, Choke Cherry, Black Cherry

Bermudagrass (*Cynodon* spp) and many other grasses are known to produce cyanogenic glycosides in immature forage. Though mentioned here, it has not been a significant problem in the southeast. African Star grass (*Cynodon nlemfluensis*) is in an example of one of the species grown in the tropics and Florida that can be a cyanide problem.

When immature and less than 0.6 m (2 ft) tall, sorghum forages such as Johnsongrass (*Sorghum halepense*), commercial sorghum hybrid forages, and sudangrass may contain toxic levels of cyanogenic glycosides. Drought stress, physical damage, or a damaging frost increases toxicity. Cyanogenic glycoside levels decrease as the plants mature. Hungry cows may begin exhibiting signs within 15 minutes after beginning to graze. Most cyanide is lost in cured hay and silage. Laurel cherry (*Prunus caroliniana*), Choke cherry (*Prunus virginiana*), Black cherry (*Prunus serotina*), and other *Prunus* spp are known for their cyanide potential. Fortunately, cyanide toxicosis is not common because the course is so fast that the opportunity to treat is limited. Carolina laurel cherry is an evergreen shrub to small tree native to the region and sometimes used as an ornamental. In winter the cyanide potential increases to highly toxic levels in the leaves. Crushing leaves with the fingers releases the "cherry coke" odor of benzaldehyde and hydrocyanic acid. Cattle, sheep, or goats fed fresh-cut or storm-downed foliage may be killed within the hour. Black cherry intoxication in a goat and diagnosis by identification of leaf fragments in rumen contents has been reported.[1]

Plant material containing more than 200 ppm cyanide potential is considered hazardous. A level of 500 ppm has been used for the sorghums. The toxic effect is to block transfer of molecular oxygen from oxyhemoglobin, leaving venous blood bright red. Signs include a marked increase in rate and depth of respiration, apparent anxiety, trembling, muscle twitches, collapse, convulsions, and death within minutes.

At necropsy soon after death venous blood is bright red, like arterial blood, because it is highly oxygenated. There is an absence of specific lesions; perhaps small hemorrhages associated with agonal death may be seen. The intravenous antidote for cyanide toxicosis is a sodium nitrite-sodium thiosulfate solution. Burroughs demonstrated the efficacy of using sodium thiosulfate alone as a 30% to 40% intravenous solution at a dose of 25 to 50 g/100 kg body weight (b.w.) in ruminants.[2]

CARDIOVASCULAR

Oleander, Gossypol, Mountain Laurel, Azaleas, Rhododendrons, Leucothea, Lyonia, Japanese Yew, Ergot, Fescue

Oleander (*Nerium oleander*), an extremely toxic ornamental shrub common to the subtropical Gulf Coast region, is not browsed when green but most animals will eat freeze-killed leaves. Most livestock and horses will consume dead leaves in lawn clippings. Perhaps a dozen 6-inch (15 cm) long leaves is a fatal dose to a cow. Cardiac glycosides similar in effect to digitalis cause depression, diarrhea, weakness and recumbency, or sudden death within hours. Auscultation may reveal bradycardia and various arrhythmias. Leaf fragments in rumen contents are easily identified. Microscopic evidence of myocardial muscle necrosis may be present.

Cottonseeds contain pigments, one of which is the toxic component gossypol, a polyphenolic compound. The solvent only method of extraction produces cottonseed meal with free gossypol content up to 0.6%. Calves in dry lot may develop pulmonary edema, ascites, diarrhea, weakness, and anemia after consuming toxic levels of gossypol in a diet containing cottonseed meal for 70 days or longer. Gossypol in the diet at 250 to 300 mg of free gossypol per day for several months apparently caused congestive heart failure in adult goats.[3] Lambs may be found dead with minimal gross lesions. Lactating Holstein cows fed high levels of cottonseed products, especially during hot humid summer weather conditions, have died suddenly. Pale areas of myocardium, liver congestion, and edema in the intestinal tract are typical lesions. Other cardiotoxic plants, ionophore toxicosis, or perhaps excessive selenium injection should be ruled out.

Japanese yew (*Taxus* spp), an evergreen along the northern border of the region, is well known for cardiotoxic effects. Bulls gathered for a sales event in North Arkansas gained access to Japanese yew clippings and some died. Others died suddenly while being driven into holding pens for examination. The needle-like leaf parts are easily identified in rumen contents.

Azaleas and rhododendrons (*Rhododendron* spp), mountain laurel (*Kalmia latifolia*), lambkill (*Kalmia angustifolia*), *Leucothoe* spp, *Lyonia* spp, and minniebush (*Menziesia pilosa*) are members of the Ericaceae family in areas within the region to the east of Arkansas and Texas. These species are highly toxic to cattle, sheep, and goats. Animals raised in contact with these evergreen plants may seem to ignore them, probably because of an earlier unpleasant experience. The toxic components are grayanotoxins, which are diterpenes that cause marked weakness, bradycardia, arrhythmias, lethargy, frothy salivation, and regurgitation of rumen contents. Poisoned goats vocalize and exhibit projectile vomiting. Inhalation pneumonia is a hazard when attempting to administer activated charcoal. Leaves can be identified in rumen contents.

Ergot (*Claviceps purpurea*) infects the flowers of many grasses and cereal grains. The fungus replaces the developing seeds with ergot bodies or sclerotia. Ergot alkaloids, primarily the ergopeptine class, cause vasoconstriction in peripheral arterioles, leading to lameness and dry gangrene in the extremities, tail, and tips of the ears. Cold weather enhances these effects. Hay is toxic. Ergot-contaminated feed containing toxic levels of ergot, perhaps below the level causing gangrene, induces a hyperthermic condition in cattle during warm months.

Tall fescue (*Festuca arundinacea*), infected with the endophyte *Neotyphodium coenophialum*, causes the same conditions as does *Claviceps purpurea*. The gangrenous form is fescue foot, which primarily affects cattle. Summer slump is a hyperthermic condition induced by ergot alkaloids that involves interference with thermoregulation. Reduced weight gain, lowered milk production, and low pregnancy rates are the largest economic impacts on cattle production. Dystocia and obstipation associated with hard masses of abdominal and pelvic fat (fat necrosis) is a condition that affects some cattle pastured on highly fertilized fescue year after year. Hay is toxic. A pigmy goat pastured on endophyte-infected fescue had abdominal fat necrosis at necropsy.[4] A great deal of scientific information is available on fescue toxicosis.

GASTROINTESTINAL

Tung Oil Tree, Buttercup, Privet, Bladderpod, Rattlebox, Tallow Tree, Nightshades, Death Camas, Pokeweed

All parts of the tung oil tree (*Aleurites fordii*) are severe gastrointestinal irritants. Tung oil tree farms were once present in the southeast. The tree is used as an ornamental, and has escaped from old farm sites to populate wooded areas. In 3 incidents, Holstein cows and heifer calves browsed leaves and stems of saplings and tungnuts on the ground in October, or leaves from trees blown down in a holding pen. In another case a group of 40 Holstein heifers, aged 4 to 10 months, ate toxic amounts of leaves and leaf stems from saplings up to 1.5 m (5 ft) tall along the fence in their pasture immediately on being returned there from holding pens. Anorexia, diarrhea (often bloody), severe dehydration, marked weight loss, and listlessness persisted for days. More than 20 affected animals died, some despite fluid therapy. Necropsies revealed a reddened and mildly edematous abomasal mucosa with several deep 2- to 4-cm abomasal ulcers, and fragments of leaves and stems.

Buttercups (*Ranunculus* spp) are common weeds with well-identified toxins that are known to irritate the gastrointestinal tract. These weeds are generally not grazed to any extent, but some may be consumed along with forage without apparent harm.

Six species of privet (*Ligustrum* spp) are established in the region. Privet is often browsed lightly by ruminants, and is an important deer browse. Cuttings from ligustrum hedges fed to hungry cattle and goats have caused anorexia, regurgitation, chronic diarrhea, and weight loss. Five cows died after being fed ligustrum hedge where clinical findings included ataxia, recumbency with an inability to stand, depression, greenish nasal discharge, cessation of rumination, normal body temperature, and increased heart and respiratory rates.[5]

Bladderpod (*Sesbania vesicara*) and rattlebox (*Sesbania drummondii*) are members of the pea family that are weeds/shrubs of up to 2.5 m (8 ft) in height. Leaves contain 20 to 40 opposite leaflets. The seedpods (legumes) of bladderpod contain 1 or 2 large seeds. Rattlebox has 4-cornered seedpods containing several small seeds. The seeds of these plants are strong irritants to the gastrointestinal tract with 1.0% b.w. being lethal. Although seldom browsed by resident animals unless there is no choice, new animals including stocker cattle, sheep, and goats have ingested toxic levels of the mature seed pods in the fall. Seeds, some sprouting, may be found in the rumen contents. Coffeeweed or danglepod (*Sesbania herbacea*, formerly *S exaltata*) has little or no significant toxicity, and is much more common than bladderpod and rattlebox.

The Chinese tallow tree (*Sapium sebiferum*), also known as the tallow tree, popcorn tree, and Florida aspen, is common in much of the region. Cattle rarely do more than lightly browse young growth unless starving. Anorexia and diarrhea are signs of ingestion of toxic amounts of leaves and fruit. Goats seem to browse tallow tree foliage without apparent harm.

The leaves, stems, and especially the root of pokeweed (*Phytolacca americana*) when ingested produce a moderate to severe gastroenteritis. Bloody diarrhea was reported in a 5-year-old Boer goat that had a history of ingesting pokeweed. It recovered in 4 days with supportive treatment.[6]

HEPATIC

Aflatoxins, Cocklebur, Crotalaria, Lantana, Moldy Forage, Bluegreen Algae

Corn, cottonseed, cottonseed meal, and peanuts grown in the southeast may contain aflatoxins when dry conditions stress these plants at critical stages of growth. See the article by Michelle Mostrom elsewhere in this issue on mycotoxins.

Cocklebur (*Xanthium* spp) in the 2-leaf stage is lethal to calves at 1% b.w. Heavily infested pastures and flood plains are potentially dangerous for cattle and calves soon after flood waters recede. Signs include spasmodic contractions of muscles and death within hours. Seeds are toxic and are potential problem in grain screenings, hay, and silage. Hepatic lesions include centrilobular necrosis.

Showy Crotalaria (*Crotalaria spectabilis*) and several other species of crotalaria are present in the region. This plant grows up to 1.3 m (4.3 ft) tall, producing showy yellow flowers in late summer followed by large inflated seed pods. Mature seeds are black or brown and look like tiny equine kidneys. Seeds can remain dormant in undisturbed soil then germinate up to 60 years later when the ground is plowed. This process may result in the reappearance of a significant toxic hazard if livestock and horses have access to the plants. All parts of showy crotalaria contain monocrotaline and other pyrrolizidine alkaloids. The seeds are a potential contaminant in corn or soybean screenings. Acute and subacute poisoning is possible, but the usual situation is ingestion of perhaps 1% to 3% b.w. over several weeks in the fall or early winter. Signs of liver failure are often delayed 6 months or longer when weight loss, rough hair coat, anorexia, diarrhea, wandering, and coma appear. Microscopic hepatic lesions in chronic cases include megalocytosis, fibrosis, and cirrhosis.

Lantana (*Lantana camara*) is a deciduous tropical-subtropical warm-season ornamental, common in southeast Texas, Louisiana, and Florida and less so elsewhere. Known in some areas as large-leaf lantana, it is one of the most toxic plants in the region. Cattle, sheep, and goats are poisoned. Lantana is an ornamental that is spread to pastures and coastal marsh levees and canal banks by birds that eat the seeds, especially mockingbirds. *L camara* is a square-stemmed shrub with or without weak thorns or prickles and dense flower clusters containing shades of yellow, orange, red, and pink petals. Other varieties and species of lantana are likely not as toxic, according to published articles. Triterpene compounds cause bile stasis due to cholangitis as well as diffuse liver changes and some degree of nephrosis. Cattle in coastal areas tend to eat lantana in the fall. Gastrointestinal mucosa irritation is moderate to severe. Ingestion of 0.1% to 0.5% b.w. by cattle is followed within 2 or 3 days by mild to severe secondary photosensitization, lethargy, dehydration, anorexia, icterus, and constipation or black diarrhea. Bloody stools may be present in calves old enough to browse. The liver is swollen and orange due to cholestasis, and the gall bladder is distended with the wall edematous. The gastrointestinal mucosa is reddened; the higher the dose, the more severe the inflammation. Death tends to occur after several days or weeks. Slow absorption of the toxins from the rumen should be countered by activated charcoal. Photosensitized animals need shade, food, and water.

Moldy forage is associated with liver necrosis, bile stasis, and secondary photosensitization. In the southeast common bermudagrass (*Cynodon dactylon*) pastures, other grasses, and clovers (*Trifolium* spp) have become toxic to cattle causing intrahepatic cholestasis, periportal fibrosis, biliary hyperplasia, and photosensitization. Hay cut from a pasture when toxic has caused liver damage when fed 6 months later.

In Louisiana, this uncommon condition tends to appear in summer during a week of clear sunny skies following 2 to 3 weeks of frequent rains. A typical case includes 20% to 30% morbidity, anorexia, weakness, icterus, photosensitization, recumbency, and death in hours to days. Toxicity seems to be lost following additional rain. Casteel[7] points out that no known toxic organism or toxin has been demonstrated, and that perhaps fungi common to pastures in the region produce toxins under these conditions that have not yet been demonstrated.

Bluegreen algae toxins are an important cause of incidents of acute hepatic congestion and necrosis in cattle in the southeast. *Microcystis aeruginosa* and *Nodularia* spp bluegreen algae are known to produce hepatotoxins. *Microcystis* is common in southeastern ponds and lakes. When conditions are right and an algae bloom occurs, windblown accumulations may be concentrated along an area of the bank in farm ponds and lakes. It is a warm-season, sunny-skies phenomenon. The history often suggests that a recent rain with runoff from fertilized pastures or crops has supplied phosphorus and nitrogen, which enhances the bloom. Morbidity may be low if only a few animals drink from the contaminated area. Laboratory confirmation of toxin is available. The green to turquoise paint-like scum may be seen on the front legs, feet, and muzzle. As an example, 6 of 16 200- to 250-kg dairy heifers placed in a pasture at 8 AM were found dead or near death at 6 PM. The abomasal mucosa was red and the liver enlarged. Two others had diarrhea, were weak, and had markedly elevated serum transaminases followed by severe secondary photosensitization in 2 to 3 days. Histopathology was consistent with *Microcystis* intoxication, and microscopic examination of algae samples confirmed the presence of *Microcystis*.

MUSCLE

Coffee Senna, Sicklepod

Coffee senna, septic weed (*Senna occidentalis*), and sicklepod (*Senna obtusifolia*) are major toxic plants known for causing myopathy in skeletal and cardiac muscle. Coffee senna is found in southeast Texas, Louisiana, Florida, and scattered locations in the other states of the region. Sicklepod is more common throughout the region. Most literature involves cattle, but other ruminants and horses are susceptible. Seeds are toxic and can be a problem when fed in contaminated grain or soybean screenings. Research points to water-soluble toxins that damage mitochondria of muscle. Coffee senna prefers sandy soils but will grow in other soil types. Pointed leaflets, 6 opposite and one at the end of the leaf, and striated seedpods that curve upward distinguish it from sicklepod, which has 6 leaflets per leaf that are rounded at the end opposite their attachment (obtuse) and sickle-shaped seedpods. Coffee senna may be ignored by cattle until shredded with a mower, trampled, or damaged by frost. Cattle held overnight in pens where it is prevalent may eat trampled plants. Yearling cattle confined to areas where sicklepod is present are likely to eat it in the fall. The author has seen more than a dozen cases where 8 to 24 heifers were down, most of which died. Both plants have been a problem as contaminants in corn and sorghum silage or green chop. Coffee senna is so toxic that it must not be included in silage at any level. The clinical signs of senna myopathy include weakness, myoglobinuria, dyspnea, and recumbency without attempts to stand. Creatine kinase levels may be elevated 10 to 1000 times above normal. Pale to almost white muscles, adjacent to normal muscles, are seen in the shoulder and pelvic limb. Mild hepatic necrosis and renal tubular necrosis are seen microscopically. Despite supportive care, shade, feed, and water, most recumbent animals die in 1 to 7 days.

NERVOUS SYSTEM

Dallisgrass, Bermudagrass, Carolina Jessamine, Phalaris, Buckeye, Water Hemlock, Poison Hemlock, Zigadenus spp, White Snakeroot

In late summer and fall a common toxicosis is paspalum staggers, caused by ingestion of Dallisgrass (*Paspalum dilatatum*) seeds infected with the fungus *Claviceps paspali*. Paspalitrem indole alkaloids similar to those reported in bermudagrass seeds (see below) are considered to be the cause. The fungus invades the grass flower and develops in the seed. The swollen, brown, or orange infected seeds are called sclerotia. When perhaps half of the seed heads in the pasture are infected, the risk is high. Outbreaks typically appear within 12 to 24 hours after cattle enter the pasture. From a distance the animals may appear normal, but they become apprehensive and signs intensify when approached. Morbidity can be 10% to 30% or higher. Tremors of the head, shoulder, and flank are accompanied by uncoordinated movement, ataxia, a stiff hopping gait, collapse, and tetanic seizures. Attempts to handle affected animals may induce severe signs. Mortality is low, and supportive care and shade is indicated for animals that remain down. Complete recovery may take days to 2 weeks. There are no specific lesions. Prevention is by mowing the pasture with blades set to remove the infected seed heads yet spare most leaves. When infected seed heads are baled in hay, sclerotia tend to drop out when the hay is unrolled and fed on the ground. Sclerotia accumulate on the floor or ground around hay feeders, where they may be ingested.

A rare condition, bermudagrass tremors, occurs in cattle when common bermudagrass (*Cynodon dactylon*) and less often coastal bermudagrass, become tremorgenic in late summer and fall. Recently in South Africa, indole-diterpene alkaloids were identified in bermudagrass seeds infected with *Claviceps cynodontis* from an outbreak of tremors in cattle.[8] Horses, sheep and goats are also susceptible. Clinical signs in cattle are identical to paspalum staggers described above. Attempts to drive or handle affected animals are met with intensification of signs. Cattle can often be lured out of a toxic pasture with feed. If necessary, an alternative is to provide feed or good-quality hay and leave them on the toxic pasture. Hay cut when the grass is toxic retains toxicity for at least 2 years. The toxicant apparently does not appear in milk.

Carolina jessamine (*Gelsemium sempervirens*) and *Gelsemium rankinii* are common evergreen vines producing clusters of yellow funnel-shaped flowers in late winter and spring. Fence lines, shrubs, trees, and the floor of forests and lightly wooded areas may be covered with jessamine, which is also used as an ornamental. Hungry cattle may ingest large amounts in late winter. Strychnine-like alkaloids cause neurologic signs including progressive weakness, recumbency, convulsions, and coma prior to death. Stems and leaves can be identified in rumen contents. A group of 5 goats confined to a fenced paddock were fed jessamine vines for 5 days, killing 3.[9]

Canarygrass (*Phalaris carolinensis*), and other *Phalaris* spp are cool-season grasses present in some fields and pastures in the southeast. In southwest Louisiana cattle and sheep have been affected, although rarely.[10] Stocker calves developed signs similar to paspalum staggers while grazing canarygrass in February, and all recovered. In one incident sheep exhibited severe tremorgenic signs and some died acutely, perhaps due to cardiotoxic effects. Then weeks after removal from the source of canarygrass, some survivors experienced a return of tremors. Bulls developed signs of rear-limb stiffness and severe weight loss caused by loss of their ability to control tongue and lip movement 2 months after last grazing canarygrass. Cows exhibited tremorgenic signs while grazing canarygrass in a field of soybean stubble, then a month later several cows became emaciated and suddenly collapsed in tetanic seizures when handled. Microscopic brain lesions reported to occur in phalaris toxicosis were seen in the fatal cases.

Red Buckeye (*Aesculus pavia*) and 5 other *Aesculus* spp inhabit forests in the southeast. These plants are small deciduous trees or shrubs that leaf out in late winter, providing an opportunity for hungry ruminants to browse the toxic green shoots. The large seeds drop to the ground in the fall. Acute onset of clinical signs soon after eating young leaves or seeds include depression, ataxia, stumbling, and tremors, with severe depression, coma, and death in some. Most affected animals survive, however. Seed fragments are recognizable in rumen contents.

Water hemlock (*Cicuta maculata*) is a perennial herb that grows up to 2 m (6.6 ft) tall and is found near streams, ponds, and wet meadows. Clusters of white flowers are arranged on stems in an umbrella fashion. The root is hollow-chambered with finger-like hollow projections that exude a yellowish liquid on the cut surface. The liquid contains an extremely toxic alcohol responsible for inducing severe muscular spasms and tetanic seizures. The early spring leaves, lower stem, and roots contain the most toxicant. These toxic parts may be pulled out of wet soil and eaten by cattle, sheep, and probably goats.

Poison hemlock (*Conium maculatum*) is a member of the parsley family. When in flower in the spring and early summer, it looks somewhat like water hemlock from a distance. Flowers are white in umbrella-shaped clusters. Stems are streaked dark red and the root is carrot-like and white. Pyridine alkaloids in the stems and leaves first stimulate then depress the central nervous system. Nervousness, tremors, salivation, and incoordination are followed by weakness, paralysis, bradycardia, coma, and death. Because the plant is not grazed, the risk of poisoning is mainly limited to ingestion in hay. Teratogenic alkaloids in the plant can cause congenital defects, including arthrogryposis when cows ingest toxic levels during gestation days 40 to 70.

White snakeroot (*Ageratina altissima* L., King & H. Rob), formerly *Eupatorium rugosum*, is a herbaceous perennial with opposite branches, leaves opposite and serrated, growing up to 1.5 m (5 ft) tall. White snakeroot is widely distributed in the region. In the fall, small clusters of white flowers are produced at the ends of branches but identification is difficult because there are several related plants blooming at the same time. The toxicant tremetone is excreted in the milk, affecting the young and sparing the dam. Suckling calves were affected when cows were confined to a lightly wooded pasture where white snakeroot was browsed. Goats unfamiliar with this plant confined where it is prevalent may eat it. Weakness, listlessness, muscle tremors, coma, and death may follow. Lesions in cattle are limited to fatty degeneration in the liver, and in goats severe centrilobular hepatic necrosis is the principal lesion reported. Tremetone analysis is available.

Nightshades (*Solanum* spp), including Carolina horsenettle, contain glycoalkaloids that cause depression, anorexia, diarrhea or constipation, weakness, and trembling. Plants are seldom grazed but are toxic and may be ingested in hay. In Florida, tropical soda apple (*Solanum viarum*), an exotic spreading in the southeast, was apparently the cause of cerebellar disease in goats.[11]

Death camas and camas (*Zigadenus* spp) have long narrow leaves, an onion-like bulb, and tall spikes with numerous small white flowers in the spring. Although not common, patches of these members of the lily family occur in damp to dry locations in the southeast. Signs in cattle and sheep include ataxia, muscular weakness, trembling, discharge of frothy saliva from the mouth and nose, regurgitation, dyspnea, collapse, and death.

NITRATES/NITRITES

Corn Stalks, Sorghum, Millet, Ryegrass, Bermudagrass, Wheat, Amaranthus, Other Grasses, Weeds

Ruminants are particularly at risk of acute, fatal, nitrate-nitrite poisoning. When nitrate levels in the diet exceed 0.5% nitrate on a dry-matter basis, the risk of abortion and possibly reduced fertility increases. Above 1.0% the risk of methemoglobinemia and death in ruminants increases. Rumen flora reduces nitrates to nitrites then ammonia for microbial growth. Excess intake of nitrates may cause toxic levels of nitrite to accumulate and be absorbed into the blood, where it oxidizes ferrous iron in hemoglobin to methemoglobin. Cattle graze a variety of grasses and weeds which, under certain conditions, especially excessive fertilization and reduced growth rate, can accumulate levels of nitrate in edible stems that may prove toxic (1.5% KNO_3; 1.0% nitrate). Excess levels of nitrate may be present in grazed forages and weeds, in hay, or in fresh-cut forage brought to the animals as greenchop. Ensiling may reduce nitrate levels by 30% or more. Goats browse leafy portions of plants and may not ingest toxic levels of nitrates in stalks and stems of forages. The major reason plants accumulate nitrates is drought, because plant growth slows or stops but nitrate transfer from roots to stems may continue. Summer temporary pastures of sorghum or millet are an example. Drought-stressed heavily fertilized common bermudagrass cut for hay while short and dark green killed 69 cows when fed as hay 6 months later.

Another important consideration is that in a field there can be areas or strips where the rate of growth of plants is slowed because the soil holds less water, has nutrient imbalance, or other factors causing plants to accumulate nitrates. Only a small percentage of hay bales from such a field may be high in nitrates. Pipeline crossings, old road beds, and previous building sites are examples of such soil conditions.

Forages and weeds growing in soil rich in manure waste or in holding pens are a potential source of poisoning. Accidental ingestion of nitrate fertilizers spilled in the field or stored within reach of cattle is possible. Nitrate accumulation in stalks and stems may follow herbicide damage or loss of leaves from hail. Plants may accumulate nitrates during periods of reduced sunlight, because sunlight is needed to drive photosynthesis and the energy-dependent nitrate reductase system in the plant. Forage or weeds growing in the shade of trees in an orchard may be subject to nitrate accumulation. Nitrate poisoning is occasionally a problem in the southeast, where winter grazing of fertilized pastures of annual grass (*Lolium multiflorum*), oats (*Avena sativa*), rye (*Secale cereal*), and the green tops and stems of turnips (*Brassica rapa*) is common. During extended periods of overcast weather when temperatures are mild (>13°C [55°F]) the nitrate content may increase in stems. At this point allowing hungry cattle to consume a large amount of green forage can have disastrous results. In general, a day or two of sunlight with temperatures above 13°C allows plant growth to resume.

Feeding hay containing increased nitrate levels to cattle grazing forages with elevated nitrate levels is additive to total nitrate intake. Nitrate in drinking water adds to dietary intake. Nitrate levels are not reduced by drying and baling as hay. Hay with high nitrate (>1.5% KNO_3; >1.0% nitrate) fed to pregnant cattle months after baling can cause multiple deaths and abortions. The ability of rumen microorganisms to safely reduce nitrate and nitrite can be increased by feeding corn-based supplements to cattle.

Clinical signs of nitrate-nitrite toxicosis become apparent when methemoglobin reaches 40% to 50%. Signs include weakness, cyanosis of mucous membranes, ataxia, collapse, and death. Increased respiratory rate may be noted in some animals.

Affected animals may remain standing, then suddenly collapse and die within minutes. The mucosa of the vulva is dark blue, and the blood is dark and may have the brown color of methemoglobin when drawn into a syringe. The clinical history may suggest nitrates and the probable source. Lesions are not diagnostic. Blood and tissues may appear brown at time of death, but this becomes less obvious as autolysis proceeds. Agonal hemorrhages in the epicardium may be present. Ocular fluid is an excellent body fluid for nitrate analysis. Plasma and serum are acceptable. The diphenylamine blue test can be used in the field for testing fluids and plant tissues.

Treatment is intravenous methylene blue in a 1% or 2% aqueous solution at a rate of 1 to 2 mg/kg b.w. Up to 10 mg/kg b.w. can be administered in severe cases. In severe cases treatment can be repeated at a lower dose. Tissues in the treated animals are stained by methylene blue and the urine becomes dark green. Treated animals should not be sold for slaughter for 180 days. See the article elsewhere by Bright and colleagues in this issue on antidotes.

PULMONARY

Perilla Mint, Sweet Potato, Pasture Forages, Peanut Hay

Perilla mint (*Perilla frutescens*) is often referred to as beefsteak plant, purple mint, or mint weed. It is a major toxic plant affecting ruminants and is widespread in the region, including northwest Florida, preferring shaded areas along creeks, the edge of woods, and fence lines. Once established perilla produces many seeds, and large colonies develop in succeeding years. Drought stress severely limits its growth. Perilla mint has a distinctive odor, square, dark green to purplish stems, and serrated leaves that are almost round with a purple tint underneath. More than one variety exists. Mature growth in late summer is 0.5 to 1.5 m (3.3–5 ft) tall, producing small white to purple flowers and numerous seeds. Toxicity is highest in the seed stage. Perilla ketone and related furan compounds are bioactivated in the lung and cause atypical interstitial pneumonia (AIP). Clinical signs are those of acute respiratory distress syndrome. Severe signs include open mouth, extended neck, tongue protruding with froth, and labored respiration. Subcutaneous emphysema may be present. Handling the animals may prove fatal to some. Less severely affected cattle have increased rate and depth of respiration. Animals that live 48 hours usually survive. The 1-mm round white seeds are easily recognized in feces and abomasal contents. Leaves and stems in rumen contents can be identified visually and by smell. Type 1 pneumocytes are destroyed and Type 2 pneumocytes are induced to proliferate. The lungs may be wet and are expanded, with rib indentations, marked interstitial and alveolar emphysema, bullae, and microscopically interstitial pneumonia.

Sweet potato (*Ipomoea batatas*) production and canning in the region creates the opportunity for cattle to eat potatoes damaged by fusarium mold (black rot) containing the toxicant 4-ipomeanol, a furan compound similar to perilla ketone, which is bioactivated in the lung. Exposure includes grazing in plowed potato fields, cannery wastes, or being fed spoiled sweet potatoes. The signs are those of acute respiratory distress syndrome. The disease is similar to other causes of AIP but in some cases the mortality is quite high, perhaps caused by the dose of lung toxicant or prolonged absorption from the rumen.

Uncommon, but not to be overlooked in the southeast, is forage-related tryptophan-induced AIP in cattle. The condition is also referred to as acute bovine pulmonary emphysema and edema (ABPEE). Lactating beef cows are usually the affected animals. Morbidity can be 30% or higher with 10% to 15% death loss. Outbreaks occur 4 to 10 days following sudden change from a diet of poor-quality forage to immature summer grass high in tryptophan. Rarely is cool-season oat forage or ryegrass involved. In this situation rumen bacteria convert tryptophan to 3-methyl indole (3-MI), a furan compound, which is further metabolized in the lung to the lung toxicant. This form of AIP can be prevented by feeding an ionophore or tetracycline for a week before pasture change until 2 weeks after the change. The incidence is so low and unpredictable in the region that few cattle owners use this approach.

Peanut hay (*Arachis hypogaea*) fed to beef cattle has caused acute respiratory distress syndrome.

RENAL

Oak, Amaranthus, Dock

Oak (*Quercus* spp) toxicosis can be a significant problem when cattle eat large amounts of acorns in the fall in some areas of the southeast. Oak buds and young leaves are readily consumed by hungry cattle when trees are downed by storms in the spring. Sheep and goats are less susceptible to oak toxicosis. Gallotannins are the chemical components that cause the gastrointestinal inflammation and tubular damage to the kidney, leading to uremia. The first indications of a problem may be finding dead cattle, or serum chemistry from a sick animal showing elevated creatinine, blood urea nitrogen, low calcium, and high phosphorus levels. Clinical signs include constipation followed by loose and sometimes bloody stools, an unkempt dry muzzle, nasal discharge sometimes blood-streaked, perineal and brisket edema, and dark then later clear urine. Necropsy reveals some or all of the following: hydrothorax, ascites, phenolic odor from kidneys, oral and esophageal ulcerations, gastroenteritis with numerous small hemorrhages on serosal surfaces, fecal balls or loose stool in colon, kidneys swollen or normal size, petecchiae on kidneys, and perirenal edema. With supportive care, some animals recover.

Redroot pigweed (*Amaranthus retroflexus*) and related *Amaranthus* spp are known for nitrate accumulation. Redroot pigweed is a palatable weed often browsed in small to moderate amounts by cattle. Severe nephrosis may develop when cattle unaccustomed to eating this weed browse it in large amounts for 1 or 2 days. Signs of intoxication include weakness and recumbency, with death in most animals after 2 to 10 days. At necropsy the outstanding lesions are perirenal edema and swollen pale kidneys. There is no inflammation in the gastrointestinal tract, as with oak toxicity. Rumen contents may contain fiber from the pigweed stems and stalks. The toxicant is unknown. Swine and probably other ruminants are susceptible.

Dock (*Rumex* spp) are common cool-season weeds, rarely consumed by ruminants, known to have potential for dangerous levels of oxalates. Two beef cows with young calves were held for 3 days in a quarter-acre pen with only curly-leaf dock, which they browsed heavily (Nicholson SS, unpublished data, February 11, 2002). On the third day the cows were down and milk fever–like, with serum calcium levels of 2.2 to 2.6 mg/dL. There was no response to intravenous calcium. Kidneys were normal at necropsy and no oxalate crystals were present.

REFERENCES

1. Radi ZA, Styer EL, Thompson LJ, et al. *Prunus* spp. intoxication in ruminants: a case in a goat and diagnosis by identification of leaf fragments in rumen contents. J Vet Diagn Invest 2004;16(6):593–9.
2. Burrows GE, Tyrl RL. Toxic plants of North America. Ames (IA): Iowa State University Press; 2001. p. 1043–56.

3. East NE, Anderson M, Lowenstine LJ. Apparent gossypol-induced toxicosis in adult dairy goats. J Am Vet Med Assoc 1994;204:642–3.
4. Smith GW, Rotstein DS, Brownie CF. Abdominal fat necrosis in a pigmy goat associated with fescue toxicosis. J Vet Diagn Invest 2004;16(4):356–9.
5. Kerr LA, Kelch WJ. Fatal privet (*Ligustrum amurease*) toxicosis in Tennessee cows. Vet Hum Toxicol 1999;41(6):391–2.
6. Smith GW, Constable PD. Suspected pokeweed toxicity in a Boer goat. Vet Hum Toxicol 2002;44(6):351.
7. Casteel SW. Forage induced photosenstization. In: Plumlee K, editor. Clinical veterinary toxicology. St Louis (MO): Mosby; 2004. p. 427–8.
8. Uhlig S, Botha CJ, Vralstad T, et al. Indole-diterpenes and ergot alkaloids in *Cynodon dactylon* (Bermuda grass) infected with *Claviceps cynodontis* from an outbreak of tremors in cattle. J Agric Food Chem 2009;57:111–29.
9. Thompson LJ, Frazier K, Stiver S, et al. Multiple animal intoxications associated with Carolina jessamine (*Gelsemium sempervirens*) ingestions. Vet Hum Toxicol 2002;44(5):272–3.
10. Nicholson SS, Olcott BM, Usenik EA, et al. Delayed phalaris grass toxicosis in sheep and cattle. J Am Vet Med Assoc 1989;195(3):345–6.
11. Porter MB, MacKay RJ, Uhl E, et al. Neurologic disease putatively associated with ingestion of *Solanum viarum* in goats. J Am Vet Med Assoc 2003;223(4):501–4, 456.

Toxic Plants of the Northeastern United States

Karyn Bischoff, DVM, MS[a,*], Mary C. Smith, DVM[b]

KEYWORDS

• Plant toxins • Ruminants • Cyanide • Nitrate

Plant poisonings in agricultural animals cause occasional catastrophic losses, however, less overt economic impact through decreased production and reproductive performance and increased veterinary and feed costs are also important considerations.[1] Most poisonous plants are not palatable and livestock will avoid consuming them, thus plant poisonings are often an indicator of other management problems, such as inadequate forage; overstocking; poor pasture management; heavy contamination of hay, silage, grain, or other feedstuffs with toxic weeds, or improper disposal of clippings from ornamental plants. Control of toxic plants is challenging; herbicides increase palatability of many plants.

Few veterinary diagnostic laboratories test for plant toxins. Diagnosis is usually based on evidence of ingestion with appropriate clinical and postmortem findings. Some phytotoxins, such as pyrrolizidine alkaloids, have chronic effects and animals often do not show clinical signs for weeks or months, after the plant is no longer present on pasture or in the current batch of hay.

Important toxic plants in the Northeastern quadrant of the United States include water hemlocks *(Cicuta* spp); poison hemlock (*Conium maculatum*); ragworts (*Senecio* spp); nightshades (*Solanum* spp); white snakeroot (*Ageratina altissima*); pigweed *(Amaranthus retroflexus);* cocklebur (*Xanthium* spp); the appellative weed marijuana (*Cannabis sativa*); pokeweed (*Phytolacca americanum*); bracken fern *(Pteridium aquilinum*); yew (*Taxus* spp); rhododendron and its relatives (*Rhododendron* spp, *Kalmia* spp, and *Pieris* spp); stone fruit trees, such as cherry (*Prunus* spp); and oak trees (*Quercus* spp).

The authors have nothing to disclose.

[a] New York State Animal Health Diagnostic Laboratory, Department of Population Medicine and Diagnostic Sciences, Cornell University, PO Box 5786, Ithaca, NY 14852, USA
[b] Ambulatory and Production Medicine, Department of Population Medicine and Diagnostic Sciences, Cornell University, Box 29, Ithaca, NY 14853, USA
* Corresponding author.
E-mail address: KLB72@cornell.edu

Vet Clin Food Anim 27 (2011) 459–480
doi:10.1016/j.cvfa.2011.02.001
0749-0720/11/$ – see front matter vetfood.theclinics.com

WATER HEMLOCKS (*CICUTA* SPP)

All 20 species of water hemlocks found throughout the world are toxic. *C douglasii* and *C bulbifera* are of interest in the Northeastern United States. As the name implies, water hemlocks are found in wet meadows or along streams, rivers, irrigation ditches, and other water sources. Plants in this genus are perennials and members of the carrot family (Apiaceae). Bulbous tubers at the base have thick bundles of long roots radiating from them. Cut sections of the tuber and stem reveals hollow chambers containing a thick, yellow, oily liquid. The cut surface has a parsniplike odor. Stems are up to 2.5 m tall, hairless, erect, and can have purple stripes. Leaves are alternate, 30 to 60 cm long, linear lanceolate, and 1 to 3 times pinnately compound with 3 to 10 cm long leaflets and serrate margins. Umbels of small white flowers are produced the second year of growth (**Fig. 1**). Seeds are small and encased in a hard, brown, flattened oval shell with prominent ribs.

The toxic principle is cicutoxin, a long-chain highly unsaturated alcohol. Spring plants are the most toxic and mature plants the least toxic. Although the highest concentrations of cicutoxin are found in the tubers and stems, all parts are toxic and flowers and seed heads have been associated with poisonings.[1] Water hemlock baled into hay can cause toxicosis.[1,2] Ingestion of 50 to 110 mg/kg body weight of green water hemlock causes toxicosis in most species.[2] A dose of 1.4 g/kg of ground *C. douglasii* tubers fed to a sheep produced clinical signs of toxicosis, 2.8 g/kg produced seizures with recovery, and 6.4 g/kg was lethal within 90 minutes.[2]

Cicutoxin acts on the central nervous system and is thought to block sodium and potassium ion channels.[3] γ-aminobutyric acid (GABA) inhibition is also suspected.[2] Absorption and action of cicutoxin are rapid, thus the plant is often identifiable in the rumen content.[2] Water hemlock is palatable. Poisonings usually occur in spring involving few or many animals, which may be found dead.[3] When observed, clinical signs occur within 15 minutes.[1] Affected animals at first appear nervous or uneasy, but signs rapidly progress to twitching of facial muscles, chewing behavior, ataxia, incoordination, generalized tremors, weakness or ataxia, and frequent urination and defecation. Some recover if left alone, others continue to progress within hours to involuntary spastic head movements, collapse, intermittent tonic-clonic seizures, bruxism, bloat, salivation, and death from respiratory failure or cardiopulmonary arrest.[1–4] Clinical pathology findings secondary to seizure activity include elevated creatinine kinase (CK), lactate dehydrogenase (LDH), and aspartate transaminase

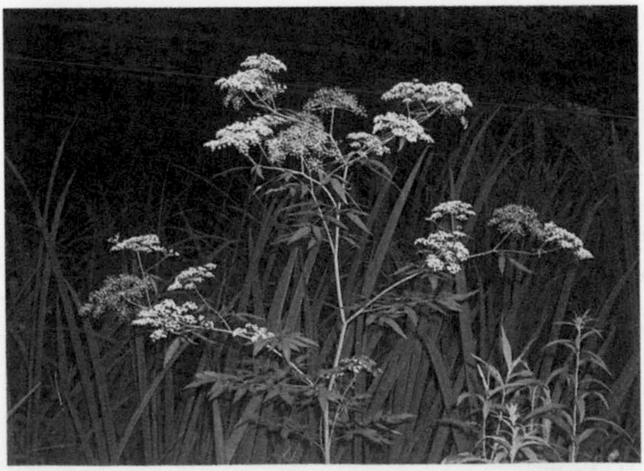

Fig. 1. *Cicuta* spp, water hemlock. (*Courtesy of* Mary C. Smith, DVM, Ithaca, NY.)

(AST), and glucose elevation caused by epinephrine release. Lesions are secondary to trauma and can include tongue lacerations and subcutaneous bruises.[3] Multifocal to coalescing myocardial and skeletal muscle degeneration are reported.[1] Tentative diagnosis is based on evidence of ingestion of water hemlock on pasture, feed, or plant material in the rumen. Some laboratories can detect cicutoxin in rumen contents.[2,3]

Because of the rapid onset of toxicosis, no effective treatment protocol has been established for field cases.[1] Restraint is likely to precipitate seizures in the animal, thus the primary goal is sedation and seizure control. Clinical signs of cicutoxin poisoning were prevented in a sheep dosed with 30 mg/kg sodium pentobarbital and 75 mg atropine.[3] Decontamination with activated charcoal and laxatives or rumenotomy is appropriate if no clinical signs are evident.[2] The prognosis is poor to grave, but animals surviving 8 hours are unlikely to be lethally poisoned.[3] Herbicides, such as 2,4-D and glyphosate, can control the plant, but there are restrictions to using these near waterways, where this plant grows, and water hemlock becomes more palatable after spraying. Manual removal and burning are other options for water hemlock infestation.[2]

POISON HEMLOCK (*CONIUM MACULATUM*)

Poison hemlock, also of the carrot family, originated in Europe but is found throughout North America. The plant grows well in moist soil along stream banks, roadside ditches, cultivated fields, and other waste areas, forming dense stands.[3,4] Poison hemlock has a large, white, carrotlike tap root with a mousy odor. The stem is erect, 2 or 3 m tall, hollow, smooth, and branched with purple spots and a similar mousy odor. Leaves are large, triangular, alternate, and 2 to 4 times pinnately compound with oblong-toothed leaflets. Inflorescences are flat-topped loose compound umbels (**Fig. 2**). The seeds are brown and ovoid with ridges.

The toxic principles are various nicotinelike pyridine alkaloids, including coniine, γ-coniceine, N-methyl coniine, conhydrine, and pseudo-conhydrine. Coniine is the primary toxin of mature plants and seeds, with a mouse median lethal dose (LD_{50}) of 11 mg/kg. Gamma-coniceine, found in the young plant, is the precursor for coniine. Plant toxicity varies. Plants in the Southern United States are more toxic than northern plants. Young plants are more toxic than mature plants and leaves and stems are the most toxic portions. Once the seeds appear, they are the most toxic part of the plant.[3,4] Dried plants remain toxic. Ingestion of as little as 0.5% body weight of

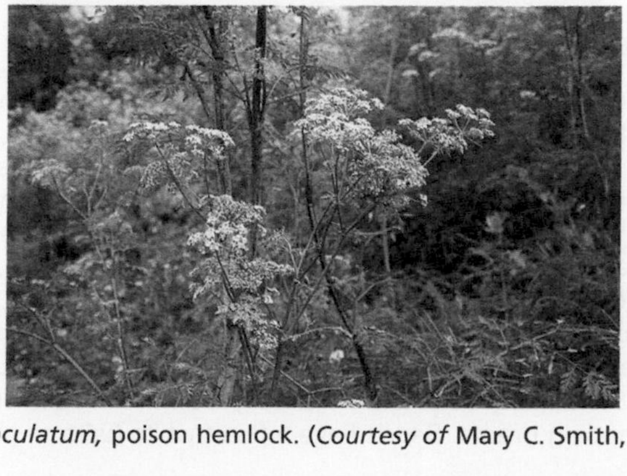

Fig. 2. *Conium maculatum,* poison hemlock. (*Courtesy of* Mary C. Smith, DVM, Ithaca, NY.)

the green plant can be lethal to cattle; sheep are less susceptible.[1,3,4] Alkaloids of poison hemlock are rapidly absorbed from the gastrointestinal tract with the maximum blood concentration achieved in 24 hours.[1] Alkaloids are excreted into milk.[4] Effects on the nicotinic receptors of γ-coniceine are stimulatory, coniine has mixed effects, and effects of N-methylconiine are inhibitory. Generally, there is an initial transient stimulatory effect at nicotinic receptors of the autonomic ganglia, neuromuscular junctions, and medulla. Large doses produce a neuromuscular blockade caused by the inability of the nerve, under constant stimulation, to repolarize.[3,4] Poison hemlock is also associated with abortion, arthrogryposis, scoliosis, torticollis, and cleft palate. Teratogenic effects, which occur if the cow is 50 to 100 days into gestation or the ewe or doe is between 30 and 60 days of gestation, are caused by decreased fetal movement. Calves are more severely affected than lambs, which often recover from the tendon contraction.[3,4]

Most species, including birds, cattle, sheep, goats, swine, horses, and people, are susceptible to poison hemlock toxicosis. Toxicosis is unlikely if animals have adequate forage but some animals develop a craving for the plant, which is palatable in early spring. Poisoning is most commonly associated with contaminated hay or green chop, affecting a large number of animals. Clinical signs are usually apparent within an hour, progressing rapidly to death in a few hours. Mild stimulation and nervousness progress to abdominal pain, groaning, muscle weakness or ataxia, trembling, loss of coordination, salivation, lacrimation, and increased urination. Signs in severely affected animals include depression, narcosis, progressive paresis, recumbency, respiratory suppression, cyanosis, weak pulse, prolapse of the nictitating membrane, hypothermia, and coma. Although most animals recover, severe respiratory suppression can be lethal.[1,3,4] Lesions are few and nonspecific. Urine and rumen contents can smell mousy and abomasal and duodenal mucosa can appear congested.[3,5] Diagnosis is based on evidence of ingestion, such as evidence of grazing the plant or plant material in the rumen, and appropriate clinical signs. Some laboratories can analyze blood, gastrointestinal contents, liver, or kidney for the alkaloids.[5]

Possible methods of gastrointestinal decontamination include rumen lavage in the asymptomatic animal with instillation of activated charcoal and a saline cathartic into the rumen.[1,2] Instillation of dilute tannic acid into the rumen will theoretically detoxifying the alkaloids from poison hemlock.[2] Assisted respiration may be required. Survivors usually make a full recovery.[1,2] Prevention is by assuring the presence of adequate, uncontaminated feed and preventing access to the plant. Destroy the plant before the seed stage by mowing or applying broadleaf herbicide.[1,2]

RAGWORTS (*SENECIO* SPP)

Senecio spp, the most common pyrrolizidine alkaloid-containing plants in the Northeastern United States, are found in woodlands, waste areas, at the edges of fields, roads, and gardens, and can survive in dry, rocky, or sandy soils. *S jacobaea*, tansy ragwort, originated in Western Europe and was brought to North America as a medicinal herb.[6] *S vulgaris*, common groundsel, and *S aureus* are also common in the northeast. *Senecio* spp, of the sunflower family Asteraceae, are difficult-to-identify biennials or perennials that bloom in the summer or autumn. First-year plants are low-to-the-ground rosettes; the next year erect, branching 0.3 to 1.2 m tall stems emerge. Leaves are simple, alternate, ovate to lanceolate, and pinnately divided with dentate margins. Stems end in clusters of dense, yellow flowers surrounded by a single layer of nonoverlapping bracts. Seeds have tufts of white hairs.

More than 150 pyrrolizidine alkaloids, varying in potency, have been identified from *Senecio* spp.[1] Highly reactive hepatotoxic pyrrolizidine alkaloids include seneciophylline and retrorsine. Other alkaloids are senecionine, jacozine, jacobine, jacoline, and jaconine.[7,8] Pyrrolizidine alkaloids are synthesized in the roots as N-oxides and transported to the rest of the plant, accumulating in flowers, stems, and leaves.[3] The highest concentrations of pyrrolizidine alkaloids are in the seeds and flowers in most *Senecio* spp, but the foliage contains higher concentrations in *S jacobaea*, the tansy ragwort.[6,7] Alkaloid concentrations vary 10-fold over the growing season and are highest during flowering and lowest over winter.[3,4] Tansy ragwort is reported to contain 0.1% to 0.9% pyrrolizidine alkaloids and common groundsel, *S vulgaris* contains 0.16% to 0.25% dry matter (dm).[3,7] These alkaloids are degraded in silage but poisonings from silage have been reported.[3] Green tansy ragwort as 4% to 8% of the diet caused acute liver necrosis in a cow, however, chronic toxicosis is more common. Clinical signs become evident when 80% of the liver is affected, which may take months.[4] Peak hepatic concentrations of pyrrolizidine alkaloids occur 2 hours after ingestion and decrease over a day or two.[3,8] Pyrrolizidine alkaloids cross the placenta and are excreted in low concentrations in milk.[3] Absorbed alkaloids are activated to pyrroles by hepatic microsomal enzymes.[1,8] Pyrroles are metabolized to less reactive water soluble compounds for urinary elimination.[3,8] The mechanism of action of pyrrolizidine alkaloids is described by Steven S. Nicholson in detail elsewhere in this issue. Briefly, pyrroles disrupt DNA-mediated RNA and protein synthesis, leading to cellular dysfunction and degeneration.[1,3] Cross-linking of DNA and other mechanisms impairs cell division leading to megalocytosis.[3,8,9] Pyrrolizidine alkaloids cause proliferation of hepatic vascular endothelium, impairing perfusion and producing portal hypertension and fibrosis.[9] Some pyrrolizidine alkaloid containing plants have extrahepatic effects.[1] Major effects of ragwort are isolated to the liver, but cerebral edema can occur secondary to hepatic encephalopathy.[1,6]

Pigs are the most susceptible agricultural species, but cattle are between 10 to 15 times more sensitive to pyrrolizidine alkaloids than goats or sheep, which may be placed on pasture first to remove the plant.[3] Deer are considered resistant, but poisoning has been reported in captive Père David's deer.[3] Young animals are more susceptible and toxicosis has been reported in neonates, whereas the lactating dams were unaffected. Poor nutritional status is a predisposing factor, in part, by depleting the glutathione reserves needed for hepatic detoxification of pyrrolizidine alkaloids.[8] Ingestion of pyrrolizidine alkaloids in the diet increases the risk for copper toxicosis in sheep.[8] Ragwort ingestion is most likely to take place in late spring or summer and when other forage is unavailable.[3] Contamination of grain by seeds from pyrrolizidine alkaloid-containing plants and feeding of contaminated hay or haylage have been associated with poisonings, although pyrrolizidine alkaloid concentrations decrease over time in haylage.[7] Clinical signs of acute toxicosis are attributable to acute liver failure: anorexia, depression, icterus, and ascites.[8] Chronic toxicosis is more common but may present acutely, precipitated by physiologic stress, such as pregnancy, lactation, transport, or nutritional stress.[3] Signs include reduced milk production, ill thrift, emaciation, depression, weakness, and recumbency. Rumen atony, abdominal pain, groaning, and diarrhea with straining and rectal prolapse are reported.[1,3,9] Ascites is caused by hypoalbuminemia and congestive heart failure.[6,9] Hepatic photosensitization is rare.[3,9] Other reported signs include icterus and hepatic encephalopathy. Ultrasound findings reported from cattle with *Senecio* spp toxicosis include ascites with edema of the omentum, gastrointestinal and gall bladder wall, generalized hepatomegaly, and heterogenous liver parenchyma with dilation of the portal vein and attenuation of the hepatic veins and caudal vena cava.[9] Elevated bilirubin is often noted. Bile acid concentrations greater than 50 μg/L are a poor prognostic indicator.[3] Transient elevation in liver enzymes, including ALT, LDH, alkaline phosphatase (ALP), and AST, are reported.[3] Although difficult to measure in the clinical setting, hyperammonemia with secondary hepatic encephalopathy can occur.[6,9] Hypoalbuminemia is caused by failure of hepatic synthesis. Impairment of bromsulphalein clearance has been used, with histopathology, to determine the degree of liver damage in pyrrolizidine alkaloid poisoning.[6] Grossly, animals usually have ascites and pleural effusions and microhepatica caused by fibrosis, although the liver is enlarged in acute toxicosis.[3] The portal vein is enlarged.[6] The gall bladder is distended secondary to anorexia with a thickened, edematous wall. Watery intestinal content with edema and petechia of the intestinal walls and omentum are reported.[3,7] Characteristic histologic lesions are hepatocyte swelling and panlobular necrosis, resulting in loss of normal architecture.[1,3,8] Bridging portal fibrosis, bile duct proliferation, megalocytosis, and nodular regeneration are common in ruminants.[3,8–10] Cerebral edema secondary to hepatic encephalopathy is reported.[6]

It is the authors' experience that by the time animals with pyrrolizidine alkaloid poisoning present with clinical signs, they have been moved off of the contaminated pasture or ragwort can no longer be observed on the pasture or in the hay. Tentative diagnosis is based on histologic lesions, history of exposure, and clinical signs. Colorimetric field tests and enzyme-linked immunosorbent assays are available for testing of plant material.[3] Blood or liver may be analyzed for pyrroles but the low concentrations bound to tissues are unlikely to be detectable.[7,8]

No effective treatment for pyrrolizidine alkaloid toxicosis has been developed. Affected animals rarely recover and are frequently culled for salvage.[6,8] Removal of ragwort from the diet and symptomatic and supportive care, such as a low protein, high energy diet to reduce ammonia production, may help for valuable livestock.[3] There could be a protective effect from sulfur-containing amino acids (methionine, cysteine) and antioxidants, such as butylated hydroxytoluene and ethoxyquin, in the diet to help scavenge reactive pyrroles.[1] *Senecio* spp are prolific and difficult to control. Biologic controls, including the cinnabar moth, *Tyria jacobaeae*, the flea beetle, *Longitarsus jacobaea*, and the ragwort seed fly, *Pegohylemyia* spp, are effective at different stages of plant growth and seeding.[3,6] Herbicides, when used, should be applied before the plants go to seed. Dicamba is effective on advanced growth, as is 2,4-D on first-year (rosette stage) growth.[6]

NIGHTSHADES (*SOLANUM* SPP)

Nightshades are annual or perennial plants that grow in disturbed areas, such as construction sites, feedlots, overgrazed pasture, and croplands. Important nightshades in the Northeast United States include *S carolinense* or horse nettle, *S dulcamara* or bittersweet, *S nigrum* or black nightshade, *S physalifolium* or hairy nightshade, *S ptychanthum* or eastern black nightshade, and *S rostratum* or buffalo bur. Green parts of the potato (*S tuberosum*) contain similar toxins.[3] Important related genera include *Lycopersicum* (tomatoes), *Nicotiana* (tobaccos), *Datura* (jimsonweeds and angel's trumpets), and *Capsicum* (peppers). Nightshades can have erect stems or vines, some with prickles. Leaves are alternate, simple or compound, and flowers are usually solitary and radially symmetric with 5 sepals and 5 petals. The berrylike fruit is usually dark red to black.

Nightshades contain steroidal alkaloids, present as glycosides. Solanine is a common glycoside and solanidine is the aglycone.[3] The solasodine glycoalkaloids of bittersweet (*S dulcamara*) have saponinlike effects, disrupting cellular membranes by detergent action thus producing severe gastrointestinal mucosal necrosis.[3] Green sprouts, vines, unripe fruit, and tubers (potatoes) contain alkaloids.[1,4] The ripe fruit of some species are also toxic.[3] Ruminants are resistant to these alkaloids. Sheep and goats may be more resistant to some species, such as *S elaeagnifolium*, than cattle.[3]

Only large nightshade ingestions produce disease. Clinical signs associated with potato sprouts or nightshades have a latent period of a few hours to a day. Animals become depressed, drowsy, weak, and uncoordinated with increased respiratory rate, abdominal pain, and bruxism. Some have constipation early and fetid diarrhea later.[3] Most animals survive. Congestion and hemorrhage of the gastrointestinal mucosa, ascites, and the presence of berries or other plant material in the rumen are reported.[3] Treatment is symptomatic and supportive.

Ingestion of jimsonweed and other *Datura* spp is associated with more severe clinical signs, beginning with central nervous system stimulation followed rapidly by depression. Inhibition of the autonomic nervous system by atropine and scopolamine presents as dry mouth, gastrointestinal stasis, dilated pupils, decreased heart or respiratory rate, muscle weakness, and gastrointestinal irritation. Animals may die of cardiac failure.[1,4] Early activated charcoal administration is recommended.[1] Cautious physostigmine use reverses competitive inhibition of acetylcholine by inhibiting acetylcholinesterase, thereby increasing the amount of acetylcholine at the synapse.[4]

WHITE SNAKEROOT (*AGERATINA ALTISSIMA*)

White snakeroot toxicosis is termed *trembles* in livestock and *milk sickness* in humans. White snakeroot is found over the eastern half of the United States and Canada in partially shaded forested areas but does not grow well in open areas. Snakeroot emerges in May or June and flowers in autumn. Apparently palatable, most poisonings occur in the fall, when other forage becomes scarce, because the plant remains green.[11] White snakeroot is a perennial herb in the family Asteraceae. Stems, 30 to 150 cm tall, are often branched. Heart-shaped leaves are simple, alternate, and serrate with 3 distinct veins and long petioles. Flat clusters of 10 to 30 white tubular flowers form at branch ends (**Fig. 3**).

The toxic principle is trematone.[12,13] Trematone is hypothesized to interfere with glucose metabolism.[11] Concentrations vary between stands of plants. Snakeroot is frost resistant and remains toxic in hay, though heat and drying do decrease the toxicity of the plant.[4,11] Snakeroot toxicosis has been reported in ruminants consuming 0.5% to 1.5% body weight of green plant (wet weight) over 1 to 3 weeks.[11]

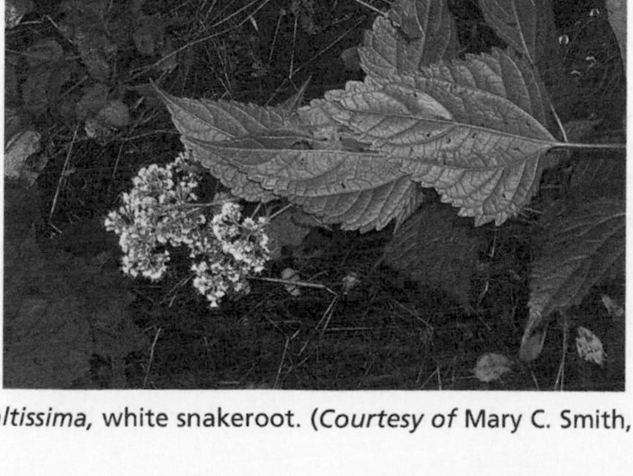

Fig. 3. *Ageratina altissima,* white snakeroot. (*Courtesy of* Mary C. Smith, DVM, Ithaca, NY.)

Toxicosis has been reported in cattle, sheep, goats, horses, and swine.[4,12] Trematone is activated to a toxic metabolite by hepatic P450 enzymes.[4,11] Lactating animals are resistant because trematone is eliminated in the milk. Milk sickness, a major historical cause of morbidity, has been reported in humans, calves, and cats that ingest the contaminated milk.[3,4,12] Toxicosis may be acute, subacute, or, most commonly, chronic. Clinical signs of chronic poisoning in ruminants include weight loss, weakness, reluctance to move, and tremors. Tremors, when animals are forced to move, are prominent and progressive and diminish with relaxation.[4,11,12] An acetone odor is sometimes detectable on the breath.[4] Sheep can have dyspnea and bruxism and usually die within a few days.[4] Goats can have hepatic necrosis, encephalopathy, and photosensitization.[4] Other reported signs include ventral edema, urinary incontinence, and abortion.[11] Serum chemistry findings include elevated CK, ALP, AST, ALT, hyperglycemia, and alkalosis.[11] Postmortem findings may be minimal and include pulmonary edema, pericardial effusion, red urine, and linear areas of myocardial pallor and hemorrhage. Microscopically, there is degeneration and necrosis of cardiac and skeletal muscle.[4,11] Renal histology is consistent with myoglobinuric nephrosis and fatty degeneration of tubular epithelium. Hepatic lesions include bile retention, centrilobular hepatocyte degeneration, and necrosis.[3,4,11]

Diagnosis of white snakeroot poisoning is usually based on history of exposure, clinical signs, and lesions. Trematone can be detected in the urine for no more than about 48 hours after ingestion. Liver and kidney from the affected animal or the aborted fetus contain detectable concentrations of trematone.[11] Treatment is supportive and symptomatic, including supplemental feeding with high-quality forage, fluid therapy with glucose and bicarbonate as needed, and rest. Exposure to the plant should stop. Frequent milking (discard the milk) will help eliminate trematone from the body. Activated charcoal and laxatives can be given soon after ingestion, with repeated doses of activated charcoal because of suspected enterohepatic cycling.[3,4,11] Recovery is possible, but it may take weeks. Prevention is more effective than treatment. Plants can be removed or sprayed with an herbicide.[3,4]

COCKLEBUR (*XANTHIUM*)

Cocklebur is a weedy herb found in flood plains and disturbed areas with rich moist soil, such as feedlots, and can form dense stands. The species most commonly found in the Northeastern United States is the invasive *X strumarium*. Cockleburs are annuals and members of the Asteraceae family. A 0.5 to 1.5 m tall, stout, erect stem with dark spots arises from the taproot. Leaves are 5 to 35 cm wide, simple, alternate, and lanceolate to triangular with entire, toothed, or lobed margins, a rough, glandular surface, and long petioles. Flowers are produced at the leaf axis. The female flower forms a 1.5 cm long oval, yellow to brown bur encasing 2 seeds.

The toxic principle is carboxyatractyloside, a water soluble glycoside.[4,14] Burs contain 0.46% carboxyatractyloside.[3,4] Poisonings follows consumption of sprouts, and, though the bur is not palatable, ingestion of heavily bur contaminated feeds.[3] Carboxyatractyloside is readily absorbed by the gastrointestinal tract and enters the liver, it's target organ, via the portal circulation.[14] Epithelial cells of the proximal convoluted renal tubules are also susceptible. Carboxyatractyloside blocks oxidative phosphorylation by competitive inhibition of a mitochondrial adenine nucleoside carrier.[4,14] Effects are not cumulative.[3] Swine and calves are most commonly affected.[4] Most poisonings occur in spring and early summer during warm, moist weather when seeds sprout en mass.[4] The presenting complaint is usually unexpected death. Progression of signs is rapid, lasting only a couple of hours, but may be protracted for up to 3 days, especially in calves with functional rumens. Clinical signs have included depression, reluctance to move, abdominal pain, hunched back, recumbency, anorexia, salivation, and dyspnea, followed by blindness, hyperexcitability, muscle fasciculation, extensor rigidity, opisthotonos, paddling, convulsions, coma, and death.[3,4,14] Serum chemistry reveals renal failure, elevated bile acids, AST, SDH, ALT, and marked hypoglycemia.[14] Lesions associated with hepatopathy predominate and include ascites; pericardial and pleural effusions; edema of the gall bladder wall; and a firm, pale liver with a pronounced lobular pattern and centrilobular hemorrhage on cut section. The predominant microscopic lesion is acute centrilobular to panlobular hepatic necrosis. Cerebral edema with neuronal degeneration is seen inconsistently, as is mild to moderate renal tubular degeneration.[3,4,14] The bur itself can cause mechanical damage to the wool or hair, eyes, and skin.[3,4]

Diagnosis of cocklebur poisoning is based on clinical signs, lesions, and evidence of ingestion of burs or dicotyledons of the plant. Analysis of gastrointestinal contents or urine for carboxyatractyloside is available only at selected laboratories.[14] Affected animals do not respond well to treatment. A high-fat diet may protect exposed animals. Activated charcoal, to prevent absorption, or mineral oil, to enhance passage and prevent absorption, can be given soon after ingestion. Clinically affected animals might respond to supportive and symptomatic care, including intravenous glucose and bicarbonate to correct hypoglycemia and acidosis, respectively. Removing mature plants by mowing or herbicides before seed production is the best method of control.[3,4,14]

PIGWEED (*AMARANTHUS* SPP)

Pigweeds are common throughout the United States. *Amaranthus retroflexus* or redroot pigweed, *A hybridus*, and *A spinosus* are found in the northeast. Pigweeds grow quickly in moist soils, invade disturbed areas rapidly, and are found between crop rows, on roadsides, in waste areas, cattle lots, and gardens.[3,4,15] Pigweeds usually have a red taproot and stout, erect, 1.0 to 1.2 m tall pubescent, branched, striated stem. Leaves are simple, alternate, and oval to lanceolate with petioles. Green flowers with long, spine-tipped bracts form dense spikes or panicles terminally or axially. Pigweeds are prolific producers of shiny dark seeds.

Toxic components of pigweed have not been fully elucidated. *A retroflexus* is known for a renal toxin that has not been isolated. Nephrosis from pigweed ingestion is uncommon but has been reported in cattle, sheep, goats, and monogastrics (primarily swine).[15] Nephrosis occurs when animals are grazed on a large stand of green pigweed for 5 to 10 days, although some animals graze pigweed with no clinical effects.[15] Death is due to secondary hyperkalemia and resulting cardiac dysfunction.[3]

A more common problem in ruminants, in the authors' experience, is nitrate toxicosis. Drought-stressed pigweed accumulates nitrate in heavily fertilized soils. Other stressors, such as injury or herbicide treatment (which increases palatability), and cool, cloudy weather contribute to nitrate accumulation.[3,4,16] Nitrate is metabolized in photosynthesis, but the enzyme required, nitrate reductase, requires heat, light, and adequate water. Nitrate concentrations are highest in roots and lower stalk and lowest in leaves, flowers, and seeds.[4,16] Concentrations in pigweed can reach 4%, dm.[3] Toxicosis is frequently associated with hay, which retains nitrate.[3,16] Nitrate concentrations are reduced by up to 60% in silage.[3] Feed nitrate concentrations of 1% are potentially toxic to mature ruminants and 0.5% might be associated with abortion.[4,16]

Ruminants are markedly more susceptible to nitrate toxicosis than monogastrics because of rapid ruminal conversion of nitrate to the more toxic nitrite for production of ammonia used in microbial protein synthesis.[4,16] Acclimation to a high-nitrate diet and the presence of a high-energy diet increase the efficiency of ammonia production.[4,16] Rumen nitrite is readily absorbed and oxidizes the iron in hemoglobin, forming methemoglobin, which does not carry oxygen.[3,4,16] Peak methemoglobin concentrations are seen in about 3 hours.[16] Conversion of 30% to 40% of hemoglobin to methemoglobin produces clinical signs and 80% methemoglobin is lethal.[4,16] Nitrite crosses the placenta and is thought to cause fetal hypoxia and abortion at any gestational stage.[4] The elimination half-life for nitrate is 9.0 hours in cattle and 4.2 hours in sheep.[16]

Pigweed also contains sodium and potassium oxalate at concentrations as high as 30%, although oxalate toxicosis from pigweed ingestion has not been documented.[3]

Clinical signs of pigweed-induced nephrosis develops 5 to 14 days after exposure.[4,15] Signs include depression, weakness, and incoordination. Knuckling of the pasterns, diarrhea, and ventral edema are reported.[3,15] Animals become recumbent and comatose, succumbing within a few days or a week, mortality reaching greater than 50% of those affected.[3,15] Animals are hypocalcemic, hyperphosphatemic, and hyperkalemic, with elevated creatine, CK, and blood urea nitrogen (BUN). Lesions noted include ascites, perirenal, perirectal, and omental edema, and large, pale kidneys with interstitial edema, renal tubular degeneration, and necrosis, most severely affecting the proximal convoluted tubules.[3,4]

Methemoglobinemia presents acutely, often as unexpected death. Clinical signs begin within a few hours of ingestion and death occurs in minutes or a few hours.[3,4,16] When evident, signs include brown mucous membranes, dyspnea, weakness, ataxia, tachycardia, tremors, staggering, collapse, and terminal convulsions, and are exacerbated by stress.[4,16] Soon after death brown mucous membranes and a brown cast to tissues can be seen caused by methemoglobinemia; however, methemoglobin reverts back to hemoglobin quickly.[4,16]

Diagnosis of pigweed toxicosis is based on evidence of ingestion and the appropriate lesions.[15] Treatment of renal disease is symptomatic and supportive, including hydration and correction of electrolyte imbalances, but response is likely to be poor with severe nephrosis.[3,15]

Nitrates can be detected in serum, plasma, or forage using the diphenylamine test or commercial test strips.[16] Nitrate toxicosis has a grave prognosis, most animals die within 8 hours, and restraint for treatment can prove fatal.[4,16] The goal is to reduce ferric iron in methemoglobin to the ferrous form in hemoglobin. Methylene blue, a reducing agent, can be given at a concentration of 1% to 4% in physiologic saline and a dose of 5 to 15 mg/kg body weight and repeated as necessary to achieve clinical response.[4,16] See the article on antidotes for information on status of methylene blue as an antidote. Rumen lavage with cold water can slow the reduction of nitrate by rumen microbes.[4,16] The prognosis is good for animals that survive 24 hours, although abortions can occur 7 days after exposure.[16] Preventing ingestion is the best way to preventing morbidity or mortality caused by pigweed, but some herbicides make pigweed more palatable.[15] Heavily contaminated hay should be discarded, but pigweed stalks can be tested for nitrate concentrations if disposal is not possible.

BRACKEN FERN (*PTERIDIUM AQUILINUM*)

Bracken fern, found throughout the United States and over most of the world, is a perennial that invades cleared agricultural lands, roads, grasslands, burned areas, and clear-cut areas and out competes other plants by sequestering soil nutrients and building dense stands. It avoids wet areas, prefers partial shade, and is associated with oaks and pines.[3,17,18] Bracken arises from a black, woody, horizontal, branching rhizome, which can extend for several meters, and has dark brown to black roots up to 50 cm long. Long shoots produce frond buds and deciduous 2 m long, triangular, and bipinnately compound fronds with brown reproductive spores developing on the underside in midsummer.

The toxic principle of primary interest is ptaquiloside. Young plants contain a high concentration, which decreases as the plant ages.[17,18] The leaves are the most dangerous part of the plant, although spores contain a unique carcinogen.[17] Mature green ferns collected in New Zealand contained, on average, 310 ppm ptaquiloside, dm, and mature brown plants contained 11 ppm, dm.[19] Other studies report ptaquiloside concentrations of nearly 13,000 ppm in fronds with 15% of the ferns containing greater than or equal to 5000 ppm and 43% containing greater than or equal to 1000 ppm ptaquiloside.[3,17,18] Ptaquiloside contaminates soil and ground water around the ferns.[18] Bracken fern remains toxic in hay.[19] Ptaquiloside is unstable under mildly acidic or alkaline conditions, producing pterosin B, which alkylates purine bases in DNA, disrupting transcription and producing strand breaks.[17,18] Furthermore, pterosin B activates the H-ras oncogene in the upper gastrointestinal tract and urinary tract.[17] Proliferation of mesenchymal cells, epithelium, and vasculature in the urinary tract and formation of friable neoplastic lesions results in the hemorrhage described clinically as bovine enzootic hematuria. Bracken fern is also associated with bone marrow suppression in ruminants. Although ptaquiloside has low cytotoxicity and adducts have not been detected in bone marrow, a calf dosed with ptaquiloside for 6 months developed pancytopenia.[17,19] Ptaquiloside is hydrophilic but approximately 8% of the ingested dose is excreted in milk as the aglycone.[18] Milk concentrations can be high enough to produce tumors in mice and aplastic anemia in calves.[3,17,19] Milk ptaquiloside concentrations are not detectable after 86 hours.[17] Pasteurizing of milk is protective.[17]

Bracken ferns also contain thiaminase 1 and 2, which destroy thiamin. A thiamin analog produced by thiaminase 1 competitively inhibits thiamin in metabolic reactions.[3] Bracken-induced thiamin deficiency has been experimentally produced in sheep, but is mostly a disease of monogastrics.[3,17] Ruminants produce ample thiamin in the rumen.[3] Bracken fern also contains cyanogenic glycosides, tannins, and phenolic acids, but these are unlikely to be of clinical significance.[17]

Acute hemorrhagic disease in cattle is the most common form of bracken fern poisoning in the United States and occurs when there is inadequate other forage, as in winter or drought conditions.[3,19] Bone marrow suppression occurs after ingestion of young fronds and rhizomes for weeks to 6 months.[3,4,17,18] Affected cattle or sheep present with thrombocytopenia and neutropenia early, followed by pancytopenia and immunosuppression.[3,17] Clinical signs include acute fever; lethargy; anorexia; and hemorrhage, which may present as bloody nasal discharge, melena, or frank blood in feces, hyphema, and conjunctival hemorrhage.[3,4,19] Clinical pathology findings that indicate a poor prognosis include total leukocyte count less than 2000/μL and a platelet count less than 50,000/μL.[4] Death resulting from anemia is caused by both bone marrow suppression and blood loss.[3,4,19]

Slow ingestion of bracken fern over months or years produces bovine enzootic hematuria.[3,4,19] Animals aged 1 to 3 years are usually affected. Bovine papilloma virus type II is associated with bovine enzootic hematuria.[19,20] Cattle present with intermittent brown urine, often precipitated by stress, and increased frequency of urination for several months. Later, individuals pass frank blood in urine, then blood clots, and affected cattle become emaciated and fail to produce milk. Although sheep are resistant, enzootic hematuria deaths in 120 out of 450 sheep were reported.[3,18] Enzootic hematuria was reported in a llama.[19] Clinical pathology findings in enzootic hematuria are typical of bone marrow suppression, with early thrombocytopenia in asymptomatic animals.[19] Coagulation times are prolonged and there is defective clot retraction.[1,3] Granulocytopenia is followed by pancytopenia.[3,17,19] Subcutaneous edema and multifocal petechia of the pleura, epicardium, and other visceral surfaces are seen post mortem.[3,19] Early urinalysis findings include epithelial cells in sediment early, proteinuria and calciuria later, and eventually the presence of erythrocytes and leukocytes in the urine.[3,18] Ultrasound of the urinary bladder reveals irregular sessile masses and increased thickening of the bladder wall in asymptomatic animals.[21] Gross urinary bladder lesions progress from mucosal proliferation and ulceration to neoplastic nodules, including hemangioma, hemangiosarcoma, squamous and transitional cell carcinoma, and adenocarcinoma.[3,18,20] Neoplasia occurs in the upper digestive tract, especially in sheep less than 4 years old, and is associated with bovine papilloma virus type 4.[3,18,19] Gastrointestinal neoplasia occurs in the United Kingdom and in 42% of bracken cases in Brazilian cattle.[19] Mandibular fibrosarcoma, papilloma, and carcinoma of the digestive tract are common.[3,19]

Diagnosis of enzootic hematuria is based on history of prolonged exposure to bracken fern, clinical signs, and lesions.[4,19] Aplastic anemia can be treated with blood or platelet transfusions and antibiotics for secondary infections but the prognosis is grave unless there is evidence of thrombocyte regeneration.[3,4,19] Neoplastic lesions are permanent. Bracken fern should be less than 50% of the diet for ruminants.[3] Supplemental feeding is required when other forage is unavailable and heavily infested pastures should not be grazed or animals should be rotated to other sources of forage every 3 weeks.[4,19] Finally, vaccination against bovine papilloma virus reduces the risk of ptaquiloside-induced neoplasia.[19]

Progressive retinal atrophy, or bright blindness, is seen in sheep more than a year old and exposed to dietary bracken fern for greater than or equal to 4 months.[3,18] Affected sheep are alert with glassy eyes, dilated pupils, and a high-stepping gait.[3,4,18] Examination of the eyes reveals a poor pupillary light reflex, a pale optic disk, narrow retinal vasculature, and light reflection from the depigmented retina.[3,19] Ocular changes are permanent.[4] Neutropenia and thrombocytopenia are reported with bright blindness.[3] Lesions in sheep with bright blindness are permanent and include degeneration of the retinal outer nuclear layer and rods and cones in the central retina.[3]

MARIJUANA (*CANNABIS SATIVA*)

Cannabis sativa has been used for more than 4000 years for its psychotropic effects.[22] Common names include marijuana, hemp or Indian hemp, weed, pot, ganja, dagga, hashish, and kief.[3] This annual plant can grow to 2 m with opposite leaves near the base and alternate leaves near the top. Leaves have 3 to 10 lanceolate leaflets with serrated margins. Each plant has green-white male or female flowers forming panicles at the leaf axil. Seeds are smooth and brown. In the authors' experience, large animals are most likely to come into contact with illegally grown marijuana planted among corn or other feed crops or possibly in the pasture. Occasionally, harvested marijuana is stored where animals have access to it.[23]

Cannabinoids of *C sativa* include more than 60 related compounds. The most important is Δ9-tetrahydrocannabinol (THC), a lipid soluble monoterpene present in all parts of the plant with highest concentrations in the flowers and leaves.[3] Cultivars grown in 1974 contained approximately 1% THC, whereas some current cultivars of sinsemilla contain greater than 6% THC.[24] THC interacts with cannabinoid receptors, CB1 and CB2.[25] CB1 receptors in the brain regulate cognitive function, emotional status, dopaminergic signaling, movement, and postural reflexes. CB1 receptors in the basal ganglia, brainstem, and autonomic nervous system regulate pain perception and cardiovascular and gastrointestinal function.[22,25] CB2 receptors in the peripheral nervous and immune systems influence inflammation and pain regulation.[2,26]

Reports of marijuana toxicosis in large animals are few. In one report, cattle presented with muscle tremors, hypersalivation, mydriasis, reluctance to move, and incoordination 20 hours after ingesting dry marijuana. None were treated, and 4 of 5 died over 3 days, although they were debilitated before exposure to marijuana.[23] Rapid onset of dyspnea, tremors, hypothermia, hypersalivation, sweating, recumbency, and death was described in 8 horses and 7 mules ingesting fresh *Cannabis* spp, again, no treatment was attempted.[27] Severe clinical signs are not expected in most cases. Gastrointestinal decontamination for large ingestions involves gastric lavage or, in cattle, rumenotomy, intraruminal instillation of activated charcoal and cathartics, monitoring, and symptomatic and supportive care. Laboratory tests are available for THC to indicate exposure and drug testing kits are available at pharmacies.[28]

POKEWEED (*PHYTOLACCA AMERICANA*)

Pokeweed is a perennial herb found across the Eastern United States and Canada, with a fleshy taproot and stem that can be 3 m tall. The green stem becomes red or purple at maturity. Leaves are ovate to lanceolate. Small flowers with 5 green-white to cream sepals form lovely drooping racemes. Pokeberries are purple-black on red stems (**Fig. 4**).

The major toxic principles are steroidal saponins found in the highest concentration in the root and during August, September, and October. Included are phytolaccagenin, phytolaccinic acid, and pokeberrygenin. Saponins irritate mucosal surfaces through detergent action. A total of 2 kg of *P americanum* plant material can cause clinical signs in cattle. Sheep dosed with 10 g/kg of leaves and sprouts from *P decandra* died within 9 hours.[3] Pokeweed can contain oxalates, histamines, GABA, a mitogen (in berries), and lectins, but these have less veterinary significance.[3]

Overt pokeweed toxicosis is rare in livestock.[3] Clinical signs include oral irritation; salivation; colic; vomiting; diarrhea, which may contain blood; depression; and temporarily reduced milk production.[3,4] Ataxia, head pressing, hyperesthesia, dyspnea, and

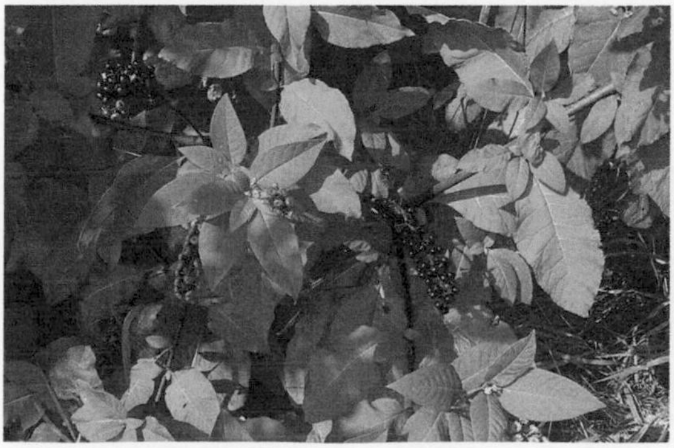

Fig. 4. *Phytolacca americanum,* pokeweed. (*Courtesy of* Mary C. Smith, DVM, Ithaca, NY.)

tremors are reported in sheep.[4] Diarrhea, which is seen 6 to 8 hours after ingestion, can be dark purple from the berries.[3] Most animals recover, but gastroenteritis with areas of mucosal necrosis and erosions have been reported on necropsy.[3,4] Treatment is supportive and symptomatic, including gastrointestinal protectants, fluid replacement, activated charcoal, atropine for severe gastrointestinal signs, and monitoring.[3,4]

YEW (*TAXUS* SPP)

T cuspidata, Japanese yew, is commonly used in landscaping in the Northeastern United States. *T canadensis,* American yew, is native to the Northeastern United States and Canada. European yew, *T baccata*, and Hicks yew, *T media*, are more common in the Southern United States. Yews are winter-tolerant evergreen shrubs with alternate branchlets and irregularly alternate twigs. Leaves are closely spaced, flexible, dark green, flat, opposite, 1 to 2 cm long, and needlelike. Flowers are inconspicuous and single, dark seeds are enclosed in a bright cup-shaped yellow to scarlet aril (**Fig. 5**).

All parts of the plant are toxic except the aril. Yews contain more than 10 alkaloids. Taxine alkaloids include taxines A, B (the most toxic), C, I, and II. Other alkaloids include taxinine, taxicatin, taxicins, and taxusin. Taxol is used as a chemotherapeutic but is of little veterinary significance.[1,4,29] Cyanogenic glycosides, lignins, ephedrine, and irritant volatile compounds have been detected in *Taxus* spp.[3] Toxin concentrations vary. *T canadensis* contains less taxine than other species. Mature leaves are less toxic in winter than summer, and dry leaves remain toxic.[3,4,29] Taxine acts in cardiac myocytes as a calcium channel antagonist and may inhibit sodium or potassium channels.[3,4] The net effect is inhibition of conduction at the atrioventricular node and depressed cardiac depolarization.[3,4,29] Alkaloids from *Taxus* spp are metabolized by the liver with some biliary excretion. Although elimination through milk has not been reported, milk from poisoned cows should probably be discarded.[3,4] The lethal dose for taxine ranges from 4 to 20 mg/kg in laboratory animals.[3] A steer died after ingesting 0.36 g/kg dry yew leaves.[4] Sheep are similarly susceptible, but goats tolerate up to about 5 times the toxic dose as sheep.[30] Although cattle are poisoned more frequently, horses are more susceptible to yew. Frequently, toxicosis is caused by livestock escaping, overgrowth of trees into pasture, or inappropriate disposal of hedge trimmings. Multiple individuals can be affected. More poisonings are expected in the winter when other green forage is unavailable.[3,4,29] Although yew poisoning is

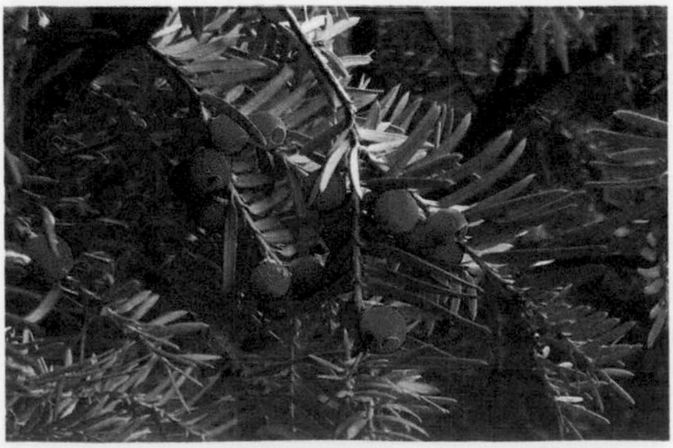

Fig. 5. *Taxus* spp, yew. (*Courtesy of* Mary C. Smith, DVM, Ithaca, NY.)

reported in captive deer and wild moose, wild ruminants regularly browse *Taxus* spp with no apparent ill effects.[3,30]

The most common presentation of *Taxus* spp poisoning is unexpected death. Most animals succumb within 4 hours, but delay for up to 3 days is reported. Clinical signs include anxiety; depression; ataxia; bradycardia; jugular distension and pulses; dyspnea; hypothermia; trembling; weakness; collapse; agonal breathing; and death, which may be hastened by restraint attempts.[3,4] Vomiting, abortion, and convulsions have been reported.[4,29] Electrocardiogram changes in people include depressed or absent P-waves, atypical bundle-branch block, and increased QRS duration.[29] Bradycardia and QRS prolongation were observed in experimentally poisoned goats.[31] Gross and microscopic lesions may be absent. Pulmonary edema, gastric mucosal congestion, and plant material in the rumen are reported.[3,29] Diagnosis is based on history and evidence of plant ingestion. Taxine is detectable in plant material and rumen contents of poisoned animals.[3,29]

If an animal is seen ingesting yew, immediate intervention could be lifesaving, but the stress of treatment could precipitate cardiac dysfunction.[3,4,29] Treatment recommendations include administration of activated charcoal mixed with palatable feed at a dose of 2 g/kg body weight, along with a cathartic, such as magnesium sulfate.[4] Rumenotomy and instillation of activated charcoal enhanced survival in goats.[29] Lidocaine is used to treat cardiac arrhythmias in humans.[3] Cautious use of atropine is suggested for bradycardia in ruminants.[3] The prognosis is good for ruminants that survive more than 3 days.[29]

RHODODENDRON AND RELATED SPECIES, (*RHODODENDRON* SPP, *KALMIA* SPP, *PIERIS* SPP)

Rhododendrons, laurels, and Japanese pieris are widely cultivated for their beautiful flowers. *Kalmia* spp, mountain laurels, are abundant in the Appalachian Mountains.[3] *Pieris* is cultivated in the Northeastern United States and found in mountain woodlands.[3,32] These plants, of the heath (Ericaceae) family, prefer moist, acidic soils. Ingestion by livestock has occurred from improper disposal of garden clippings and inadequate alternative forage.[32] Rhododendrons and related species are shrubs or small trees. Leaves are simple, elliptical to lanceolate, and usually alternate with pinnate venation. Rhododendron leaves can appear in false whorls at branch ends. *Kalmia* leaves can be opposite, whorled, or alternate. Clusters of showy flowers are white or pink, although rhododendrons can be other colors (**Fig. 6**A). *Kalmia* flowers form umbels (see **Fig. 6**B) and *Pieris* flowers form drooping panicles or racemes. All produce seeds in elongated 5-sectioned capsules.

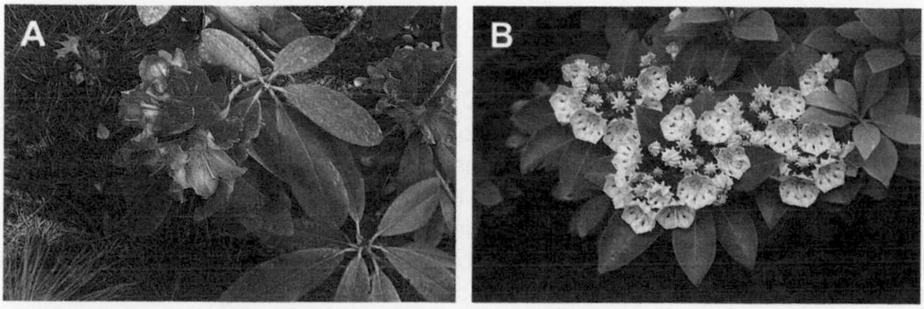

Fig. 6. (*A*) *Rhododendron* spp, (*B*) *Kalmia* spp, mountain laurel. (*Courtesy of* Mary C. Smith, DVM, Ithaca, NY.)

Grayanotoxins are present in all parts of the plants, with the highest concentration in leaves.[3,32] Honey made from the flowers can cause mild to moderate clinical signs in people.[32] The intraperitoneal mouse LD_{50} of grayanotoxin is approximately 0.1 mg/kg.[3,32] The toxic dose of fresh foliage for sheep or cattle is about 0.2% body weight.[4,32] Grayanotoxin binds to voltage-dependent cell membrane sodium channels, causing them to open and close slowly, which results in persistent activation and increased axon permeability to sodium by almost 100 fold.[3] Decreased sodium channel selectivity allows potassium ions to cross. The net effect is persistent depolarization.[4] Neurotransmitter release is also altered.[3,32] Cardiac effects include prolonged depolarization of Purkinje fibers and arrest at the sinoatrial node.[3] Water soluble grayanotoxins are rapidly absorbed and eliminated.[32]

Goats are the most susceptible and commonly poisoned domestic ruminants.[3,4,32] Sheep are commonly affected, and poisonings have been reported in cattle, llamas, kangaroos, and monogastrics.[3,32] Rhododendron, an evergreen, is most commonly ingested in the winter.[3,4] Because grayanotoxins are not accumulated, the clinical presentation is acute with an onset usually within a few hours.[3,32] Clinical signs include depression; marked salivation; repeated swallowing; anorexia; colic; bruxism; bellowing; bloat; vomiting and regurgitation, often projectile; secondary aspiration pneumonia; and rarely diarrhea.[3,4,32] Diarrhea is an indicator of a good prognosis in sheep.[3,32] More severe clinical signs include irregular respiration, muscle weakness, inability to stand, paralysis, blindness, convulsions, hypotension, tachycardia or bradycardia, and fever up to 106°F (41°C).[3,4,32] Some pregnant goats abort. Dehydration, acidosis, and other electrolyte imbalances are reported.[4,32] Grayanotoxin poisoning is rarely fatal, but uncontrolled convulsions and aspiration pneumonia have a poor prognosis.[32] Lesions are nonspecific and can include mild hemorrhagic enteritis, degeneration of hepatic and renal tubular epithelium, aspiration pneumonia, and plant material in the rumen.[3,32] Tentative diagnosis is based on clinical signs and evidence of yew ingestion.[4] Some laboratories analyze urine, gastrointestinal contents, and suspect plant material for grayanotoxins.[3,30] Grayanotoxins are detectable in urine for up to 5 days after exposure.[32]

Treatment is based on detoxification and supportive care. Early rumenotomy is appropriate only for large ingestions and before onset of clinical signs.[4,32] Activated charcoal and sorbitol or saline cathartic can be given early to asymptomatic animals. A stomach tube for relief of bloat, analgesics for pain, atropine for bradycardia, other antiarrhythmic drugs as needed, and oral or intravenous fluid and electrolyte replacement might be needed for affected livestock.[3,4,32] Aspiration pneumonia is treated with antibiotics.[32] Poison prevention is achieved through removal of these plants from the pasture, supplemental feeding as needed, and proper disposal of hedge clippings.[4,32]

OAK TREES (*QUERCUS* SPP)

All species of oak are potentially toxic.[33] Oaks in the Northeastern United States are deciduous with alternate, dark green, glossy, and usually deeply pinnately lobed leaves. Male flowers form pendulous catkins in the spring. Oaks produce subspherical to oblong acorns with a scaly base cap in the autumn.

The toxic principle of oak has not been definitively determined. Gallotannins, tannic acid, pyrogallol, and phenolic acid have been implicated.[3,4,33] Tannins and related compounds are astringents and denature cell proteins, causing coagulative necrosis of cells on contact.[3,4] However, an attempt to replicate oak poisoning experimentally using tannic acid failed.[33] Although gallotannins are present in the leaves, bark, and acorns, they are concentrated in new spring growth, and poisonings are common in the spring or after green or mature acorn ingestion in autumn. Ruminal hydrolysis of gallotannins to gallic acid, pyrogallol, and resorcinol may be responsible for the clinical effects, but acorn poisoning has also been reported in monogastric species.[4] Oak toxicosis requires that 50% or more of the diet be acorns or oak buds for at least several days.[1,3] Oak poisoning most commonly affects cattle, but sheep are susceptible. Toxicosis has been reported in goats, which are less susceptible and commonly browse oak.[3] Wild deer consume acorns with impunity because of a tannin binding protein in their saliva.[3] Oak is unpalatable and poisonings are most often associated with late snow storms or drought conditions when other forage is not available, but some animals develop a taste for acorns.[3,4,33]

Clinical signs of oak toxicosis can begin soon after exposure or up to 18 days later.[33] Anorexia and constipation within 48 hours followed by transient elimination of red or brown urine occurs early but these signs are often missed.[34] After 6 days of exposure, cattle become progressively more depressed and can exhibit abdominal pain, nasal discharge, polydipsia, polyuria, increased respiratory rate, and fever.[1,33,34] Later, diarrhea (possibly bloody), dehydration, colic, dependent subcutaneous edema, weakness, emaciation, hypothermia, and sometimes icterus develop.[1,3,4] Clinical pathology findings can include elevated BUN, creatinine, AST, and transiently elevated sorbitol dehydrogenase. Electrolyte abnormalities include hypocalcemia, hyperphosphatemia, hypochloremia, hyponatremia, and acidosis.[3,33,34] Urinalysis reveals proteinuria soon after exposure and hematuria, glycosuria, and low specific gravity later.[3,33,34] Postmortem findings are subcutaneous edema, peritoneal and pleural effusions, multifocal ulceration from the oral cavity through the intestines, and edema and inflammation of the mesentery.[34] Nephritis is characterized grossly by perirenal edema; hemorrhage; enlarged perirenal lymph nodes; and pale, enlarged kidneys with small, white cortical foci or, in chronic cases, a roughened cortical surface.[3,33] Microscopically, there is diffuse tubular necrosis, with interstitial fibrosis in chronic cases.[3,33] Diagnosis is based on evidence of oak ingestion, acorns, oak leaves, or oak buds in the rumen contents by gross or microscopic examination, history, clinical signs, and lesions. Pyrogallol is briefly detectable in the serum or urine, but is no longer present when clinical signs become evident.[33]

Supplemental feeding to prevent ruminants from consuming more than 50% of the diet as acorns should prevent oak poisoning. Alfalfa hay or a high-energy feed composed of 30% alfalfa meal, 54% cottonseed or soybean meal, 6% vegetable oil, and 10% calcium hydroxide might be protective against oak poisoning in cattle.[1,3] Calcium hydroxide binds tannins in the rumen but decreases feed palatability at concentrations greater than 10% in the diet.[3] Clinically affected cattle should not have further access to oak. Treatment is supportive and symptomatic, including access to adequate good quality water and hay.[3,4] Acidosis, dehydration, and electrolyte imbalances are treated with intravenous fluids.[3] Recovery is prolonged and the prognosis is poor for cattle with markedly elevated BUN and creatinine, but good for young cattle and those that continue to eat. Some will make a complete recovery, others will remain debilitiated.[3,4,33]

CHERRIES, PEACHES, AND OTHER STONE FRUITS (*PRUNUS* SPP)

The most important members of the genus *Prunus* in the Northeastern United States are cherry laurel (*P laurocerasus*), wild red or bird cherry (*P pensylvanica*), choke cherry (*P virginiana*), black cherry (*P serotina*), peach (*P persica*), and apricot (*P armeniaca*). These trees prefer the rich, moist soils of forests and floodplains. Toxicosis in livestock is usually associated with ingestion of leaves, but there have been cases in animals fed *Prunus* spp pits in bakery waste.[35] *Prunus* is part of the rose family, Rosaceae. Some species can form large thickets by sprouting from existing roots. The trees or shrubs may have thorns. The bark is smooth or forms smooth plates. Leaves are simple, alternate, and oval to lanceolate with serrate or entire margins. Fragrant flowers grow in racemes or clusters, or occasionally as solitary blossoms in early spring and may be white, pink, red, or green with 5 or 10 petals. Fruits are drupes and include cherries, choke cherries, apricots, and plums, each containing a stone or pit.

Cyanogenic glycosides are the major toxic concern. Amygdalin is a cyanogenic diglycoside found within the seeds. Prunasin is a monoglycoside found in the leaves, bark, and shoots.[3,35] These glycosides are located within cell vacuoles and are nontoxic unless the cell is damaged by freezing, wilting, or crushing, as occurs with mastication. Then glycosides are released and acted upon by cellular glycosidases, which rapidly release free cyanide.[2,4,35] Beta-glycosidases from rumen microbes also hydrolyze cyanogenic glycosides, making ruminants particularly susceptible to poisoning from cyanogenic plants, such as *Prunus* spp.[35,36]

Cyanide reversibly inhibits mitochondrial cytochrome c oxidase, preventing electron transfer and thus inhibiting cellular respiration. Consequently, hemoglobin cannot release oxygen resulting in supersaturation of the blood with oxyhemoglobin and the characteristic cherry red blood associated with cyanide poisoning.[3,4,36] Animals are exposed to low dietary concentrations of cyanide, which are detoxified by the mitochondrial enzyme rhodanese, through the formation of thiocyanate, and excreted in the urine.[3] The capacity of rhodanese is overwhelmed after ingestion of a large cyanide dose, and the central nervous system only has limited rhodanese activity.[3,4] Cyanide also alters release of calcium-dependent neurotransmitters and metabolism of catecholamines.[36]

The concentration of cyanogenic glycosides in *Prunus* spp varies. High soil nitrogen and phosphorus and cool moist weather promote glycoside accumulation, but there is increased cyanide release when leaves wilt, as occurs in drought. Young, spring leaves are more toxic than mature leaves, but toxicosis can occur later in the year.[3] Leaves of *P persica* contain approximately 100 ppm potential hydrogen cyanide based on glycoside concentration, and seeds contain 450 ppm potential hydrogen cyanide.[3] Leaves from *P serotina* contain 25,000 ppm potential hydrogen cyanide in the early spring, 500 ppm after 6 weeks, and 40 ppm after several months.[3] Black cherry is the species of most concern in the Northeastern United States.[37] Fruits of wild black cherries and choke cherries also contain cyanide.[3] The minimum toxic dose of cyanide is near the lethal dose.[4] Plants containing 200 ppm potential hydrogen cyanide are considered hazardous to livestock and those containing greater than or equal to 2% prunasin, dm, can be lethal to cattle and other species.[3,4] Ingestion of 2 kg apricot pits containing at least 100 ppm free hydrogen cyanide and 300 ppm cyanide potential caused severe toxicosis and death in cattle.[33] There is little risk associated with ingestion of seeds from cultivated cherries.[3] Most of the cyanide is lost in hay, haylage, and silage; plant material containing 25,000 ppm potential hydrogen cyanide when fresh contained only 200 ppm after 24 hours and 40 ppm after 48 hours, but the decline is slow under cool, humid conditions.[4] The authors have seen cyanide poisoning from hay. Cyanide is not a cumulative toxin and there is no evidence of tolerance.[4]

Leaves from *Prunus* spp are palatable. Ruminants have increased susceptibility to cyanide toxicosis because of the alkaline environment in the rumen compared with the stomach of monogastrics and the ability of rumen microflora to hydrolyze cyanogenic glycosides. The acidic rumen pH in cattle on high-concentrate diets makes them less susceptible.[3,4] Wild ruminants are also susceptible to cyanogenic plant poisoning.[3] Ingestion of water soon after ingestion of the plants enhances their toxicity.[4] Cyanide toxicosis commonly presents as unexpected death affecting multiple animals. Onset of clinical signs is usually between 15 minutes and an hour after ingestion of the plant, and death usually occurs rapidly but may be delayed for up to 48 hours.[3,35,38] Clinical signs begin with distress, ataxia, weakness, rapid and labored breathing, frothing at the mouth, dilated pupils, decreased blood pressure, increased heart rate, arrhythmias, urination attempts, and recumbency. Some ruminants bloat and regurgitate because of rumen stasis. Hypoxia-induced signs include nystagmus, muscle tremors, fasciculations, tonic-clonic convulsions, and opisthotonos. Animals rapidly become comatose and die of respiratory failure. Mucous membranes are bright red but can appear cyanotic at the time of death.[4,35,36] Necropsy findings are nonspecific and include slow blood coagulation, generalized congestion, froth in the airways, and multifocal petechia on the heart and viscera caused by agonal stress, and *Prunus* spp leaves in the rumen.[3,4,37,38] Centrilobular hepatic necrosis secondary to hypoxia is common. Rumen contents can have a bitter almond smell, which dissipates rapidly and many people are unable to detect it.[35]

Tentative diagnosis of *Prunus* spp toxicosis is based on clinical signs, evidence of plant ingestion, response to treatment, or the bitter-almond odor detected in rumen contents. Species of leaves from rumen contents can be determined using microscopy.[37] Plant material or rumen contents can be analyzed for cyanide release using picrate papers, commercial test kits, or other analyses.[3,4] A blood cyanide concentration of 0.53 mg/L is reported with toxicosis in cattle. Rumen content and whole blood should be collected from the carcass and fresh plant material from the environment.[35] Testing must be done within hours of death and collection or samples must be immediately placed in airtight containers and frozen to prevent dissipation of the cyanide.[3,36] Serum thiocyanate concentrations remain elevated briefly after exposure to cyanide; the half-life is 3 days in humans. Thiocyanate concentrations ranging from 145 to 211 μmol/L were detected in serum of cows with cyanide toxicosis and decreased to between 50 and 60 μmol/L after recovery. The concentration in an unaffected cow was 52 μmol/L.[35]

Cyanide toxicosis usually progresses too rapidly for effective treatment. The rationale for treatment is to produce methemoglobinemia, which removes cyanide from cytochrome oxidase by producing cyanmethemoglobin. Methemoglobinemia is reduced by rapid intravenous infusion of sodium thiosulfate, which binds the cyanide to form thiocyanate. Induction of methemoglobinemia is not required for treatment of ruminants because of their high rhodanese activity, but methemoglobinemia can be induced by cautious rapid administration of sodium nitrite in 20% solution at a dose of 10 to 20 mg/kg or to response, or of methylene blue (but not both) in 1% to 4% solution at a dose of 2 to 3 g/200 kg body weight. Sodium thiosulfate is given as a sulfur donor at a 20% solution for a dose of 6 mL/100 kg body weight, repeated as needed.[3,4] A total of 30 g of sodium thiosulfate can be dosed via stomach tube to detoxify cyanide in the rumen even before clinical signs are evident.[4] A gallon of vinegar diluted in 3 to 5 Gal of water will decrease the pH of the rumen to slow hydrolysis of cyanogenic glycosides.[4] Hydroxocobalamin is used to successfully treat poisoning in humans and experimental dogs. Hydroxocobalamin binds to cyanide, forming cyanocobalamin (vitamin B12), which is eliminated in the urine. Hydroxocobalamin is safer than inducing methemoglobinemia and has few side effects; however, the expense of treatment limits its veterinary use.[39,40]

The prognosis for cyanide toxicosis is grave because of the rapid onset of clinical signs, particularly labored respiration and seizures, but response is good if treatment is initiated rapidly. The prognosis is good if the animal survives for more than an hour after onset of signs.[3,36] It is by far better to prevent animals from having access to cyanogenic plants.

SUMMARY

Livestock are at risk for ingestion of toxic plants. Some plants, such as the cyanogenic *Prunus* spp (cherry, apricot, and peach trees) and cardiotoxic *Taxus* spp (yews) can affect a large number of animals and cause rapid mortality. Others, such as *Quercus* spp (oak) and *Senecio* spp (ragworts) cause chronic, debilitating conditions that adversely affect production. Still others, such as *Rhododendron* spp and pokeweed (*Phytolacca americanum*) cause dramatic clinical signs and short-term production losses but are rarely lethal.

Plant poisonings are most likely underdiagnosed because tests for plant toxins are not routinely available at veterinary diagnostic laboratories. Tentative diagnosis is usually based on evidence of toxic plant ingestion, such as evidence of grazing or the presence of plant material in the rumen, and appropriate clinical signs and lesions. Prevention of access to poisonous plants is more effective and economical than treatment of plant poisonings. Use of herbicides, biologic controls, or hand removal of plants is the best way to prevent animals from accessing poisonous plants.

REFERENCES

1. Panter KE, Gardner DR, Lee ST, et al. Important poisonous plants of the United States. In: Gupta RC, editor. Veterinary toxicology: basic and clinical principals. New York: Elsevier; 2007. p. 825–72.
2. Knight AP. Cicutoxin. In: Plumlee KH, editor. Veterinary clinical toxicology. St Louis (MO): Mosby; 2004. p. 338–40.
3. Burrows GE, Tyrl RJ. Toxic plants of North America. Ames (Iowa): Iowa State Press; 2001.
4. Knight AP, Walter RG. A guide to plant poisoning of animals in North America. Jackson (MS): Teton NewMedia; 2001.
5. Panter KE. Piperidine alkaloids. In: Plumlee KH, editor. Veterinary clinical toxicology. St Louis (MO): Mosby; 2004. p. 365–9.
6. Walsh RB, Dingwell RT. Beef herd poisoning due to ingestion of tansy ragwort in southwestern Ontario. Can Vet J 2007;48:737–40.
7. Crews C, Driffield M, Berthiller F, et al. Loss of pyrrolizidine alkaloids on decomposition of ragwort (*Senecio jacobaea*) as measured by LC-TOF-MS. J Agric Food Chem 2009;57:3669–73.
8. Stegelmeier B. Pyrrolizidine alkaloids. In: Plumlee KH, editor. Veterinary clinical toxicology. St Louis (MO): Mosby; 2004. p. 370–7.
9. Braun U, Linggi T, Pospischil A. Ultrasonographic findings in three cows with chronic ragwort (*Senecio alpines)* poisoning. Vet Rec 1999;144:122–6.
10. Bondan C, Soares JC, Cecim M, et al. Oxidative stress in the erythrocytes of cattle intoxicated with *Senecio sp*. Vet Clin Pathol 2005;34:353–7.
11. Meerdink GL, Fredrickson RL Jr, Bordson GO. Trematone. In: Plumlee KH, editor. Veterinary clinical toxicology. St Louis (MO): Mosby; 2004. p. 349–50.
12. Lee ST, Davis TZ, Gardner DR, et al. Trematone and structurally related compounds in white snakeroot (*Ageratina altissima*): a plant associated with trembles and milk sickness. J Agric Food Chem 2010;58:8560–5.
13. Stegelmeier BL, Davis TZ, Green BT, et al. Experimental rayless goldenrod (*Isocoma pluriflora*) toxicosis in goats. J Vet Diagn Invest 2010;22:570–7.

14. Pickrell JA, Oehme FW, Mannala SA. Carboxyatractyloside. In: Plumlee KH, editor. Veterinary clinical toxicology. St Louis (MO): Mosby; 2004. p. 385–6.
15. Nicholson SR. Pigweed. In: Plumlee KH, editor. Veterinary clinical toxicology. St Louis (MO): Mosby; 2004. p. 437.
16. Casteel SW, Evans TJ. Nitrate. In: Plumlee KH, editor. Veterinary clinical toxicology. St Louis (MO): Mosby; 2004. p. 127–30.
17. Alonso-Amelot ME, Avendano M. Human carcinogenesis and bracken fern: a review of the evidence. Curr Med Chem 2002;9:675–86.
18. Vetter J. A biological hazard of our age: bracken fern (*Pteridium aquilinum* (L.) Kuhn)–a review. Acta Vet Hung 2009;57:183–96.
19. Plumlee KH, Nicholson SR. Ptaquiloside. In: Plumlee KH, editor. Veterinary clinical toxicology. St Louis (MO): Mosby; 2004. p. 402–3.
20. Karimuribo ED, Swai ES, Kyakaisho PK. Investigation of a syndrome characterized by passage of red urine in smallholder dairy cattle in East Usambara Mountains, Tanzania. J S Afr Vet Assoc 2008;79:89–94.
21. Hoque M, Somvanshi R, Singh GR, et al. Ultrasonographic evaluation of urinary bladder in normal, fern fed, and enzootic bovine hematuria-affected cattle. J Vet Med 2002;9:403–7.
22. Di Marzo V, De Petrocellis L. Plant, synthetic, and endogenous cannabinoids in medicine. Annu Rev Med 2006;57:17, 1–17. 22.
23. Driemeier D. Marijuana (*Cannabis sativa*) toxicosis in cattle. Vet Hum Toxicol 1997;39:351–2.
24. Anonymous. Street drugs a drug identification guide. Plymouth (UK): MN. Publishers Group, LLC; 2005.
25. Ashton CH. Pharmacology and effects of cannabis: a brief review. Br J Psychiatry 2001;178:101–86.
26. Vomer PA. Recreational drugs. In: Peterson ME, Talcott PA, editors. Small animal toxicology. 2nd edition. Philadelphia: Saunders; 2005. p. 273–311.
27. Cardassis J. Intoxication des équidés par *Cannabis indica*. Rec Méd Vét 1951; 127:971–3.
28. Janczyk P, Donaldson CW, Gwaltney S. Two hundred and thirteen cases of marijuana toxicosis in dogs. Vet Hum Toxicol 2004;46:19–21.
29. Casteel SW. Taxine alkaloids. In: Plumlee KH, editor. Veterinary clinical toxicology. St Louis (MO): Mosby; 2004. p. 379–81.
30. Handeland K. Acute yew (*Taxus*) poisoning in moose (*Alces alces*. Toxicon 2008; 52:829–32.
31. Van Gelder GA, Buck WB, Osweiler GD, et al. Research activities of a veterinary toxicology laboratory. Clin Toxicol 1972;5:271–81.
32. Puschner B. Grayanotoxins. In: Plumlee KH, editor. Veterinary clinical toxicology. St Louis (MO): Mosby; 2004. p. 412–5.
33. Plumlee KH. Tannic acid. In: Plumlee KH, editor. Veterinary clinical toxicology. St Louis (MO): Mosby; 2004. p. 346–8.
34. Plumlee KH, Johnson B, Galey FD. Comparison of disease in calves dosed orally with oak or commercial tannic acid. J Vet Diagn Invest 1998;10:263–7.
35. Kupper J, Schuman M, Wennig R, et al. Cyanide poisoning associated with the feeding of apricot kernels to dairy cattle. Vet Rec 2008;162:488–9.
36. Pickrell JA, Oehme F. Cyanogenic glycosides. In: Plumlee KH, editor. Veterinary clinical toxicology. St Louis (MO): Mosby; 2004. p. 391–2.
37. Radi ZA, Styer EL, Thompson LJ. *Prunus* spp intoxication in ruminants: a case in a goat diagnosed by identification of leaf fragments in the rumen. J Vet Diagn Invest 2004;16:593–9.

38. Sargison ND, Williamson DS, Duncan JR, et al. *Prunus padus* (bird cherry) poisoning in cattle. Vet Rec 1996;138:188.
39. Borron SW, Baud FJ, Megarbane B, et al. Hydroxocobalamin for severe acute cyanide poisoning by ingestion or inhalation. Am J Emerg Med 2007;25:551–8.
40. Borron SW, Stonerook M, Reid F. Efficacy of hydroxocobalamin for the treatment of acute cyanide poisoning in adult beagle dogs. Clin Toxicol 2006;44:5–15.

Treatment of Animal Toxicoses: A Regulatory Perspective

Susan J. Bright, DVM[a,*], Michael J. Murphy, DVM, JD, PhD[b], Janice C. Steinschneider, MA, JD[c], Randall A. Lovell, DVM, PhD[d], Lynn O. Post, DVM, PhD, CAPT, USPHS[d]

KEYWORDS

• Toxicoses • Antidotes • Regulatory

Veterinarians are frequently called upon to treat known or suspected animal toxicoses in clinic, farm, or field situations. A definitive diagnosis is not always established at the time of clinical presentation. Many of these toxicoses are a diagnostic and therapeutic challenge for veterinary practitioners yet early diagnosis and treatment are often key to a successful outcome. Useful diagnostic and treatment information may be obtained from a variety of sources. These sources include poison control centers, such as the ASPCA Animal Poison Control Center (http://www.aspca.org/pet-care/poison-control/) (888-426-4435); Pet Poison Helpline (800.213.6680, www.petpoisonhelpline.com); veterinary diagnostic laboratories (www.aavld.org); veterinary toxicologists (www.abvt.org); and colleges of veterinary medicine (http://www.avma.org/education/cvea/colleges_accredited/colleges_accredited.asp). Veterinary diagnostic laboratories are also useful for testing samples from animals and from suspected toxin sources, such as feed samples or plants.

When a toxicosis is suspected by a veterinary practitioner, obtaining a detailed clinical history is of prime importance, particularly to determine if administration of

No official support or endorsement by the Food and Drug Administration is intended or should be inferred.

The authors have nothing to disclose.

[a] Division of Veterinary Product Safety, Office of Surveillance & Compliance, Center for Veterinary Medicine, Food and Drug Administration, 7519 Standish Place, Rockville, MD 20855, USA
[b] Division of Surveillance, Office of Surveillance & Compliance, Center for Veterinary Medicine, Food and Drug Administration, 7519 Standish Place, Rockville, MD 20855, USA
[c] Office of Surveillance & Compliance, Center for Veterinary Medicine, Food and Drug Administration, 7529 Standish Place, Rockville, MD 20855, USA
[d] Division of Animal Feeds, Office of Surveillance & Compliance, Center for Veterinary Medicine, Food and Drug Administration, 7519 Standish Place, Rockville, MD 20855, USA
* Corresponding author.
E-mail address: susan.bright@fda.hhs.gov

Vet Clin Food Anim 27 (2011) 481–512
doi:10.1016/j.cvfa.2011.02.002
0749-0720/11/$ – see front matter. Published by Elsevier Inc.

a specific antidote is indicated. Prognosis of animals in the same herd may vary considerably depending on the toxin, exposure dose, length of time between exposure and treatment, and availability of drugs to treat an animal. Treatment generally requires stabilization of vital signs, institution of supportive care, decontamination to prevent further toxin absorption, and/or administration of compounds to enhance the elimination of absorbed toxins.

This article is not intended to provide an in-depth discussion of the diagnosis or treatment of animal toxicoses. Several publications provide this information.[1–9] Rather, this article focuses on the regulatory considerations of treating animals with toxicoses, in particular food animals, because virtually all of the drugs used to treat animals with toxicoses are not Food and Drug Administration (FDA) approved for that use. Because the drugs actually used are not approved to treat toxicoses, extra-label drug use (ELU) regulations may be of interest to practitioners. Consequently, in this article, the prevalence of toxicoses is discussed briefly, followed by a discussion of drugs that are commonly used to treat these toxicoses, categorized by a drug's regulatory status: approved use, ELU, and unapproved use. Hopefully, this information is useful to practicing veterinarians as a reminder of the regulatory status of drugs used in these emergency situations.

PREVALENCE OF ANIMAL TOXICOSES

The prevalence of toxicoses in dogs and cats is reasonably well known. This prevalence was reported in 1990[10] and has been frequently updated.[11–15] Although new toxicoses, such as those due to lilies (*Lilium spp*), xylitol, and melamine-cyanuric acid, are discovered with some frequency, the majority of drugs needed to treat toxicoses in companion animals are reasonably well known.

Unfortunately, the prevalence of toxicoses in food animals is less well known. **Table 1** summarizes toxicoses listed in referenced texts[8] for food animal practitioners by page number and the results of a recent survey. The toxin topics in the Current Veterinary Therapy (CVT) texts are largely empirical based on the authors' experience and informal surveys of those familiar with animal toxicoses (periodic informal surveys of American Board of Veterinary Toxicology, American Academy of Veterinary and Comparative Toxicology and American Association of Veterinary Laboratory Diagnosticians [AAVLD] member, conducted by and for those members). In addition, a survey of 41 veterinary diagnostic laboratories was undertaken to determine the prevalence of feed-related toxicoses that occurred between 2003 and 2007 in the United States (Animal Feed Safety System [AFSS] survey of 41 AAVLD laboratories conducted by Dr Gary Osweiler as reported to the Center for Veterinary Medicine [CVM]). Sixteen laboratories provided data on 504 incidences, many of which are listed in **Table 1** under the AFSS column. Consequently, many drugs used to treat food animals are borrowed from companion animal use or are based on empirical data. Prevalence data of toxicoses in food animals may be useful to pharmaceutical companies to know which drugs, and in what amounts, may be needed to treat food animal toxicoses, when considering drug development needs (see **Table 1**).

DRUGS USED TO TREAT ANIMAL TOXICOSES

This article includes information on the treatment of both companion animal toxicoses and food animal toxicoses, because (1) the authors anticipate that some readers are in a mixed animal practice and (2) illustration of the added ELU and compounding considerations that should be addressed when treating food animals versus nonfood animals may be useful.

The Federal Food, Drug, and Cosmetic Act (FFDCA) (Section 201 [21 U.S.C. 321(g)(1)]) defines a "drug" as:

(A) Articles recognized in the official United States Pharmacopeia, official Homoeopathic Pharmacopoeia of the United States, or official National Formulary, or any supplement to any of them; and
(B) Articles intended for use in the diagnosis, cure, mitigation, treatment, or prevention of disease in man or other animals; and
(C) Articles (other than food) intended to affect the structure or any function of the body of man or other animals; and
(D) Articles intended for use as a component of any articles specified in clause (A), (B), or (C)...

Drugs administered to animals to treat (diagnose, cure, mitigate, treat, or prevent a disease or to affect the structure or any function of the body) a toxicosis are regulated by the FDA under the FFDCA and its implementing regulations, published in Title 21 of the Code of Federal Regulations (available on-line at http://www.gpoaccess.gov/cfr/). Practicing veterinarians often place drugs used in treating an animal toxicosis into 3 categories—general treatment, supportive treatment, and specific treatment. This article does likewise.

General Treatment

General treatment is normally given irrespective of the toxin, unless a contraindication exists. General treatment is often intended to induce emesis, reduce absorption, or enhance elimination of toxins. Commonly used emetics in dogs and/or cats include apomorphine, xylazine, salt, syrup of ipecac, and hydrogen peroxide. (See Refs.[5–7] for some of the contraindications to inducing emesis.) Activated charcoal is often used orally to reduce further absorption of toxins from the gastrointestinal tract, whereas soap and water are often used dermally to remove a toxin from the skin and/or reduce toxin absorption through the skin. Mineral oil, sodium sulfate, and other laxatives are often used to enhance elimination of toxins still present in the gastrointestinal tract. Gastric lavage may be used to enhance removal of toxins still present in the stomach.

Supportive Treatment

A myriad drugs are given to animals with toxicoses with the intention of providing supportive treatment. Supportive treatment is often also given irrespective of the specific toxin. These drugs are normally given to correct an abnormal physiologic state of the animal. For example, fluids may be given to treat dehydration, bicarbonate may be given to treat acidosis, and furosemide may be given to treat edema.

Specific Treatment

A few drugs are indicated when a specific toxin is known or suspected. These specific treatment agents are often called antidotes. (The definition of antidote used in this article is not as defined by the FDA but rather as presented in different veterinary texts.) An antidote is a substance that can counteract the activity or effect of a known or suspected poison. Antidotes may be classified according to their mechanism of action: chemical or pharmacologic. Chemical antidotes interact specifically with a toxicant or neutralize a toxicant. For example, chelators combine with elements (especially heavy metals) to form complexes that can then be eliminated (eg, molybdenum and sulfate for copper toxicity or calcium disodium EDTA for lead

Table 1
Toxicoses in food animals

Toxin	AFSS (No. of Cases)	CVT–FA-1	CVT–FA-2	CVT–FA-3	CVT–FA-4
Feed-Associated Toxicoses					
Gossypol	2	—	—	p. 331	p. 245
Iodine	—	p. 398	p. 357	—	—
Ionophore	46	p. 400	p. 359	p. 329	p. 244
Selenium	4	p. 436	p. 394	—	p. 252
Sulfur	—	—	—	—	p. 280
Trichloroethylene extracted soybean oil meal	—	p. 514	p. 450	—	—
Urea and other nonprotein nitrogen sources	35	p. 393	p. 354	p. 327	p. 242
Industrial Chemicals					
Chlorinated napthalenes	—	p. 516	—	—	—
Coal tar and phenols	—	p. 521	p. 454	p. 409	—
Crude oils, fuel oils, and kerosene	1	p. 517	p. 451	p. 407	—
Hexachlorobenzene	—	p. 510	p. 447	—	—
Polybrominated biphenyls	—	p. 511	p. 448	p. 403	—
Inorganic Toxins					
Arsenic	3	p. 493	p. 435	p. 394	—
Copper-molybdenum	113	p. 495	p. 437	p. 396	—
Fluorides	2	p. 504	p. 442	p. 398	—
Iron	—	p. 502	—	—	—
Lead	3	p. 498	p. 439	—	p. 251
Mercury	—	p. 500	p. 440	—	—
Miscellaneous Toxins					
Animal waste and sewage sludge	—	—	—	—	p. 249
Iodine	—	p. 398	p. 357	—	—
Toxic gases	—	p. 523	p. 456	—	p. 247
Zootoxins	—	p. 533	p. 463	p. 411	—
Mycotoxins					
Aflatoxins	16	p. 401	p. 363	—	p. 254
Citrinin	—	p. 403	p. 367	p. 337	—
Ergot	7	p. 404	p. 367	p. 334	p. 261
Fescue toxicosis	—	—	p. 389	—	p. 263
Fumonisins	35	—	—	—	p. 258
Ochratoxin	—	p. 407	p. 369	p. 336	—
Rubratoxin	—	p. 408	p. 370	—	—
Slaframine	—	p. 411	p. 373	p. 338	—
Sporodesmins	—	p. 414	p. 375	—	—

(continued on next page)

Table 1 (*continued*)					
Toxin	**AFSS (No. of Cases)**	**CVT–FA-1**	**CVT–FA-2**	**CVT–FA-3**	**CVT–FA-4**
Stachbotrytoxicosis	—	p. 417	p. 379	p. 340	—
Tremorgenic mycotoxins	3	p. 415	p. 378	—	p. 260
Trichothecenes	67	p. 410	p. 372	p. 332	p. 256
Zearalenone	3	p. 419	p. 380	—	p. 257
Pesticides					
Fumigants	—	p. 491	—	—	—
Fungicides	—	p. 487	—	—	—
Insecticides	26	p. 475	p. 424	p. 380	—
Organic herbicides	—	p. 481	p. 429	p. 386	—
Rodenticides	—	p. 478	p. 426	p. 383	—
Plants					
Cyanogenic plants	—	p. 430	p. 390	p. 367	—
Nitrate accumulator plants	26	p. 433	p. 392	—	p. 278
Other toxic plants	8	p. 438–71	p. 396–420	p. 343–72	p. 264–78
Water					
Geothermal water	—	p. 424	p. 384	p. 377	—
Salt-poisoning water deprivation	1	p. 396	p. 356	p. 328	—
Water quality	—	p. 420	p. 381	p. 375	—

Data from Howard JL, Smith RA. Current Veterinary Therapy—Food Animal Practice (editions 1–4). Philadelphia: WB Saunders; 1981, 1986, 1993, 1999.

toxicity). Pharmacologic antidotes may neutralize or antagonize the effects of a toxicant. This type of antidote may act by preventing the formation of toxic metabolites (eg, 4-methylpyrazole for ethylene glycol toxicity), by competing with a toxicant's action at a receptor site (eg, naloxone for opioid toxicity), by facilitation of more rapid or complete elimination of a toxicant (eg, bicarbonate to alkalinize the urine for salicylate, phenobarbital, and 2,4-D poisoning or ammonium chloride or chlorethamine to acidify the urine for amphetamine, phencyclidine, and strychnine poisoning), by blocking receptors responsible for the toxic effect (eg, atropine for organophosphate toxicity), or by aiding in the restoration of normal detoxification mechanisms (eg, N-acetylcysteine for acetaminophen toxicity).[5] In addition, specific antidotes may act directly on the toxin (eg, antitoxins).

Animal Drugs that are Biologics

Some drugs used to treat toxicoses are licensed by the US Department of Agriculture (USDA) under the Virus-Serum-Toxin Act and not approved by the FDA under the FFDCA. The Virus-Serum-Toxin Act is implemented by the Center for Veterinary Biologics of the USDA Animal and Plant Health Inspection Service. Examples of such products include antivenins and antitoxins. Animal drugs produced and distributed in full conformance with the animal, virus, serum, and toxin law have a USDA code rather than an FDA-assigned New Animal Drug Application [NADA] or Abbreviated New Animal Drug Application [ANADA] number. Examples include botulinum antitoxin (USDA Code 6400), tetanus antitoxin (USDA Code 6302.00 & 6302.01), and Crotalidae antivenin (USDA Code 6101.00). Antivenoms for animals that are licensed as biologics by USDA are a unique form of legally marketed animal drugs.[a,b] More information about the USDA Center for Veterinary Biologics and a listing of licensed veterinary biologics are available at http://www.aphis.usda.gov/animal_health/vet_biologics/.

Drugs Approved to Treat Toxicoses

The limited availability of drugs approved to treat toxicoses is a long-standing problem in veterinary medicine. The drugs listed in **Table 2** are approved by the FDA for use in animals with toxicoses. Use of these drugs, as indicated on the label, does not give rise to the ELU issues (discussed later). Other than the 7 drugs listed in **Table 2**, any drug used to treat animal toxicoses is likely done so in an extralabel, or an unapproved, manner. Consequently, review of ELU regulations may be of value to practicing veterinarians.

ELU IN TREATING ANIMAL TOXICOSES

The Animal Medicinal Drug Use Clarification Act (AMDUCA) of 1994 (Pub. L. 103-396) allows veterinarians to legally administer or prescribe any drug approved for use in humans or animals in an extralabel manner ("Extralabel Drug Use in Animals; Final Rule," published in the Federal Register 1996;61[217]:57732–46).[16] AMDUCA and the regulations that implement it, however, require that such ELU conform with several conditions and comply with several limitations (described later). Because of the need to avoid potentially harmful tissue residues in food derived from food-producing animals, there are additional conditions and limitations that apply when food animals are treated with a drug in an extralabel manner.

ELU: Definition

ELU use is defined in 21 CFR § 530.3 as

> actual use or intended use of a drug in an animal in a manner that is not in accordance with the approved labeling. This includes, but is not limited to, use in species not listed in the labeling, use for indications (disease or other conditions) not listed in the labeling, use at dosage levels, frequencies, or routes of administration other than those stated in the labeling, and deviation from the labeled withdrawal time based on these different uses.

According to 21 CFR § 530.2, ELU is

> limited to treatment modalities when the health of an animal is threatened or suffering or death may result from failure to treat.

When considering an ELU of an approved drug, veterinarians are encouraged to keep in mind that ELU is permitted only for such therapeutic uses. In the authors' view, treating animals with a toxicosis is a case in which the health of the animals is threatened or suffering or death may result from a failure to treat the animal. Consequently, treatment of animals with a toxicosis often meets the purpose of the regulation implementing the ELU statute.

---

[a] 21 CFR § 510.4 Biologics; products subject to license control. An animal drug produced and distributed in full conformance with the animal, virus, serum, and toxin law of March 4, 1913 (37 Stat. 832; 21 U.S.C. 151 *et seq.*) and any regulations issued thereupon shall not be deemed to be subject to section 512 of FFDCA.

[b] Blood and blood products are unique animal drugs. Although animal blood and blood products, such as fresh or frozen plasma, whole blood, or blood cell products, are drugs under the FFDCA, the FDA is not currently regulating blood and blood products for animals.

Only veterinarians may authorize or prescribe ELU. Laypersons may administer an approved animal or human drug in an extralabel manner only under the supervision of a licensed veterinarian.

ELU: Responsibilities and Limitations

ELU privileges come with many responsibilities for the veterinary profession. These responsibilities include establishing a valid veterinarian-client-patient relationship (VCPR), establishing extended withdrawal times when the use is in food animals, providing labeling that meets the ELU requirements, and keeping records of the ELU. In addition, veterinarians need to know when ELU is not permitted and the responsibilities and limitations of using drugs compounded from approved products. Each of these responsibilities and limitations is discussed in turn.

Responsibilities

Valid VCPR Both the scope of the ELU regulation and the provisions permitting it require that ELU be within the context of a valid VCPR. Most practicing veterinarians are aware of what constitutes a valid VCPR under their state practice act or the American Veterinary Medical Association Principles of Veterinary Medical Ethics. These requirements may not align exactly with the requirements under the FFDCA. For purposes of ELU that is permitted under the FFDCA, a VCPR requires that a veterinarian has assumed responsibility for making medical judgments, the client has agreed to follow the veterinarian's instructions, the veterinarian has made a preliminary diagnosis, and the veterinarian is readily available for follow-up.[c]

Extended withdrawal times When an ELU is for a food animal, the prescribing veterinarian must establish a substantially extended withdrawal period before marketing of

[c] Provision permitting ELU of animal drugs. An approved new animal drug or human drug intended to be used for an extralabel purpose in an animal is not unsafe under section 512 of the act and is exempt from the labeling requirements of section 502(f) of the act if such use is (a) by or on the lawful written or oral order of a licensed veterinarian within the context of a valid VCPR and (b) in compliance with this part. 21 CFR § 530.10.
Scope: This part applies to the ELU in an animal of any approved new animal drug or approved new human drug by or on the lawful order of a licensed veterinarian within the context of a valid VCPR. 21 CFR § 530.1. Definition of a valid VCPR(i): a valid VCPR is one in which
(1) A veterinarian has assumed the responsibility for making medical judgments regarding the health of (an) animal(s) and the need for medical treatment, and the client (the owner of the animal or animals or other caretaker) has agreed to follow the instructions of the veterinarian;
(2) There is sufficient knowledge of the animal(s) by the veterinarian to initiate at least a general or preliminary diagnosis of the medical condition of the animal(s); and
(3) The practicing veterinarian is readily available for follow-up in case of adverse reactions or failure of the regimen of therapy. Such a relationship can exist only when the veterinarian has recently seen and is personally acquainted with the keeping and care of the animal(s) by virtue of examination of the animal(s), and/or by medically appropriate and timely visits to the premises where the animal(s) are kept. 21 CFR § 530.3(i).

Table 2
Drugs approved by the US FDA/CVM to treat animal toxicoses

Proprietary Name (Established Name)	Dose (Consult Labeling for Full Information)	Indication	CFR Citation and NADA or ANADA No.
Antisedan (atipamezole hydrochloride)	Inject intramuscularly the same volume as that of dexmedetomidine or medetomidine used	For reversal of the sedative and analgesic effects of dexmedetomidine hydrochloride or medetomidine hydrochloride in dogs	21 CFR § 522.147[a] NADA 141-033
Cuprate (cupric glycinate)	200 mg (1 mL) for calves 300 lb and under; 400 mg (2 mL) for calves over 300 lb and adult cattle. For subcutaneous use.	For beef calves and beef cattle for the prevention of copper deficiency or, when labeled for veterinary prescription use, for the prevention and/or treatment of copper deficiency alone or in association with molybdenum toxicity. **Note: slaughter withdrawal time = 30 days**	21 CFR § 522.518 NADA 031-971
Antizol-Vet (fomepizole)	20 mg Intravenously per kg initially, 15 mg intravenously per kg at 12 and 24 hours, and 5 mg intravenously per kg at 36 hours	As an antidote for ethylene glycol (antifreeze) poisoning in dogs that have ingested or are suspected of having ingested ethylene glycol	21 CFR § 522.1004 NADA 141-075, ANADA 200-472
Narcan injection (naloxone hydrochloride)	It is administered by intravenous, intramuscular, or subcutaneous injection at an initial dose of 0.04 mg per kg of body weight. When given intravenously, the dosage may be repeated at 2- to 3-minute intervals as necessary. Onset of action by intramuscular or subcutaneous injection is slightly longer than it is by intravenous injection, and repeated dosages must be administered accordingly	As a narcotic antagonist in dogs	21 CFR § 522.1462 NADA 035-825

Protopam (pralidoxime hydrochloride)	It is administered as soon as possible after exposure to the poison. Before administration of the sterile pralidoxime chloride, atropine is administered intravenously at a dosage rate of 0.05 mg per lb of body weight, followed by administration of an additional 0.15 mg of atropine per lb of body weight administered intramuscularly. Then the appropriate dosage of sterile pralidoxime chloride is administered slowly intravenously. **See labeling for further dosage information**	For use in horses, dogs, and cats as an antidote in the treatment of poisoning due to those pesticides and chemicals of the organophosphate class, which have anticholinesterase activity in horses, dogs, and cats	21 CFR § 522.1862 NADA 039-204
Tolazine (tolazoline hydrochloride)	100 mg per mL. Administer slowly by intravenous injection 4 mg per kg of body weight or 1.8 mg per lb	For use in horses when it is desirable to reverse the effects of sedation and analgesia caused by xylazine	21 CFR § 522.2474 NADA 140-994
Yobine Antagonil (yohimbine hydrochloride)	0.05 mg per lb (0.11 mg per kg) of body weight intravenously	To reverse the effects of xylazine in dogs	21 CFR § 522.2670 NADA 140-866, NADA 140-874

[a] 21 CFR § 522.147 = Title 21 of the Code of Federal Regulations, part 522, section 147.

milk, meat, eggs, or other edible products from the animal to be treated. The time should be supported by appropriate scientific information (**Table 3**).[d]

If there is no scientific information on the human food safety aspect of using the drug in food-producing animals, the veterinarian must take appropriate measures to assure that treated food animals and food derived from them do not enter the food supply.

Labeling ELU requires special labeling by the practitioner. Specifically, the veterinarian's name and address, established name of the ingredients, directions for use, cautionary statements, and withdrawal time for milk, eggs, or meat must be included on the label.[e] Adequate directions for use include the species, dosage, frequency, duration of treatment, and route of administration.

Records Veterinarians are required to keep records as a condition of ELU. These records are required to contain the established name of the ingredients, condition

---

[d] Food Animal Residue Avoidance Database (FARAD): veterinarians may be able to obtain information regarding withdrawal times by consulting the FARAD. The veterinarians and staff of FARAD are available to assist veterinarians in determining appropriate withdrawal times for drugs used as antidotes in food animals. FARAD has published withdrawal times for some commonly known drugs that are used extralabelly as antidotes for food animals. For most of these antidotes, limited information is actually available concerning tissue residues, so withdrawal recommendations are normally made for many antidotes based on pharmacokinetic principles. Complex interactions may occur between the toxicant and antidotal agent also affecting the withdrawal time. For these reasons, practitioners are advised to contact FARAD for specific advice on a case-by-case basis, for specific withdrawal recommendations. FARAD may be contacted at 888-873-2723 or at the FARAD Web site: www.farad.org.

[e] Any human or animal drug prescribed and dispensed for ELU by a veterinarian or dispensed by a pharmacist on the order of a veterinarian shall bear or be accompanied by labeling information adequate to assure the safe and proper use of the product. Such information shall include the following:

(a) The name and address of the prescribing veterinarian. If the drug is dispensed by a pharmacy on the order of a veterinarian, the labeling shall include the name of the prescribing veterinarian and the name and address of the dispensing pharmacy and may include the address of the prescribing veterinarian;

(b) The established name of the drug or, if formulated from more than one active ingredient, the established name of each ingredient;

(c) Any directions for use specified by the veterinarian, including the class/species or identification of the animal or herd, flock, pen, lot, or other group of animals being treated, in which the drug is intended to be used; the dosage, frequency, and route of administration; and the duration of therapy;

(d) Any cautionary statements; and

(e) The veterinarian's specified withdrawal, withholding, or discard time for meat, milk, eggs, or any other food, which might be derived from the treated animal or animals. 21 CFR § 530.12.

Table 3
Withdrawal times published by the Food Animal Residue Avoidance Database

		Withdrawal Times	
Antidote	**Toxicity**	**Milk**	**Meat**
Atropine sulfate	Organophosphate toxicosis	3 Days (at 0.1 mg/kg dose) 6 Days (at 0.2 mg/kg dose)	14 Days (at 0.1 mg/kg dose) 28 Days (at 0.2 mg/kg dose)
Epinephrine	Anaphylaxis	0 Days	0 Days
Vitamin K_1	Anticoagulant rodenticides, sweet-clover toxicosis	0 Day	0 Day
Pralidoxime hydrochloride (2-PAM)	Organophosphate toxicosis	6 Days	28 Days
Dimercaprol	Arsenic, lead, and mercury toxicoses	5 Days	5 Days
Copper glycinate	Molybdenum toxicosis	Not for use in dairy cattle	30 Days
Calcium disodium EDTA	Lead toxicosis	2 Days	2 Days
Activated charcoal	Adsorbent	0 Days	0 Days
D-Penicillamine	Lead and mercury toxicoses	3-Day minimum	21-Day minimum
Sodium nitrite, sodium thiosulfate, sodium sulfate	Cyanide toxicosis	2 Days (48 h)	1 Day (12 h)

Data from Haskell SR, Payne M, Webb A, et al. FARAD Digest: antidotes in food animal practice. J Am Vet Med Assoc 2005;226(6):884–7.

treated, species, dosage, duration, number of animals treated, and the withdrawal time provided. These records are to be kept for a minimum of 2 years or longer if required by state law or another federal law. The FDA is to be provided access to these records on request.[f]

[f] (a) As a condition of ELU permitted under this part, to permit FDA to ascertain any ELU or intended ELU of drugs that the agency has determined may present a risk to the public health, veterinarians shall maintain the following records of ELU. Such records shall be legible, documented in an accurate and timely manner, and be readily accessible to permit prompt retrieval of information. Such records shall be adequate to substantiate the identification of the animals and shall be maintained either as individual records or, in food animal practices, on a group, herd, flock, or per-client basis. Records shall be adequate to provide the following information:
(1) The established name of the drug and its active ingredient, or if formulated from more than one ingredient, the established name of each ingredient;
(2) The condition treated;
(3) The species of the treated animal(s);
(4) The dosage administered;
(5) The duration of treatment;
(6) The numbers of animals treated; and
(7) The specified withdrawal, withholding, or discard time(s), if applicable, for meat, milk, eggs, or any food, which might be derived from any food animals treated. (b) A veterinarian shall keep all required records for 2 years or as otherwise required by federal or state law, whichever is greater. (c) Any person who is in charge, control, or custody of such records shall, upon request of a person designated by FDA, permit such person designated by FDA to, at all reasonable times, have access to, permit copying, and verify such records. 21 CFR § 530.5.

Limitations and prohibitions

Approved drugs ELU is permitted only if there is no approved new animal drug that is labeled for such use and that contains the same active ingredient in the required dosage form and concentration except where a veterinarian finds, within the context of a valid VCPR, that the approved new animal drug is clinically ineffective for its intended use.[g,h] Few approved animal drugs meet this requirement for food animals. Only Cuprate (cupric glycinate) is approved for treatment of molybdenum toxicosis. Dextrose, furosemide, gelatin solution, and neostigmine are approved for use in food animals although not approved to treat toxicoses (**Table 4**).

Specific drugs Some approved drugs may not be used in food-producing animals in an extralabel manner. Drugs for which ELU is not permitted in food-producing animals are published in 21 CFR § 530.41 (a) (see http://www.access.gpo.gov/nara/cfr/waisidx_10/21cfr530_10.html). These drugs include chloramphenicol, clenbuterol, diethylstilbestrol, dimetridazole, ipronidazole, other nitroimidazoles, furazolidone, nitrofurazone, sulfonamide drugs in lactating dairy cattle (except approved use of sulfadimethoxine, sulfabromomethazine, and sulfaethoxypyridazine), fluoroquinolones, glycopeptides, and phenylbutazone in female dairy cattle 20 months of age or older. Many of these prohibited drugs are antibiotics; however, phenylbutazone should not be used in female dairy cattle 20 months of age or older, even in a toxicosis case

[g] In addition to uses which do not comply with the provision set forth in Sec. 530.10, the following specific ELUs are not permitted and result in the drug being deemed unsafe within the meaning of section 512 of the act:
(a) ELU in an animal of an approved new animal drug or human drug by a lay person (except when under the supervision of a licensed veterinarian);
(b) ELU of an approved new animal drug or human drug in or on an animal feed;
(c) ELU resulting in any residue which may present a risk to the public health; and
(d) ELU resulting in any residue above an established safe level, safe concentration or tolerance. 21 CFR 530.11.

[h] Conditions for permitted extralabel animal and human drug use in food-producing animals:
(a) The following conditions must be met for a permitted ELU in food-producing animals of approved new animal and human drugs:
  (1) Prior to prescribing or dispensing an approved new animal or human drug for an ELU in food animals, the veterinarian must
    (i) Make a careful diagnosis and evaluation of the conditions for which the drug is to be used;
    (ii) Establish a substantially extended withdrawal period prior to marketing of meat, milk, eggs, or other edible products supported by appropriate scientific information, if applicable;
    (iii) Institute procedures to assure that the identity of the treated animal or animals is carefully maintained; and
    (iv) Take appropriate measures to assure that assigned timeframes for withdrawal are met and no illegal drug residues occur in any food-producing animal subjected to extralabel treatment.
(b) The following additional conditions must be met for a permitted ELU of in food-producing animals an approved human drug, or of an animal drug approved only for use in animals not intended for human consumption:
  (1) Such use must be accomplished in accordance with an appropriate medical rationale; and
  (2) If scientific information on the human food safety aspect of the use of the drug in food-producing animals is not available, the veterinarian must take appropriate measures to assure that the animal and its food products do not enter the human food supply.
(c) ELU of an approved human drug in a food-producing animal is not permitted under this part if an animal drug approved for use in food-producing animals can be used in an extralabel manner for the particular use. 21 CFR § 530.20 (a)(2) (b) and (c).

(see 21 CFR § 530.41 [a][12]). Adamantanes and neuraminidase inhibitors are approved for treating or preventing influenza A but are prohibited from ELU in chickens, turkeys, and ducks (see 21 CFR § 530.41 [d]).

Animal feed ELU is not permitted in animal feed. This prohibition of using drugs in an extralabel manner in animal feed is worth remembering in cases of copper toxicosis and perhaps other toxicoses of food animals.

Residues ELU should not result in a residue that may present a risk to public health or that exceeds established safe levels or tolerances. Tolerances for residues of approximately 109 new animal drugs are published by the FDA in 21 CFR § 556 (see http://www.access.gpo.gov/nara/cfr/waisidx_10/21cfr556_10.html for a list of drug tolerances) and tolerances of residues for approximately 381 pesticides are published by the EPA in 40 CFR § 180 (http://www.access.gpo.gov/nara/cfr/waisidx_09/40cfr180_09.html). When treating a toxicosis in food animals, a practitioner should consider both residues of the drugs used therapeutically and residues of the toxin being treated.

Compounding

Compounding of drugs from approved, finished animal, or human drugs is permitted as an ELU of approved drugs. Such compounding is permitted only when the available dosage form or concentration of the approved animal or human drug does not treat the condition diagnosed (see **Table 4** and **Table 5**). Compounding of drugs from bulk chemicals is not permitted under the ELU regulations (discussed later).[i]

Approved animal or human drugs that are commonly recommended to treat animal toxicoses but are not approved to treat a toxicosis Drugs that are commonly recommended to treat animal toxicoses and that are approved for use in animals or humans, but are not approved to treat a toxicosis per se, are listed, respectively, in **Tables 4** and **5**.

---

[i] Definition: animal drug compounding is defined as a process by which a person combines, mixes, or alters ingredients to create a new animal drug that is not the subject of an application that has been approved under §512 of the FFDCA. Requirements: (a) This part applies to compounding of a product from approved animal or human drugs by a veterinarian or a pharmacist on the order of a veterinarian within the practice of veterinary medicine. Nothing in this part shall be construed as permitting compounding from bulk drugs. (b) ELU from compounding of approved new animal or human drugs is permitted if

(1) All relevant portions of this part have been complied with;
(2) There is no approved new animal or approved new human drug that, when used as labeled or in conformity with criteria established in this part, will, in the available dosage form and concentration, appropriately treat the condition diagnosed. Compounding from a human drug for use in food-producing animals will not be permitted if an approved animal drug can be used for the compounding;
(3) The compounding is performed by a licensed pharmacist or veterinarian within the scope of a professional practice;
(4) Adequate procedures and processes are followed that ensure the safety and effectiveness of the compounded product;
(5) The scale of the compounding operation is commensurate with the established need for compounded products (eg, similar to that of comparable practices); and
(6) All relevant state laws relating to the compounding of drugs for use in animals are followed. (c) Guidance on the subject of compounding may be found in guidance documents issued by FDA. 21 CFR § 530.13.

Table 4
Extralabel drug use—drugs approved for use in animals but not approved to treat a toxicosis per se

Established Name	Indication	CFR Citation and NADA or ANADA No.	Examples of Toxicoses	References
Acepromazine maleate	Used as a tranquilizer in dogs, cats, and horses	21 CFR § 522.23 NADA 015-030; ANADA 200-319; ANADA 200-361	Sympathomimetics (eg, pseudoephedrine, phenylpropanolamine) Ammoniated feed syndrome (imidazoles)	7,9
	Used as a tranquilizer in dogs and cats	21 CFR § 520.23 NADA 032-702		
	Used in dogs as an aid in tranquilization and as a preanesthetic agent in dogs	21 CFR § 522.23 NADA 117-531; NADA 117-532		
Dextrose	Dextrose/glycine/electrolyte is indicated for use in the control of dehydration associated with diarrhea (scours) in calves. It is used as an early treatment at the first signs of scouring. It may also be used as follow-up treatment after intravenous fluid therapy. Cattle and calves. **Note: withdrawal times not reported in the CFR**	21 CFR § 520.550 NADA 125-961	—	—
Furosemide	Used for the treatment of edema (pulmonary congestion and ascites) associated with cardiac insufficiency and acute noninflammatory tissue edema in dogs, cats, and horses	21 CFR § 522.1010 NADA 034-478; ANADA 200-293	Toxins causing pulmonary edema (eg, Japanese yew) Cholecalciferol	9 7,9
	For treatment of edema (pulmonary congestion and ascites) associated with cardiac insufficiency and acute noninflammatory tissue edema in dogs and cats	21 CFR§ 520.1010 NADA 034-621; NADA 129-034		
	For treatment of edema (pulmonary congestion and ascites) associated with cardiac insufficiency and acute noninflammatory tissue edema in dogs	21 CFR § 520.1010 NADA 102-380; ANADA 200-373; ANADA 200-382		
	Used for treatment of acute noninflammatory tissue edema in horses	21 CFR § 520.1010 NADA 118-550; NADA 127-034		
	Used for the treatment of physiologic parturient edema of the mammary gland and associated structures in cattle. **Note: 48 hours for milk and slaughter withdrawal**	21 CFR § 520.1010 NADA 045-188		

Gelatin solution	Used to restore circulatory volume and maintain blood pressure in animals being treated for shock. Horse, small animals, cattle, sheep. **Note: withdrawal times not reported in the CFR**	21 CFR § 522.1020 NADA 006-281	—	—
Methocarbamol	As an adjunct for treating acute inflammatory and traumatic conditions of the skeletal muscles and to reduce muscular spasms in dogs, cats, and horses	21 CFR § 522.1380 NADA 038-838	Strychnine, metaldehyde, pyrethrins (cats), some mycotoxins	7,9,17
	As an adjunct to therapy for acute inflammatory and traumatic conditions of the skeletal muscles to reduce muscular spasms in dogs and cats	21 CFR § 520.1380 NADA 045-715		
Neostigmine	The drug is intended for use for treating rumen atony; initiating peristalsis, which causes evacuation of the bowel; emptying the urinary bladder; and stimulating skeletal muscle contractions. It is a curare antagonist in horses. Sheep, cattle, swine, horses. **Note: not for use in animals producing milk**	21 CFR § 522.1503 NADA 008-097	Larkspur, neuromuscular blockers (curare and others), ivermectin (cats)	7,17
Pentobarbital	The drug is indicated for use as a general anesthetic in dogs and cats. Although it may be used as a general surgical anesthetic for horses, it is usually given at a lower dose to cause sedation and hypnosis and may be supplemented with a local anesthetic. It may also be used in dogs for the symptomatic treatment of strychnine poisoning	21 CFR § 522.1704 NADA 004-536; NADA 045-737	Strychnine, chlorinated hydrocarbons	17
	Used as an anesthetic for intravenous administration to dogs during short to moderately long surgical procedures in dogs and cats	21 CFR § 522.2444b NADA 010-346		
	For humane, painless, and rapid euthanasia	21 CFR § 522.900 NADA 119-807; ANADA 200-071: ANADA 200-280		
	General anesthesia and as a sedative-relaxant in horses and cattle	21 CFR § 522.380 NADA 046-789	—	—

(*continued on next page*)

Table 4
(continued)

Established Name	Indication	CFR Citation and NADA or ANADA No.	Examples of Toxicoses	References
Prednisone	Used for conditions requiring an anti-inflammatory agent in dogs, cats, and horses	21 CFR 522.1890	Cholecalciferol	7,17
	Used for conditions requiring an anti-inflammatory agent in dogs, cats, and horses	21 CFR § 522.1881 NADA 010-312		
	Used for conditions requiring an anti-inflammatory agent in dogs, cats, and horses	21 CFR § 522.1885 NADA 011-080		
Prednisolone	Inflammatory, allergic, or other stress conditions in horses, dogs, or cats	21 CFR § 522.1884 NADA 011-593		
Methylprednisolone	For use as an anti-inflammatory agent in dogs and cats	21 CFR § 520.1408 NADA 011-403		
	Treatment of inflammation and related disorders in dogs; treatment of allergic and dermatologic disorders in dogs; and as supportive therapy to antibacterial treatment of severe infections in dogs	21 CFR § 522.1410 NADA 012-204		
Xylazine	Dogs: to produce sedation, as an analgesic, and as a preanesthetic to local or general anesthesia Cats: the drug is used in cats to produce sedation, as an analgesic, and a preanesthetic to local anesthesia. It may also be used in cats as a preanesthetic to general anesthesia.	21 CFR § 522.2662	As an emetic in cats	9,17

To produce sedation, as an analgesic, and as a preanesthetic to local or general anesthesia in dogs and cats	21 CFR § 522.266 NADA 047-955; ANADA 200-184
To produce sedation, as an analgesic, and as a preanesthetic to local or general anesthesia in dogs, cats, and horses Fallow deer (*Dama dama*), mule deer (*Odocoileus hemionus*), sika deer (*Cervus nippon*), white-tailed deer (*Odocoileus virginianus*), and elk (*Cervus canadensis*)— indications: to produce sedation, as an analgesic, and as a preanesthetic to local anesthesia. To produce sedation, accompanied by a shorter period of analgesia. May be used to calm and facilitate handling of fractious animals for diagnostic procedures, for minor surgical procedures, for therapeutic medication, for sedation and relief of pain following injury or surgery, and as a pre–anesthetic to local anesthetic. At the recommended dosages, can be used in conjunction with local anesthetics, such as procaine or lidocaine	21 CFR § 522.2662 NADA 047-956; NADA 139-236; ANADA 200-088; ANADA 200-139;
To produce sedation, as an analgesic, and as a pre-anesthetic to local or general anesthesia	NADA 140-442

Withdrawal times are based on use at the label dosage. Longer withdrawal times may be required if higher or longer dosages are used.

Table 5
Extralabel drug use: established names of drugs approved for use in humans but not in animals

Active Ingredient	Dosage Form/Route	Concentration	Potential Use in Animals with Toxicosis	Examples of Toxicoses
Acetic acid, glacial	Solution, drops/otic	2%	Acidify	Ammonia and other alkylinating agents
Acetic acid, glacial	Solution/irrigation, urethral	250 mg/100 mL (0.25%)	Acidify	Ammonia and other alkylinating agents
Aminophylline	Enema/rectal	300 mg/5 mL[a]	Bronchodilator	Fog fever
Aminophylline	Injectable/injection	25 mg/mL	Bronchodilator	Fog fever
Aminophylline	Solution/oral	105 mg/5 mL[a]	Bronchodilator	Fog fever
Aminophylline	Suppository/rectal	250[a] mg and 500[a] mg/suppository	Bronchodilator	Fog fever
Aminophylline	Tablet, delayed release/oral	100[a] and 200[a] mg/tablet	Bronchodilator	Fog fever
Aminophylline	Tablet, extended release/oral	225 mg/tablet[a]	Bronchodilator	Fog fever
Aminophylline	Tablet/oral	100 and 200 mg/tablet	Bronchodilator	Fog fever
Aminophylline in sodium chloride 0.45%	Injectable/injection	100[a] mg and 200[a] mg and 400[a] mg and 500[a] mg/100 mL	Bronchodilator	Fog fever
Ammonium chloride	Injectable/injection	900 mg/100 mL (0.9%)[a]; 40 mEq/100 mL (2.14% or 21.4 mg/mL)[a]; 3 mEq/mL (160.5 mg/mL)[a]; and 5 mEq/mL (267.5 mg/mL)	Urine acidification	—
Apomorphine hydrochloride	Injectable/SC	20 mg/2 mL[a] and 30 mg/3 mL (note: both products 10 mg/mL)	Emetic	Many

Atropine	Injectable/injection	Eq to 0.5-mg sulfate/0.7 mL (0.71 mg/mL); Eq to 0.25-mg sulfate/0.3 mL (0.83 mg/mL); Eq to 1-mg sulfate/0.7 mL (1.43 mg/mL); Eq to 2-mg sulfate/0.7 mL (2.86 mg/mL)	Anticholinergic	Cholinesterase inhibitors, pyrethroids
Atropine and pralidoxime chloride	Injectable/IM	2.1-mg atropine/0.7-mL and 600-mg pralidoxime chloride/2 mL	Reactivation of cholinesterase activity	Cholinesterase inhibitors
Atropine sulfate	Aerosol, metered/inhalation	Eq to 0.36-mg base/inh[a]	Anticholinergic	Cholinesterase inhibitiors, pyrethroids
Atropine sulfate	Injectable/IM-IV-SC	0.05 mg and 0.1 mg/mL	Anticholinergic	Cholinesterase inhibitiors, pyrethroids
Calcitonin human	Injectable/injection	0.5 mg/vial[a]	Hypercalcemia	Hypervitaminosis D
Calcitonin salmon	Injectable/injection	400 IU/vial,[a] 100 IU/mL,[a] and 200 IU/mL	Hypercalcemia	Hypervitaminosis D
Calcitonin salmon	Metered spray/nasal	200 IU/spray	Hypercalcemia	Hypervitaminosis D
Calcitonin salmon recombinant	Metered spray/nasal	200 IU/spray	Hypercalcemia	Hypervitaminosis D
Calcium chloride	Injectable/injection	100 mg/mL	Hypocalcemia	Oxalis
Cholestyramine	Powder/oral	Eq to 4-g resin/packet and equivalent to 4-g resin/scoopful	Hypercholesterolemia	—
Cholestyramine	Chewable bar/oral	Equivalent to 4-g resin/bar[a]	Hypercholesterolemia	—
Cholestyramine	Tablet/oral	Equivalent to 1-g resin/tablet[a] and Eq to 800-mg resin/tablet[a]	Hypercholesterolemia	—

(*continued on next page*)

Table 5
(continued)

Active Ingredient	Dosage Form/Route	Concentration	Potential Use in Animals with Toxicosis	Examples of Toxicoses
Cimetidine	Tablet/oral	100 mg,[a] 200 mg, 300 mg, 400 mg, and 800 mg/tablet	Gastric protectant	NSAID/vitamin D
Cimetidine	Suspension/oral	200 mg/20 mL[a]	Gastric protectant	NSAID/vitamin D
Cimetidine HCl	Solution/oral	Eq to 300-mg base/5 mL	Gastric protectant	NSAID/vitamin D
Cimetidine HCl	Injectable/injection	Eq to 90-mg base/100 mL[a]; Eq to 120-mg base/100 mL[a]; Eq to 180-mg base/100 mL[a]; Eq to 240-mg base/100 mL[a]; Eq to 360-mg base/100 mL[a]; Eq to 480-mg base/100 mL[a]; Eq to 6-mg base/mL; and Eq to 300-mg base/2 mL (150 mg/mL)	Gastric protectant	NSAID/vitamin D
Cyanocobalamin	Gel, metered/nasal	0.5[a] mg/inh	Vitamin B_{12}	Cyanide
Cyanocobalamin	Injectable/injection	0.03[a] mg/mL and 0.05[a] mg/mL and 0.1[a] mg/mL and 0.12[a] mg/mL and 1 mg/mL	Vitamin B_{12}	Cyanide
Cyanocobalamin	Spray, metered/nasal	25[a] g/spray and 0.5 mg (500 g)/spray	Vitamin B_{12}	Cyanide
Cyanocobalamin	Tablet/oral	1[a] mg/tablet	Vitamin B_{12}	Cyanide
Cyproheptadine HCl	Tablet/oral	4 mg/tablet	Antihistamine	Serotonin syndrome
Cyproheptadine HCl	Syrup/oral	2 mg/5 mL	Antihistamine	Serotonin syndrome
Dantrolene sodium	Capsule/oral	25 mg, 50 mg, and 100 mg/capsule	Muscle relaxant	Black widow spider
Dantrolene sodium	Injectable/injection	20 mg/vial	Muscle relaxant	Black widow spider

Dapsone	Gel/topical	5%	Antimycobacterial	Brown recluse spider
Dapsone	Tablet/oral	25 mg and 100 mg/tablet	Antimycobacterial	Brown recluse spider
Deferoxamine mesylate	Injectable/injection	500 mg/vial and 2 g/vial	Chelate divalent cations	Iron, aluminum
Digoxin	Capsule/oral	0.05[a] mg/capsule, 0.1 mg/capsule, 0.15[a] mg/capsule, and 0.20 mg/capsule	Cardiac glycoside	—
Digoxin	Injectable/injection	0.1 mg/mL and 0.25 mg/mL	Cardiac glycoside	—
Digoxin	Tablet/oral	0.0625[a] mg/tablet, 0.125 mg/tablet, 0.1875[a] mg/tablet, 0.25 mg/tablet, 0.375[a] mg/tablet, and 0.5[a] mg/tablet	Cardiac glycoside	—
Dimercaprol	Injectable/injection	10% (100 mg/mL)	Sulfhydryl group binding	Arsenic, mercury
Diphenhydramine HCl	Syrup/oral	12.5 mg/5 mL[a]	Muscle fasciculations	Nicotine
Diphenhydramine HCl	Elixir/oral	12.5 mg/5 mL	Muscle fasciculations	Nicotine
Diphenhydramine HCl	Capsule/oral	25 mg[a] and 50 mg/capsule	Muscle fasciculations	Nicotine
Diphenhydramine HCl	Injectable/injection	10 mg/mL and 50 mg/mL	Muscle fasciculations	Nicotine
D-Penicillamine	Capsule/oral	125 mg[a] and 250 mg/capsule	Chelate divalent cations	Lead
Edrophonium chloride	Injectable/injection	10 mg/mL	Anticholinesterase	Reversal of nondepolarizing agents (eg, tubocurarine)
Epinephrine	Aerosol, metered/inhalation	0.25[a] mg/inh	Anaphylaxis	—
Epinephrine	Injectable/IM-SC	0.15 mg and 0.3 mg/delivery	Anaphylaxis	—
Epinephrine	Injectable/injection	1.5[a] mg/amp and 5[a] mg/mL	Anaphylaxis	—
Epinephrine	Injectable/intramuscular	0.15[a] mg and 0.3[a] mg/delivery	Anaphylaxis	—

(continued on next page)

Table 5
(continued)

Active Ingredient	Dosage Form/Route	Concentration	Potential Use in Animals with Toxicosis	Examples of Toxicoses
Epinephrine bitartrate	Aerosol, metered/inhalation	0.3[a] mg/inh	Anaphylaxis	—
Etidronate disodium	Injectable/injection	50 mg/mL[a]	Hypercalcemia	—
Etidronate disodium	Tablet/oral	200-mg and 400-mg/tablet	Hypercalcemia	—
Ferric hexacyanoferrate (II) (Prussian Blue)	Capsule/oral	500 mg/capsule	—	Toxic effects of cesium or thallium
Flumazenil	Injectable/injection	0.5 mg/5 mL and 1 mg/10 mL (both 0.1 mg/mL)	—	Benzodiazepene antagonist
Folic acid	Injectable/injection	5 mg/mL	Folic acid deficiency	—
Folic acid	Tablet/oral	1 mg/tablet	Folic acid deficiency	—
Glucagon HCl	Injectable/injection	Eq to 1-mg[a] and 10-mg[a] base/vial	Hypoglycemia	—
Glucagon HCl recombinant	Injectable/injection	Eq to 1-mg base/vial	Hypoglycemia	—
Glucagon recombinant	Injectable/injection	1 mg/vial	Hypoglycemia	—
Hydroxocobalamin	Injectable/injection	2.5 g/vial and 2.5 g/vial (5 g kit) and 1 mg/mL	Vitamin B_{12} precursor	Cyanide
Lactated Ringer solution	Injectable/injection AND solution/irrigation	Calcium chloride—20 mg/100 mL; potassium chloride—30 mg/100 mL; sodium chloride—600 mg/100 mL; sodium lactate—310 mg/100 mL	Dehydration, diuresis	Many

Leucovorin calcium	Injectable/injection	Eq to 3[a]-mg base/mL and 5[a]-mg base/mL and 50-mg base/vial and 100-mg base/vial and 350-mg base/vial	Reduced form of folic acid	Folic acid antagonist toxicity (eg, methotrexate, trimethoprim)
Leucovorin calcium	(For) solution/oral	Eq to 60[a]-mg base/vial	Reduced form of folic acid	Folic acid antagonist toxicity (eg, methotrexate, trimethoprim
Leucovorin calcium	Tablet/oral	Eq to 5-mg base/tablet and 10-mg base/tablet and 15-mg base/tablet and 25-mg base/tablet	Reduced form of folic acid	Folic acid antagonist toxicity (eg, methotrexate, trimethoprim)
Levoleucovorin calcium	Powder/IV (infusion)	Eq to 50-mg base/vial	Reduced form of folic acid	Folic acid antagonist toxicity (eg, methotrexate, trimethoprim)
Magnesium sulfate	Injectable/injection	4 g/100 mL (40 mg/mL), 4 g/50 mL (80 mg/mL), 2 g/50 mL (40 mg/mL), and 500 mg/mL	Hypomagnesemia	Oxalate toxicity, grass tetany
Magnesium sulfate in dextrose 5%	Injectable/injection	1 g/100 mL (10 mg/mL), and 2 g/100 mL (20 mg/mL)	Hypomagnesemia	Oxalate toxicity;, grass tetany
Mannitol	Injectable/injection	5 g/100 mL (50 g/mL or 5%; 10 g/100 mL (100 mg/mL or 10%), 15 g/100 mL (150 mg/mL or 15%), 20 g/100 mL (200 mg/mL or 20%), 12.5 g/50 mL (250 mg/mL or 25%)	Osmotic diuretic	—
Mannitol	Solution/irrigation	5 g/100 mL (50 g/mL or 5%)	Osmotic diuretic	—
Misoprostol	Tablet/oral	0.1 mg and 0.2 mg/tablet	Prostaglandin deficiency	NSAID

(*continued on next page*)

Table 5
(continued)

Active Ingredient	Dosage Form/Route	Concentration	Potential Use in Animals with Toxicosis	Examples of Toxicoses
N-Acetylcysteine	Injectable/IV	6 g/30 mL (200 mg/mL)	Donate sulfhydryl groups, maintain cellular glutathione, reduced organ damage	Acetaminophen, other toxins that deplete glutathione
N-Acetylcysteine	Solution/inhalation, oral	10% and 20%	Donate sulfhydryl groups, maintain cellular glutathione, reduced organ damage	Acetaminophen, other toxins that deplete glutathione
Norepinephrine Bitartrate	Injectable/injection	Eq to 1-mg base/mL	Cardiac arrest, septic shock	—
Pamidronate disodium	Injectable/injection	30 mg/10 mL (3 mg/mL), 60 mg/mL (6 mg/mL), 90 mg/10 mL (9 mg/mL), 30 mg/vial, 60 mg/vial, and 90 mg/vial	—	Hypercalcemia—especially associated with hypervitaminosis D
Phentolamine mesylate	Injectable/injection	0.4 mg/1.7 mL and 5 mg/vial	Hypertensive episodes	—
Phytonadione (vitamin K_1)	Injectable/injection	1 mg/0.5 mL (2 mg/mL) and 10 mg/mL	Hypovitaminosis K	Anticoagulant rodenticides
Phytonadione (vitamin K_1)	Tablet/oral	5 mg/tablet	Hypovitaminosis K	Anticoagulant rodenticides
Pilocarpine	Insert, extended release/ophthalmic	5 mg[a] and 11 mg[a]/insert	Parasympathomimetic	—
Pilocarpine HCl	Gel/ophthalmic	4%	Parasympathomimetic	—
Pilocarpine HCl	Solution/ophthalmic	1%, 2%, and 4%	Parasympathomimetic	—
Pilocarpine HCl	Tablet/oral	5 mg and 7.5 mg/tablet	Parasympathomimetic	*Datura spp*

Pralidoxime chloride	Injectable/injection	300 mg/mL and 1 g/vial	Reactivate Acetylcholinesterase enzyme	Organophosphates
Pralidoxime chloride	Tablet/oral	500[a] mg/tablet	Reactivate Acetylcholinesterase enzyme	Organophosphates
Protamine sulfate	Injectable/injection	10 mg/mL; and 50 mg[a] and 250[a] mg/vial	Complexes with heparin	Heparin overdose, bracken fern
Pyridostigmine bromide	Injectable/injection	5 mg/mL	Anticholinesterase agent	Myasthenia gravis, curariform drug toxicity
Pyridostigmine bromide	Syrup/oral	60 mg/5 mL (12 mg/mL)	Anticholinesterase agent	Myasthenia gravis, curariform drug toxicity
Pyridostigmine bromide	Tablet, extended release/oral	180 mg/tablet	Anticholinesterase agent	Myasthenia gravis, curariform drug toxicity
Pyridostigmine bromide	Tablet/oral	30[a] and 60 mg/tablet	Anticholinesterase agent	Myasthenia gravis, curariform drug toxicity
Pyridoxine HCl	Injectable/injection	50[a] and 100 mg/mL	Vitamin B_6	Isoniazid, crimidine, doxorubicin
Ranitidine	Solution/oral	15 mg/mL[b]	Reduce gastric acid secretion	NSAID, vitamin D
Ranitidine	Syrup/oral	15 mg/mL[b]	Reduce gastric acid secretion	NSAID, vitamin D
Ranitidine bismuth citrate	Tablet/oral	400 mg/tablet[a]	Reduce gastric acid secretion	NSAID, vitamin D
Ranitidine HCl	Capsule/oral	Eq to 150-mg and 300-mg base/capsule	Reduce gastric acid secretion	NSAID, vitamin D
Ranitidine HCl	Granule, effervescent/oral	Eq to 150-mg base/packet[a]	Reduce gastric acid secretion	NSAID, vitamin D
Ranitidine HCl	Injectable/injection	Eq to 1-mg and 25-mg base/mL; Eq to 50-mg base/100 mL[a] (0.5 mg/mL)	Reduce gastric acid secretion	NSAID, vitamin D
Ranitidine HCl	Syrup/oral	Eq to 15-mg base/mL	Reduce gastric acid secretion	NSAID, vitamin D

(*continued on next page*)

Table 5
(continued)

Active Ingredient	Dosage Form/Route	Concentration	Potential Use in Animals with Toxicosis	Examples of Toxicoses
Ranitidine HCl	Tablet/oral	Eq to 150-mg base/mL and 300-mg base/mL	Reduce gastric acid secretion	NSAID, vitamin D
Ranitidine HCl	Tablet, effervescent/oral	Eq to 25-mg, 75-mg,[a] and 150-mg[a] base/tablet	Reduce gastric acid secretion	NSAID, vitamin D
Salt (sodium chloride)	Injectable/injection	450 mg/100 mL (4.5 mg/mL), 45 mg/50 mL and 112.5 mg/125 mL and 900 mg/100 mL and 9 mg/mL (all equal to 9 mg/mL), 3 g/100 mL (30 mg/mL), 5 g/100 mL (50 mg/mL), 2.5 mEq/mL (146.1 mg/ml), 20 g[a] /100 mL (200 mg/mL), and 234[a] mg/mL	Hyponatremia	Water deprivation–sodium ion intoxication
Salt (sodium chloride)	Solution/irrigation	450 m/100 mL (4.5 mg/mL); 900 mg/100 mL (9 mg/mL)	Hyponatremia	Water deprivation-sodium ion intoxication
Sodium bicarbonate	Injectable/injection	0.9 and 1 mEq/mL	Alkalinize blood	Acidosis
Sodium polystyrene sulfonate	Powder/oral, rectal	453.6 g and 454 g/bottle	Hyperkalemia	—

Sodium polystyrene sulfonate	Suspension/oral, rectal	15 g/60 mL (250 mg/mL)	Hyperkalemia	—
Sodium thiosulfate	Injectable/injection	250 mg/mL[a] (note: 7 drugs already marketed but without an approved NDA)	Sulfur donor	Cyanide, arsenic
Succimer (*meso*-dimercaptosuccinic acid)	Capsule/oral	100 mg/capsule	Chelate divalent cations	Lead, other metals
Sucralfate	Suspension/oral	1 g/10 mL (100 mg/mL)	Reduce gastric acid secretion	NSAID, vitamin D
Sucralfate	Tablet/oral	1 g/tablet	Reduce gastric acid secretion	NSAID, vitamin D
Thiamine HCl	Injectable/injection	100 and 200 mg/mL	Thiamine deficiency	Bracken fern
Trientine hydrochloride	Capsule/oral	250 mg/capsule	Chelating agent	Copper chelation

Note: established names of drugs in this table are based on an approved product at http://www.accessdata.fda.gov/scripts/cder/drugsatfda/index.cfm. The site should be consulted to determine whether a given product has been discontinued. Dosage form and concentration are based on all approved products whether or not they have become discontinued.

Abbreviations: amp, ampule; Eq, equivalent; IM, intramuscular; inh, inhalation; IV, intravenous; NSAID, nonsteroidal anti-inflammtory drug; SC, subcutaneous.

[a] Marketing status is discontinued.

[b] Tentative approval with a marketing status of none.

Data from Refs.[1–9,11,15–20]

BEYOND ELU—UNAPPROVED DRUGS

The limited availability of approved safe and effective drugs to treat animal toxicoses has been a long-standing problem for food animal veterinarians. This almost complete lack of approved drugs is in part due to the cost incurred to provide the evidence required to adequately evaluate human food safety concerns and to a small and unpredictable market for the finished products. Consequently, practitioners have few legal treatment options when treating animals with a toxicosis, in particular food animals. Unfortunately, the economic impact of exposure of an entire herd to a toxicant can be devastating to food animal owners and veterinarians, and large amounts of antidotes may be needed to treat an entire herd. A great need exists for drugs approved for use in food animals to treat toxicoses.

This article identifies chemicals and other products that contemporary veterinary reference texts recommend for use to treat toxicoses for which no FDA human or animal approval currently exists. These products are presented in 3 broad categories: drugs that were approved but have been withdrawn, bulk chemicals for which enforcement discretion[j] has historically been exercised by FDA, and bulk chemicals for which enforcement discretion has not historically been exercised. This list of products is not exhaustive. Because the chemicals or other products listed are commonly recommended in contemporary veterinary texts to treat toxicoses, the authors hope that inclusion of them in this article illustrates to practitioners the limit of the ELU regulations as a legal foundation for the treatment of animals with toxicoses.

Withdrawn Drugs

Drug approvals may be voluntarily withdrawn by a sponsor. If a drug is withdrawn, it is no longer an approved new animal drug. An example of a withdrawal relevant to this article is calcium disodium EDTA, formerly approved as Havidote Injection (NADA 010-540). If an animal drug approval is withdrawn and no human approval exists, the drug is then outside the scope of the ELU regulations (discussed previously).

Bulk Chemicals with Historic Enforcement Discretion

Box 1 lists bulk chemicals commonly recommended for the treatment of animals with toxicoses for which no animal or human drug approval by FDA exists but for which enforcement discretion has historically been exercised by FDA. Veterinary practitioners should be aware that use of these chemicals is outside the scope of the federal ELU regulations (discussed previously). These chemicals do, however, fall within the scope of a Compliance Policy Guide (CPG) published by FDA.

CPGs are policy documents issued by the FDA that describe the agency's enforcement approach to a particular set of products or activities that violates the FFDCA. CPG section 608.400, entitled "Compounding of Drugs for Use in Animals," explains the FDA's policies with regard to compounding of animal drugs by veterinarians and pharmacists that violate the FFDCA (http://www.fda.gov/ICECI/ComplianceManuals/CompliancePolicyGuidanceManual/ucm117042.htm). Because drugs compounded from bulk chemicals do not have approvals, their manufacture, distribution, and use

[j] For a variety of reasons, agencies do not enforce laws in all instances; enforcement discretion is a phrase used to refer to those particular times when an agency makes a choice to not fully enforce the law. Agencies' exercise of enforcement discretion does not make the product or activity legal and may be reversed at any time.

Box 1
Unapproved drugs: bulk chemicals included in Appendix a of compliance policy guide 608.400

Ammonium molybdate
Ammonium tetrathiomolybdate
Methylene blue
Picrotoxin
Pilocarpine
Sodium nitrite
Sodium thiosulfate
Tannic acid

violate the FDCA (as discussed previously, drugs compounded from approved, finished drugs may meet the requirements for legal ELU). There is a potential for causing harm to public health and to animals when drug products are compounded, distributed, and used in the absence of adequate and well-controlled safety and effectiveness data or adherence to the principles of contemporary pharmaceutical chemistry and current good manufacturing practices. Use of compounded drugs in animals can result in adverse reactions and animal deaths. Furthermore, because the pharmacokinetics and depletion times for residues from compounded products intended for use in food-producing animals are not known, the assignment of an extemporaneous withdrawal time may result in potentially harmful residues in food. Inactive ingredients, such as excipients and vehicles, from unapproved or unknown origins may also pose additional risk (eg, Freund adjuvant, a carcinogen).

The FDA recognizes, however, that in some circumstances compounded animal drugs are important to veterinary practice and are necessary to prevent the suffering and death of animals. The FDA's CPG on compounding of animal drugs describes factors the FDA considers in deciding whether to take enforcement action against illegally compounded drugs. In addition, Appendix A of the CPG includes a list of substances for compounding and subsequent use in animals to which the FDA has not normally objected. These bulk chemicals are listed in **Box 1**. The FDA periodically revisits and updates such guidance, particularly as new information comes to the attention of the agency, so enforcement discretion may not be applied in the future in the same way it has in the past. Also, the CVM has recently requested public comment on a potential policy change regarding unapproved animal drugs (http://www.regulations.gov/#!documentDetail;D=FDA-2010-N-0528-0001).

Bulk Chemicals Without Historic Enforcement Discretion

Table 6 lists some bulk chemicals identified by veterinary texts as useful treatments for which enforcement discretion has not historically been exercised by the CVM.

The Unique Status of Epinephrine and Atropine

Epinephrine and atropine have historically been marketed without approval. They are two examples of a very few drugs that FDA has exempted from certain labeling requirements generally applicable to animal drugs and instead provided the labeling by regulation. See **Table 7** for the specific indications for epinephrine and atropine.

Table 6
Unapproved drugs: bulk chemicals not in appendix a of compliance policy guide 608.400

General Treatment	
Adsorbent	Activated charcoal
Emetics	Syrup of ipecac Hydrogen peroxide
Laxatives	Mineral oil Sodium sulfate
Demulcents	Egg whites Milk
Supportive Treatment	
—	Methylthionium chloride
Ammonium acetate	Milk thistle
Amyl nitrite	Oxygen
Ascorbate	—
Calcium gluconate	Pentylenetetrazol
Calcium lactate	Physostigmine salicylate
Calcium phosphate	Sterile saline
Diphenylthiocarbazone	—
Specific Treatment	
Ethanol	
Calcium disodium EDTA	

Data from Refs.[1–9,11,15–20]

OPTIONS

Practicing veterinarians may have an interest in potential solutions to the problem of scarcity of legal drugs to treat animals with toxicoses. Several options exist under, or related to, the Minor Use and Minor Species Animal Health Act of 2004 (MUMS)

Table 7
Drugs exempted from some labeling requirements when used to treat animal toxicoses

Established Name	Indication	Code of Federal Regulations
Atropine sulfate	As an injectable, should not be in excess of 15 mg per dosage unit for cattle, goats, sheep, horses, and pigs and not in excess of 0.6 mg per dosage unit for dogs and cats	21 CFR § 500.55
Epinephrine	Injection should be at the concentration of 1:1000 for cats, dogs, cattle, goats, horses, pigs, and sheep	21 CFR § 500.55
	Epinephrine 1:1000 in 10-mL containers for emergency treatment of anaphylactoid shock in cattle, horses, sheep, and swine can be made available for over-the-counter sale	21 CFR § 500.65

(see http://www.fda.gov/AnimalVeterinary/NewsEvents/CVMUpdates/ucm048420.htm) to potentially alleviate this problem. These options include conditional approval, indexing, designation, and National Research Support Project 7 (NRSP-7). Only conditional approval and designation are currently potential options for food animals.[k]

SUMMARY

When faced with the need to treat a toxicosis, veterinary practitioners may legally use drugs approved for that use in the species to be treated (see **Table 2**). If an approved drug is not clinically effective, practitioners may consider ELU of a drug approved for use in humans or animals, as long as that use meets the conditions of the FDA's ELU regulations (see **Tables 4** and **5**). Treatments that must be compounded from bulk chemicals are often recommended, but such compounding violates the FFDCA, although the FDA does not always take action when animal drugs are compounded from bulk (see **Box 1**).

The authors recommend that veterinarians become aware of the FDA's stated enforcement policies regarding animal drug compounding. At present, obtaining treatment for companion animal toxicoses may be accomplished through judicious ELU and compounding as needed.[l] In contrast, no single solution for increasing the availability of antidotes for food animals is apparent. The situation is different for food animals because sufficient information to set science-based withdrawal times to avoid tissue residues is generally lacking, precluding the use of approved human or animal drugs that may be

---

[k] MUMS of 2004. This legislation helps make more medications legally available to veterinarians and animal owners to treat minor animal species and uncommon diseases in major animal species. It is found in Sections 571, 572, and 573 of the FFDCA. Minor use drugs are drugs for use in major species (cattle, horses, swine, chickens, turkeys, dogs, and cats) that are needed for diseases that occur infrequently or in limited geographic areas. Minor species are defined by exclusion, as any species other than the major species listed above. Because of the small market shares, low-profit margins involved, and capital investment required, it is generally not economically feasible for pharmaceutical firms to pursue approvals for minor species, and/or uncommon diseases and conditions of major animal species. Three mechanisms are possible for improving the availability of new animal drugs under the MUMS legislation: (a) conditional approval—a sponsor of a veterinary drug can request conditional approval for the drug, which allows the sponsor to make the drug available before collecting all necessary effectiveness data, but after proving the drug is safe for its intended use. The drug sponsor can keep the product on the market for up to 5 years while collecting the required effectiveness data. (b) Indexing—the Index is limited to non–food-producing minor species, with a limited exception for some early life stages of food animals, such as fish eggs. (c) Designation—this section of the MUMS is similar to the Orphan Drug Act for humans, which provides incentives to pharmaceutical firms that develop drugs for rare diseases or conditions.
The NRSP-7 is a program that provides funds for research to generate data in support of drug approvals for minor uses. NRSP-7 submits data from research projects to the FDA-CVM for inclusion in a public master file. Once accepted, the data are available for sponsors to refer to, in support of an NADA for minor use. Further information is available at http://www.nrsp-7.org.

[l] (a) The following conditions must be met for a permitted ELU in food-producing animals of approved new animal and human drugs and in nonfood animals of an approved animal drug.

(1) There is no approved new animal drug that is labeled for such use and that contains the same active ingredient which is in the required dosage form and concentration, except where a veterinarian finds, within the context of a valid VCPR, that the approved new animal drug is clinically ineffective for its intended use. 21 CFR § 530.20(a)(1) and last sentence of 21 CFR § 530.30(a). Because ELU of animal and human drugs in non–food-producing animals does not ordinarily pose a threat to the public health, ELU of animal and human drugs is permitted in non–food-producing animal practice except when the public health is threatened.

legally compounded or used in an extralabel manner for many toxicoses. For producers, however, the economic impact is great when there is loss of multiple animals in a herd due to poisoning. Every effort should thus be made to increase the availability of life-saving antidotal therapies for these animals. When possible, use of MUMS regulatory pathways to increase the availability of antidotal therapies may be considered.

REFERENCES

1. Anderson DE, Rings DM. Current veterinary therapy: food animal practice. 5th edition. Philadelphia: WB Saunders; 2008.
2. Firth A. Treatments used in small animal toxicoses. In: Bonagura JD, editor. Current veterinary therapy—small animal practice XIII. Philadelphia: WB Saunders; 2000. p. 207.
3. Ford M, Delaney K, Ling L, Erickson T, editors. Clinical toxicology. Philadelphia: WB Saunders; 2001.
4. Murphy MJ. A field guide to common animal poisons. Ames (IA): Iowa State University Press; 1996.
5. Osweiler GD. Antidotes. In: Osweiler GD, editor. Toxicology. Philadelphia: Williams & Wilkins; 1996.
6. Peterson ME, Talcott PA, editors. Small animal toxicology. 2nd edition. Philadelphia: WB Saunders; 2005.
7. Plumlee KH. Clinical veterinary toxicology. St Louis (MO): Mosby; 2004.
8. Howard JL, Smith RA. Current veterinary therapy—food animal practice. 1–4 editions. Philadelphia: WB Saunders; 1981, 1986, 1993, 1999.
9. Gupta RC, editor. Veterinary toxicology. New York: Elsevier; 2007.
10. Hornfeldt CS, Murphy MJ. 1990 Report of the American Association of poison control centers: poisoning in animals. J Am Vet Med Assoc 1992;200:1077–80.
11. Buck WB. Current veterinary therapy—small animal practice XII. Philadelphia: WB Saunders; 1995. p. 210.
12. Hornfeldt CS, Murphy MJ. Poisonings in animals: the 1993–1994 report of the American association of poison control centers. Vet Hum Toxicol 1997;39(6):361–5.
13. Hornfeldt CS, Murphy MJ. Summary of small animal poison exposures in a major metropolitan area. In: Bonagura JD, editor. Current veterinary therapy—small animal practice XIII. Philadelphia: WB Saunders; 2000. p. 206.
14. Hovda LR. Toxin exposures in small animals. In: Bonagura JD, editor. Kirk's current veterinary therapy—small animal practice XIV. Philadelphia: WB Saunders; 2009. p. 92.
15. Hall K. Toxin exposures and treatments: a survey of practicing veterinarians. In: Bonagura JD, editor. Kirk's current veterinary therapy—small animal practice XIV. Philadelphia: WB Saunders; 2009. p. 95.
16. Extralabel Drug Use in Animals; Final Rule, published in the Federal Register 1996;61[217]:57732–46.
17. Plumb DC. Plumb's veterinary drug handbook. 6th edition. Stockholm (WI): PharmaVet; 2008.
18. Kirk RW, Bonagura JD, editors. Current veterinary therapy IX (1986), X (1989), XI (1992), XII (1995), XIII (2000) and XIV (2008): Small Animal Practice. Philadelphia: WB Saunders.
19. Radostits OM, Gay CC, Blood DC, et al. Veterinary medicine—a textbook of the diseases of cattle, sheep, pigs, goats and horses. 9th edition. London: WB Saunders; 2000.
20. Roder JD. Veterinary toxicology. Woburn (MA): Butterworth-Heinemann; 2001.

Index

Note: Page numbers of article titles are in **boldface** type.

Vet Clin Food Anim 27 (2011) 513–523
doi:10.1016/S0749-0720(11)00026-0

O

P

Printed and bound by CPI Group (UK) Ltd, Croydon, CR0 4YY
03/10/2024
01040461-0011